BACCHIC MEDICINE

WINE AND ALCOHOL THERAPIES FROM NAPOLEON TO THE FRENCH PARADOX

THE WELLCOME SERIES IN THE HISTORY OF MEDICINE

Forthcoming Titles:

Turquet de Mayerne as Baroque Physician: The Art of Medical Portraiture
Brian Nance

The Road to Medical Statistics
Edited by Eileen Magnello and Anne Hardy

The Biographies of Remedies
Edited by Marijke Gijswijt-Hofstra, Godelieve van Heteren and E. M. Tansey

The Wellcome Series in the History of Medicine editors are H. J. Cook, C. J. Lawrence and V. Nutton.
Please send all queries regarding the series to Michael Laycock, The Wellcome Trust Centre for the History of Medicine at UCL, 24 Eversholt Street, NW1 1AD, UK.

BACCHIC MEDICINE

WINE AND ALCOHOL THERAPIES FROM NAPOLEON TO THE FRENCH PARADOX

Harry W. Paul

Amsterdam – New York, NY 2001

First published in 2001
by Editions Rodopi B. V., Amsterdam – New York, NY 2001.

Design and Typesetting by Michael Laycock,
The Wellcome Trust Centre for the History of Medicine at UCL.
Printed and bound in The Netherlands by Editions Rodopi B. V.,
Amsterdam – New York, NY 2001.

Index by Dr. Laurence Errington.

British Library Cataloguing in Publication Data
A catalogue record for this book is available from the British
Library
ISBN 90-420-1111-4 (Paper)
ISBN 90-420-1121-1 (Bound)

Bacchic Medicine
Wine and Alcohol Therapies from Napoleon to the French Paradox
Amsterdam – New York, NY
Rodopi. – ill.
(Clio Medica Series No. 64/ ISSN 0045-7183;
The Wellcome Series in the History of Medicine)

Front cover:
A Parisienne liqueur label from the 1800s, surrounded by ancient
drinking vessels (wood engravings by J. T. Balcomb, c. 1873)
Images courtesy, the *Wellcome Library*, London,
Montage by Michael Laycock

Printed in The Netherlands

All titles in the Clio Medica series (from 1999 onwards) are available to
download from the CatchWord website: http://www.catchword.co.uk

CONTENTS

Preface

Dr. Georges Portmann (1889-1985) was a well known ear, nose, and throat specialist in the faculty of medicine in Bordeaux with a general practice in surgery from the 1920s to the 1960s. He eventually became dean of the medical faculty, a member of the French Senate, Grand Maître de la Chaîne des Rôtisseurs, and a superb propagandist for French wines. While monkishly preparing his *agrégation de médecine* he was afflicted with stomach pains. He consulted his colleagues. Professor Pierre Mauriac diagnosed cholecystitis and advised surgical removal of the gall bladder. An alarmed Portmann got a second opinion from Chavannaz, professor of clinical surgery, whose careful examination revealed chronic appendicitis, also requiring excision of the offending organ. Frightened by this prospect of the knife, Portmann went to Paris to consult his friend Dr. Pierret, who discovered a new problem, tubercular peritonitis; confirmation of this diagnosis would have required exploratory surgery. A depressed Portmann returned to Bordeaux to relate his adventures to his father-in-law, Professor Moure, an old fashioned doctor 'for whom human contact had as much importance as scientific methods.' Moure recognised that Portmann, exhausted from overwork, simply needed a long rest and good wine. His prescription was a month of absolute rest and a glass of mature Château Latour with each meal. After a month Portmann's stomach pains disappeared along with a few bottles from Moure's cellar, and he was never sick again in his life. He consequently became a fervent medical advocate of moderate wine consumption and with a fellow physician, Max Eylaud, founded the Association des médecins amis du vin. There was a long hard struggle ahead as they tried to get wine taken seriously in the practice of medicine.[1]

The medicinal use of wine was one of the oldest 'therapeutic traditions' in western medicine, including popular medicine, which sometimes overlapped with professional medicine and sometimes went its own therapeutic way.[2] *Bacchic Medicine* is about the alcohol and wine therapies of the nineteenth and twentieth centuries, when an increasingly scientific medicine tested the theories and practices of the great doctors of earlier periods. Wine therapy involved treating sick people rather than keeping healthy people healthy. A concern with the potential of wine as preventive medicine makes it easy to ignore the historical role of wine as a cure for disease. There were very few diseases, whether classified as somatic or mental, in which one of the many kinds of wines could not speed the patient's recovery -- even from love. In Jane Austen's *Sense and Sensibility* when Marianne was suffering from the pains of unrequited love and faint and giddy from lack of sleep and food, with 'an aching head, a weakened stomach, and general nervous faintness,' her sister Elinor gave her a glass of wine. The lovelorn maiden soon became more comfortable and talkative. Later in the novel, Elinor drank a glass of fine old Constantia wine to try 'its healing powers on a disappointed heart' (her own). And according to a dual system of wine therapy, poor people could do nearly as well on cheaper wines as rich people could do on expensive *crus.*

In the early-nineteenth century Xavier Bichat, a star of the Paris school of clinical medicine, dreamed that his analytically-based pathological anatomy would enjoy a success in medicine comparable to that of Lavosier's analytical chemistry.[3] Etienne Lancereaux, a well known Parisian doctor and faculty man, was still expressing the same hope towards the end of the century.[4] Scientific medicine was the *ignus fatuus* of the medical elite. And we find that Eduard Loebenstein-Loebel, professor of medicine at Jena and famous practitioner, did not escape being lured by the certainties and professional popularity of the scientific model when he wrote his manual on wine therapy in 1816. There is no other work before the appearance of French manuals in the twentieth century that shows in such detail the clinical value of wine. Its significance is enhanced by the fact that it integrated German wines into its therapeutic repertory.[5]

W. F. Bynum has convincingly argued that 'science was one of the important influences shaping the structure of medicine in the nineteenth century.'[6] Increasing scientific knowledge of the nature of alcohols corresponded to a growing role for alcohol in internal medicine. Distillation of wine had been used to produce alcohol since the middle ages, with alcohol becoming an important part of the doctor's therapeutic baggage. The vehicle for alcohol could be brandy, whisky, and beer as well as wine. Or if the doctor believed that medical virtue resided exclusively in the alcohol, the product could be administered in a pure ethyl form. So after an analysis of an early nineteenth-century German–French model of wine therapy this book deals with the emergence and decline of alcohol as 'a remarkable medicine.'[7] Part of the story of the role of alcohol in orthodox medical practice centres on its being prescribed excessively by many doctors, especially in London. No good medicine seems to escape abuse by doctor and patient. The decline of alcohol therapy in the late nineteenth century was also due to serious doubts about its efficacy and to the development of new pharmaceutical products. New products, new therapies, and even a new paradigm in medicine.

Wine continued to enjoy a privileged place in therapy, partly because doctors have always been prominent among the privileged consumers of good wines. The medical role of wine grew when chemists identified many of its complex of ingredients, to which doctors quickly assigned specific therapeutic properties, much in the fashion of contemporary doctors optimistically finding cardiac virtues in wine phenols. As alcoholism came to be more and more identified as a distinguishing characteristic of the working class poor, ordinary wine, having a low alcohol content compared with hard liquor, was increasingly touted by paternal protectors of working class virtue as a more acceptable drug than whisky, gin, and the new products of the powerful alcohol industry. Preventive medicine in two ways.

After mid-nineteenth century wine came increasingly under the scrutiny of science, eventually having to depend on it for the survival of the vine and for the production of a liquid of consistent quality. Pasteur's work on wine diseases and their prevention established the dominant oenological paradigm, which lasted into the 1930s.[8] Wine had always been a product particularly subject to adulteration, and advances in chemistry made it easier to adulterate as well as easier to detect the adulteration. Even traditional practices such as plastering and sulphuring came under governmental and medical scrutiny. Wine could be dangerous medicine in more ways than one.

Like any other medicine, wine has its iatrogenic tales, especially in France, where debates over the dangers of additives to wine run through much of the late nineteenth and early twentieth centuries. Newspaper revelations identifying sherry as a dangerous drink, adulterated by chemical practices essential to its commercial viability, led to a mild tempest in English wine circles. But the big debates took place in France, where the medical community played a prominent role in a national debate over the safety of the 'national drink.' The state had long accepted the idea that sick subjects or citizens should be cured of their diseases in order to exercise their full productive capacity. By the late-nineteenth century, governments, especially at the municipal level, began to take preventive measures to protect citizens from adulterated food and drink.[9] Doctors necessarily played an important role in the debates over the dangers of the use of a wide array of chemicals in food production. We are still debating some of these issues and even quibbling over some of the same products, though these days the threat is more likely to be from contamination of wines by pesticides and herbicides. We are fortunate in having governmental agencies to assure us of the innocuity of residual traces of dangerous chemicals.[10]

Whether wine has a role in modern medicine became the subject of a twentieth century French debate unequalled in intensity and extent since the much earlier quarrels over the comparative medicinal virtues of burgundy and champagne. In the early part of the century some French doctors, especially in the Bordelais, were keen to establish the clinical basis of the therapeutic role of wine and to show that moderate wine consumption has a place in good preventive medicine. The enthusiasm of Bordeaux's doctors in giving wine a role in preventive medicine and therapy might seem to justify Erwin Ackerknecht's view of local medicine as a cultural system. In spite of its clinically demonstrated positive results in both preventive medicine and therapy, wine enjoyed only a modest success in getting integrated into French medical practice. Even the considerable scientific support given by laboratory work in the 1920s and 1930s did little to put wine into the place in the therapeutic repertory that a small but active group of doctors believed it deserved. An entente cordiale developed between the wine industry and doctors in the 1930s; it flowered into an alliance after World War II, when doctors organized in defence of wine as an essential element of civilisation – the physician had become a guardian of western civilisation – and as a useful therapeutic product.

It is tempting to argue, though perhaps with more enthusiasm than accuracy, that using wine as medicine constitutes what might be called a 'distinctly conceptualised system of therapy.'[11] But the fact is that even with some very good evidence and more good press, wine has had only a peripheral role in modern medicine; it might be regarded as a kind of 'marginal medicine,' a medicine on the fringe.[12] Which does not mean it is ineffective. A good medical case has been made for using wine in fighting infectious diseases, heart disease, and cancer. Whether the French paradox – defined as an apparent compatibility of a high fat diet with a low incidence of coronary atherosclerosis – exists or not is a subject of intense medical debate. Many doctors accept the view that drinking in moderation –

unfortunately, a word defined in many ways – produces cardiovascular, renal, and neurological benefits. (None of this is true in Scotland.[13]) Convincing consumers or patients to be moderate drinkers is another matter. It seems reasonable to conclude that a glass or two of wine will make it unnecessary for us to join Will Lightbody on the road to Wellville.[14] Of course, wine cannot provide us with an escape from the diseased medical system itself, which, 'faced with a healthier population, is driven to medicalizing normal events ... converting risks into diseases, and treating trivial complaints with fancy procedures.'[15] We escape Dr. Kellogg only to fall into the welcoming arms of *le docteur* Knock.[16]

Notes

1. Georges Portmann, *Contacts et pensées. Souvenirs recueillis par René Massot et Anne Portmann* (Bordeaux: Editions Bière, 1982), 139–40. Before becoming indignant over the mistaken diagnoses of Portmann's doctors, we should consider the difficulty of arriving at a diagnosis, even in our enlightened age. For example: 'Of 788 patients referred to a Lyme disease clinic in a university hospital during a four and one half year period who were thought by the referring physician to have Lyme disease, 20 percent had previous Lyme disease, 23 percent had active Lyme disease and other current illness, and 57 percent did not have Lyme disease.' Letter by David J. Herman, M.D., director of the Lyme Disease Center, Somerville, N.J., to *The New York Times* (21 Feb. 1995).
2. On 'the concept of therapeutic traditions,' see Steven Feierman and John M. Janzen, eds, *The Social Basis of Health & Healing in Africa* (Berkeley, CA: University of California Press, 1992).
3. Michel Foucault, *The Birth of the Clinic – An archaeology of Medical Perception* (Paris: Presses Universitaires de France, 1963; New York: Vintage Books, 1975), 131. Translated by A. M. Sheridan Smith.
4. Etienne Lancereaux, *Leçons de clinique médicale,* (Paris: A. Delahaye, 1883; 2 vols., 1892-94), i, 281.
5. German wines were also dealt with favorably in previous works by other great doctors. Prominent among them were Friedrich Hoffmann, Edward Barry, and Robert James. Compared with Thomas Sydenham (1624-89), these eighteenth century doctors were enthusiastic about wine therapy. The case for wine therapy, including praise of German Wines, was superbly summed up in Robert James, *A Medicinal Dictionary* (London: T. Osborne, 1743-5, 3 vols). An expanded and corrected French translation came out in six volumes, 1746-48; the work, but not the translation, was done

by Julien Busson, Docteur-Régent de la Faculté de médecine de Paris.

6. W. F. Bynum, *Science and the Practice of Medicine in the Nineteenth Century* (Cambridge: Cambridge University Press, 1994), xii.
7. Bert L. Vallee gives a quick survey of the role of 'Alcohol in the Western World,' in *Scientific American* (June 1998), 80–5.
8. See ch. 6 ('Louis Pasteur') of Harry W. Paul, *Science, Vine, and Wine in Modern France* (Cambridge: Cambridge University Press, 1996), 155–93.
9. See Harry W. Paul, *From Knowledge to Power – The Rise of the Science Empire in France, 1860-1939* (Cambridge: Cambridge University Press, 1985), 211–20.
10. On a recent coverup of the presence of the pesticide chlorophenol in high quality French wines, see Frank J. Prial, 'Sommelier, what's that smell?,' *The New York Times* (13 Jan. 1999), B11.
11. The phrase quoted is from Paul U. Unschuld, *Medicine in China – A History of Ideas* (Berkeley, CA: University of California Press, 1985), 2.
12. For a development of this concept, see Roy Wallis and Peter Morley (eds), *Marginal Medicine* (London: Owen, 1976).
13. Carole L. Hart and others, 'Alcohol consumption and mortality from all causes, coronary heart disease, and stroke: results from a prospective cohort study of Scottish men with 21 years of follow up,' *British Medical Journal*, 318 (26 June 1999), 1725–9. No positive effects were found for drinkers of spirits, beer, and wine. Worse, drinkers of more than 22 units a week increased their mortality risk – a bottle of wine equals 6 units.
14. T. Coraghessan Boyle, *The Road to Wellville* (New York: Penguin, 1993).
15. Roy Porter, *The Greatest Benefit to Mankind. A Medical History of Humanity* (London: HarperCollins, 1997), 717–18
16. Jules Romains, *Knock ou le triomphe de la médecine* (Paris: Gallimard, 1924), staged for the first time in 1923.

Acknowledgements

Acknowledgements remind me of F. M. Cornford's definition of propaganda, which can be found in the preface to the 1922 edition of *Microcosmographia Academica*: 'that branch of the art of lying which consists in very nearly deceiving your friends without quite deceiving your enemies.' And though reviewers are not necessarily disarmed by the author's feint, the formality has its place in our academic rituals. I wish to thank the National Endowment for the Humanities and the National Science Foundation for supporting the early stages of *Bacchic Medicine.* Over the years the University of Florida has been generous with research help, and the department of history has always supported my research and scribbling. I also wish to thank the personnel of the Archives de l'Assistance publique -- Hôpitaux de Paris, the Bibliothèque nationale de France, the Bibliothèque de l'Académie nationale de médecine, the Archives départementales de la Gironde (Bordeaux), and the department of viticulture and enology of the University of California at Davis, where Linda Bisson, Susan Ebeler and Andy Waterhouse gave me advice and materials. Among many people who helped me in various ways are Elisabeth Crawford, Antoinette Emch-Deriaz, Nancy Green, Jan Goldstein, Louis Latour, Matthew Ramsey, Allister and Jeanette Paul, Pascal Ribéreau-Gayon, Guenter B. Risse, and George Weisz and, above all, Mike Laycock. Larry Jennings, Terry Shinn, Claire and Homer Orologas, and Vassiliki Betty Smocovitis cheerfully consented to be among the subjects for some of my experiments in wine therapy; they all agreed with one of Louis Pasteur's most comforting dogmas: 'Le bon vin peut être à bon droit considéré comme la plus saine, la plus hygiénique des boissons' (*Etudes sur le vin,* 2d edn, 1873, p. 53).

PART I

POPULAR AND PROFESSIONAL WINE THERAPIES

1

People's Stories: Wine in Popular Medicine

Disease and medicine, its faithful companion, existed long before the human race invented doctors, though healers of many sorts have always been with us. Popular medicine, like the professional medicine founded by Asclepius, has divine roots. Christians continued the tradition of a medical connection with a higher power. Jeremy Taylor (1613-67) stated the basic axiom: 'God plants remedies there where the diseases are most popular.'[1] Speaking in a secular and anthropological vein more appropriate to a twentieth-century thinker, Charles Talbot found it striking that 'Wherever we look in folk medicine we find the traditions, the customs, the remedies, the whole corpus of doctrine drawing substance and vigor from an almost timeless source, as if they belonged to the very nature of man himself.'[2]

In a pioneering study of folk medicine, published in 1883, William George Black introduced the idea of an archaeology of the mind, which included as a tacit sub-category the archaelogy of popular medicine.[3] Historians and the organizers of their research categories seem to have taken a serious interest in constructing the literary text of popular medicine much later. A historical dig I carried out in the *Catalogue Matières Ouvrages* of the Bibliothèque nationale de France revealed that its librarians invented the category of popular medicine, with cross references to popular belief and superstitions, in cataloguing works of the period 1960-1979. I did not find a category of popular medicine for the periods before 1960. Suddenly, it seemed, anthropologists, ethnologists, doctors, folklorists, and local historians had created a body of literature, a new scholarly category in the history of medicine.[4] The Hegelian owl of Minerva had taken flight.

Marcelle Bouteiller was a bit optimistic in noting that 'the fashion of popular medicine, in full flower in the eighteenth and nineteenth centuries, progressively weakened' in the twentieth century.[5] The foundations had been sapped earlier. In Enlightenment France, as in Georgian England, popular thinking about diseases and cures seemed 'increasingly to have come adrift from its traditional cosmological moorings,' with devils and witches losing 'their cultural legitimacy.'[6] Historians, great cultural conformers, were long uninterested in studying what they regarded as phenomena of the diseased mind. Popular medicine could even be excluded from a historical construct called 'the old art of curing,' a humane medicine that looked at the whole person.[7] But in our enlightened age we are finding that looking at 'the social world of [past] medical practice,' both professional and popular, can be intellectually satisfying as well as entertaining.[8]

If one considers popular medicine within a system of analysis emphasizing such things as medical acts undertaken by unlicensed healers and the use of 'remèdes de bonne femme', then it is difficult to understand its survival in that useful construct we call the modern world. Merely mentioning the survival of residual magical practices is hardly enlightening. So commentators have drawn on ethnological-anthropological systems of analysis to explain the continued strength of various types of medicine. It seems that just as there are several types of logic, there are several kinds of rationality – at least in anthropology. This mental flexibility is very useful in trying to understand popular medicine. And it certainly sounds scientifically kosher to deal with 'the mechanisms of the logic of myth.' Following Lévi-Strauss, Bouteiller points out that one of the basic steps of 'primitive'– and also 'civilized' – thought is to establish 'relationships of resemblance'. So in a therapeutic system plants with yellow flowers would be used to treat urinary disorders, and the necessary extrapolation being made, also to treat ailing male organs. A reciprocal mental act gives to artemisia or wormwood a nocturnal, moon-related feminine association. So in Anjou a jaundiced person would drink macerated cornflowers in white wine or Indian chestnuts in red wine. 'The magical equivalent of the same being the opposite,' the Baugeois ate hare's brains to cure fear. Wine too could help a timid person face the dragons of daily life. But practices such as the application of pigeons that are split open alive and putting a piece of raw meat on the table for cancer to devour have to be explained by the fact that mythic thought is also based on 'relations of contiguity.'[9]

In addition to the associations of popular medicine with certain so-called magical processes, there was its more evident connection with religion, especially the Catholic dogma of transubstantiation. This connection could manifest itself in various unusual popular ways. In Anjou it was a traditional practice to put bottles of wine at the foot of the altar when Mass was celebrated on the Sunday following the feast (February 3) of Saint-Blaise de Corné, the saint who cured sore throats. As soon as the bottles of wine were blessed, the faithful rushed forward, grabbed them, and guzzled generous amounts even before leaving the church.[10] The post-Revolutionary clergy ended the practice. Perhaps collective action that had seemed harmless or even devotional in the old regime seemed dangerous, especially for religion, after popular power had been brutally demonstrated in the Revolution. Or the new Vatican-oriented clergy no longer retained faith in the old medicine. In any case, the connection of popular medicine with mainline religion clearly weakened in the nineteenth century.

The nineteenth century saw a striking decline in mortality from the leading infectious diseases (whooping cough, measles, scarlet fever, diphtheria, smallpox, typhoid, typhus, and tuberculosis). At the present time the strongest explanation of this decline is that preventive medicine or public health measures (general sanitary improvements, slum clearance, improved water supply and sewerage systems, and increased cleanliness) were strikingly effective in reducing deaths from the mainly adult diseases of smallpox, typhoid fever, typhus, and tuberculosis. By contrast, preventive medicine seems to have had 'little direct influence on the prevalence of the childhood infections of whooping cough, measles, scarlet fever, or diphtheria.'[11] An antitoxin for diphtheria was aided by the appearance of milder strains of the disease. Declining mortality is a complex historical phenomenon unamenable to simple explanations based on public health, or improved nutrition, or treatment of disease by doctors and other healers.[12]

For a simple understanding of the modern conceptual and practical transformation of medicine, there is no better tool than the Whig model, which encompasses the triumphs of Pasteur and Knock.[13] Danielle Voldman gave us a typical summary in beginning a survey of the state of medicine in France about 1900.[14] By the beginning of the twentieth century medicine had made enormous progress, meaning that new sciences had sprouted from the old ones and that biology, chemistry, physics, and pathological anatomy now fed directly into the doctor's art and the healing machine. Or at least we can admit that they did eventually and that there was hope for better care than before and, through the use of vaccines and serums, hope for cures and even the elimination of certain diseases that had seemed to be an inevitable ingredient of civilisation. Man's view of disease necessarily became more optimistic. People and patients took a friendlier view of doctors, whose social status was slowly improving. Using the new tool of extended male suffrage, the physician became a familiar figure in national politics. By the 1890s doctors made up between ten and twelve per cent of parliamentary deputies and some climbed to the highest political levels.[15] Popular or family medicine, often castigated now as illegal medicine, was considerably weakened by the onslaught of official scientific medicine supported by the political and bureaucratic powers.

The resilience of some parts of popular medicine, especially in the nineteenth and early-twentieth century countryside, may be seen in the formation of a sort of symbiosis with official medicine through the 1930s. But for most commentators the striking thing was the transformation of medicine in the period 1880-1905 – a spectacular transformation, Bouteiller calls it. The old, largely woman-dominated medicine could not survive the transformation of the rural environment itself, which had provided the support system for the basic ideas on which popular medicine rested. Whatever it means, modernization is the only word that we have to describe the 'principal stages of the evolution' of France after 1850 that are presented in all the textbooks. The context of modernization includes going from the closed economy to the exchange economy with its new modes of transport and travel, its stores and shops, its new professions and expanded old ones, its burgeoning bureaucracy, its PTT (communications), its new laws, and new schools. After 1872 compulsory military service affected (and infected) the male population in many ways. With public education and the spread of the idea of secular progress through an expanded teaching corps and newspapers there was also a transformation of religious practice.[16] 'Thanks to modern medicine,' according to one doctor writing in 1984, 'humanity has entered into a true civilisation of health.'[17] The popularization of this modern or professional medicine further reduced but did not eliminate the field of popular medicine. Professionalization and popularization, Ramsey notes, may not be 'fully compatible enterprises,' but they did coexist, and 'that story forms a crucial chapter in the history of modern medicine.'[18] And in the history of that amorphous entity we call popular medicine itself.

Since popular medicine provided remedies for various common ailments it may be considered simply as an emergency medicine. To treat wounds: the Samaritan balm of red wine and oil, which was historically part of the repertory of official medicine. To prevent a cold: hot mulled wine (red wine boiled with five pieces of sugar and a scraped nutmeg, then filtered). To treat ulcerated varicose veins: compresses made with 200 grams of agrimony and a liter of alcoholic red wine, prepared in a cassserole for five minutes. Hypertension required strong stuff, namely, a garlic alcoholate made with 150 grams of garlic macerated for six weeks in a liter of eau-de-vie, then strained and bottled. This product was similar to the different alcohol-based products that were one of the mainstays of the older pharmacy.[19] A peeled clove of garlic was recommended as a suppository, which the patient kept in his rectum overnight. Gout and rheumatism could be helped by drinking an apertif glass of *vin de bleuet* twice a day before meals. (The medicine was made by macerating a handful or so of cornflowers for a week in a bottle of bordeaux; the bottle was shaken daily, finally filtered, and put into another bottle.) Lemon juice also had a good medical reputation in the treatment of gout and acute articular rheumatism.[20] This is the sort of common sense approach we find in recipes supplied by Jacques Veissid in a treatise on popular medicine published in the series Guides pratiques Vermot.[21] (The *Almanach Vermot* had started spreading the rational gospel of simple medical knowlege in rural areas in the nineteenth century.)

Popular medicine did not forget sexual problems; even ordinary people had them. (In the United States at present forty three per cent of females and thirty one per cent of males experience some sort of sexual dysfunction.[22]) Frigidity required fennel seeds: 100 grams in a bottle of port, shaken daily for three weeks and strained; as the prelude to amorous play, a liqueur glass of the stimulant was to be drunk after the evening meal. The aperitif glass also carried the cure for impotence, *Heracleum sphondylium.* The hopeful male downed a glass of cow parsnip wine before lunch and dinner. Sunburn could be cured with juniper boiled in wine, which would be drunk hot three glasses at a time, with a *pater* recited after each glass, over a period of three evenings. The wine had to be prepared with juniper picked during full moon when the last stroke of midnight sounded. Wines made with ginger (*Zingiber offinale*) or ginseng (*Panax ginseng*, whose forked root gave it a psychological advantage) were reputed to possess aphrodisiacal powers. Throughout much of their sexually-charged history the Chinese do not seem to have included either of these items in their long lists of aphrodisiacs.[23] M. F. K. Fisher reminds us of the importance of 'the mysterious truffle, the purportedly potent crayfish, and the symbolism of the eel' in the 'Receipt for la cuisine d'Amour,' with the baked eel and the truffles served 'on a bed of crayfish tails which have been stewed in dry white wine and well seasoned with cayenne.'[24] Popular medicine had become complex since the days when, according to Pliny, just eating basil could excite the coupling desire; this erotic herb was also given to asses and horses before they mounted the females of their species.[25]

Early-nineteenth century medicine seemed to have been required to kill sexual desire as much as to stimulate it. Anti-aphrodisiacs were used to keep satyriasis and nymphomania under control and perhaps to counter excessive stimulation from erotic plant products. Two of the standard anti-erotic items were nenuphar and camphor. Nenuphar or water lily is a plant of the genus Nymphaea whose roots and flowers were processed to produce a calming, anti-spasmodic, and anti-aphrodisical medicament. A dose of this plant, sacred to nymphs, was given in an infusion of 150 grams per liter of water. Camphor, a beloved ketone of nineteenth-century pharmacy, had a reputation as an effective agent of detumesence. Raspail touted it as a panacea.[26] Cantharides, a dried insect preparation with toxic and vesicant or blistering properties, traditionally used as an aphrodisiac, was so powerful that it was mixed with camphor to modify or even neutralize its action on the sexual and urinary organs. To combat superfluous erections, which presumably arose from the irritant action of cantharidin on the genito-urinary tract, the sufferer took twenty pills containing three grams of camphor each, with four pills required at the fall of night.[27]

In spite of the ambitious universal therapy it often proclaimed, popular medicine was largely a rural phenomenon, dealing with health problems that could be treated without going on a long journey to the doctor or even summoning health officer Bovary: colds, sore throats, corns, warts, minor injuries and wounds, small burns, and so on. Jacques Veissid, a sympathetic commentator on the non-magical kind of popular medicine, noted its limitations; though it worked in most cases, it was hardly more than a *pis-aller*.[28]

Veissid's analysis does not get us as far in understanding popular medicine as does the analysis of eighteenth-century English doctoring done by the Porters. First, 'the aura of magic' provided 'an endorsement of regular herbalism and kitchen physic,' thus enhancing the efficacy of any treatment through the power of a comforting system of belief, which we might be tempted to see as related to a powerful placebo effect.[29] Even if one sticks to a positivistic position, popular medicine stands up well under modern scrutiny, for its 'lore dictated, above all, a familiar therapeutic battery of medicaments, each to be tried in appropriate circumstances.' Since many herbal medicines worked, as their modern derivatives do, 'in that sense, they possessed an empirical authenticity.' People also got a certain satisfaction from their belief that there was an overarching cosmic rationality into which popular medicine fitted. The efficacy of their remedies was guaranteed by a higher harmony, whose authority was made clear in the theory or doctrine of signatures. Each disease had its own cure not far from the place in which it originated: the bark of the weeping willow contained the substance needed to counter the rheumatism afflicting people in marshy regions, and a plant that resembled a particular body organ showed that it was intended to treat that disease. So 'the fact that eyebright (*Euphrasia officinalis*) had a bloom so marked as to resemble an eye, demonstrated it to be a specific for eye disease.' In fact many of the plants and herbs used in popular medicine had a quite respectable pedigree in professional medicine. Porter points out that Robert Burton 'pooh-poohed his mother's quaint herbal lore ... until he discovered similar ideas in ...the great classical herbalist Theophrastus.' Many of the post-moderns, preferring St. John's wort to Prozac and horny goat weed (*Epimedium*) to Viagra, seem to have taken to this medicine of 'the green pharmacy' with considerable enthusiasm.[30]

Now it is precisely the type of enumeration we have indulged in here that has been partly responsible for the low scientific status of popular medicine; the fact that it may or may not work does not give it more than placebo status or change the 'heterogeneous image' that it has acquired chiefly from its 'incoherent borrowings from all sorts of sources.'[31] For Loux this disorder was only apparent; beneath the seething caldron of facts was a perfectly coherent foundation, on interrelated empirical and symbolical levels. (Loux sternly warns us that the important thing for the ethnologist is to reconstitute the meaning of these prescriptions, not to judge their efficacy, on which opinion changes over time.) To show the importance of this way of looking at things, Loux analyzed the Norman practice of adding apple brandy or Calvados to the baby's bottle, a practice often seen as evidence of an alcoholism-tainted culture and also condemned as evidence of the selfishness of parents who prefer a sleeping to a squealing baby even at the risk of injury to the child.

How can we understand this practice? First we invoke history, always a useful relativiser. Up to the eighteenth century, 'Calva dans le biberon' was a recommendation made by eminent official authorities, including those in medicine. Calvados was a preventive medicine used to kill worms, which were believed to generate spontaneously in sweet foods such as milk. Buffon could be quoted on a related practice, that of letting children drink a little wine from time to time because alcohol was thought to hinder the development of worms once they had gotten into the child's system. So here we have a coherent alcohol-based system of prevention and therapy for dealing with a common children's problem. The harmfulness of the practice is another matter, which Loux recognizes as a legitimate subject to be discussed after an ethnological understanding of the problem has been achieved. A collar of garlic hanging from the neck was supposed to prevent 'parasites' from rising and even force them to go down again into 'the lower part of the body' and presumably to exit. The essential thing is to understand that these practices were based on 'a pathological reality very different from our own.'[32] Our therapeutic uses of the same substances, based on their bactericidal and antioxidant properties, may have little to do with that world.

Wine occupied a position of considerable significance within the therapeutic arsenal of popular medicine; it was nearly as importance as shit, and was, indeed, often used as a vehicle for this valuable item of popular *materia medica.* To understand this old therapeutic grammar, one must keep in mind that 'the body itself possesses the faculty of curing itself,' a faculty based on a 'complex process of relations between the different parts of the body, between animal and man, and between the body and its excretions.'[33] So within this conceptual framework one would also expect saliva and urine to work wonders. And they did. The urinal was the classic emblem of the doctor, symbolizing the diagnostic knowledge revealed by an analysis of urine, but this liquid was also a remedy. Nowadays urine therapy is likely to be viewed as an exotic import from ancient tantric and yogic techniques, a footnote to Indian medicine – *The Golden Fountain – The Complete Guide to Urine Therapy* by Coen an der Kroon is advertised on the Net – but urine long enjoyed an important role in western popular medicine. 'A person who drinks the urine of a young man in perfect health can be assured that there is no better remedy in the world.' Pulmonary congestion was treated In the Haute-Loire by having a woman drink the urine of a boy of seven years and a man drink that of a girl of seven years. Here we have opposites in sex and a powerful number, which may or may not imply that the growing boy possesses 'the seven spirits of God and the seven stars' (*Revelation,* 3: 1). In Provence forcing an alcoholic to smell his own urine was held to cure alcoholism. Urine was reputed 'to cure ringworm, suppurating ulcers in the ears, and wounds that won't heal.'[34] (Red wine mixed with an equal amount of olive oil was a more common remedy for wounds.)

Complex preparations were not uncommon in shit therapy. To treat burns an ointment could be composed of ingredients including five ounces of cow dung, one ounce of *eau-de-vie*, five ounces of pork grease, three ounces of celery, and two ounces of soap. In cow-rich Normandy the gout called for an early morning shot of steaming cow urine, preferably from a black bovine. 'An infallible remedy for pleurisy' would include in its composition two handfuls of horse shit that had just been dropped, powered ginger root, two pints of white wine, all of which would be put in a cloth and boiled down to one-half to one-third its original volume before consumption.[35] Anyone objecting to an enema of red wine for diarrhea could take powdered dog shit with wine (kept in a container with river stones as ballast) three times a day for three days; in Maine-et-Loire the residue of three burnt corks in red wine worked equally well. In the Lorraine, cow shit diluted in *eau-de-vie de marc* was a treatment for alcoholism. In cultures unfortunate enough to be without wine, shit alone could be applied to wounds: 'in the south of Hampshire a plaster of warm cowdung' used to be 'applied to open wounds.'[36]

The therapeutic use of the faeces and urine of various animals is not a modern cultural innovation. When Aristophanes described doctors as shit-eaters he got a laugh from the audience (male, it seems), just like when he used the term 'little pigs' for female genitals, because he was drawing on a common body of phallic culture.[37] In his famous book on the scatologic rites now so remote from our sanitized minds, J. C. Bourke enumerated the learned doctors and other distinguished minds who prescribed and believed in the medicinal properties of faeces and urine.[38] Hippocrates prescribed dung of the hawk, a bird of virile appearance and behavior, to help the foetus emerge from the womb and also to cure sterility. Xenocrates (presumably the one from Aphrodisias, not Ephesus) prescribed women's urine and their catamenia, among other animal and human secretions. And Pliny presented a 'catalogue raisonné' of the uses of urine. The famous and influential *De materia medica* (c. AD 77) of Dioscorides expounded their virtues, though nowadays we praise the text because it dealt with the simple drugs and herbals and chemical drugs that were the foundation of western medical practice. Even Galen was cited as having often cured tumors and hard lumps on the knees by using a poultice containing goat turds among its ingredients. Julius Ausonius, the doctor who was the father of the Bordelais wine-estate owning poet Ausonius, acquired a certain notoriety for his pills capable of curing sciatica and arthritis in five days. The pills were based on turds of the wild goat (*chamois*) of the Pyrenees gathered on the seventeenth day of the moon's cycle.[39] Excremental medicine did not lack authorities.

The importance of wine as a vehicle for waste products was clearly stated in later texts. Some of the authorities, clerks great in their day, are now silent in our standard histories of medicine: Daniel Beckherius, author of *Medicus Microcosmus* (London, 1660), keen on excremental remedies; Christian Franz Paullini, whose *Pharmacopée excrémentielle* (1696, in German) listed diseases with the appropriate excremental medication; and Martin Schurig, author of *De Stercoribus Brutorum – Chylologia historico-medica* ... (1725). Schurig's work was full of useful remedies, though some of the droppings he prescribed might not be found on every farm. The treatment for jaundice was to give the patient a drink of wine mixed with human excrement. For vertigo and epilepsy the treatment required the consumption of wine containing cat shit; this feline ingredient was also recognised as effective in ointments used to treat such male tragedies as baldness. (Pigeon droppings – in pure form or made suitably palatable – were regarded as a good stimulant for moustache growth.) Cat shit in white wine would work well against a bout of fever. Horse dung juice, preferably from the droppings of a stallion fed on oats, mixed with warm beer helped cramps and colic go away. Anyone fortunate enough to be able to use the dung of a lionness took it in spirit of wine; wolf droppings (preferably from a white wolf) required red wine. Other authorities recommended rat droppings to counteract constipation. Young goose shit, 'warm and drying in its effects,' given with wine, was prescribed for jaundice, scurvy, and dropsy; it was also valuable in controlling the menses. In fact it seems difficult to find any authority who did not recognize the medicinal power of body products, especially urine and faeces. The authorities often cited included Sextus Placitus, Avicenna, von Helmont, Paracelsus, and Bayle.

The famous poem *Regimen Sanitatis Salernitanum*, which presumably embodied some of the wisdom of the Salerno school of medicine of the eleventh and twelfth centuries, devotes some attention to maintaining a healthy stomach, including a recommendation for people to piss six times a day and to have two of three bowel movements with the biggest possible stools. Nor was farting while pissing much of a mystery, but an old practice very healthy for the kidneys. ('Pratiquez-le sans honte, ou bien, dans l'intestin/Reste un gaz malfaisant rapporté du festin.') Not many practitioners of popular medicine knew the famous Salernitan *Rule of*

Health, but like the toffs of official medicine, its popular if poor relations also liked to cite the classic authorities.[40]

As was often the case, the medicinal uses of a product sometimes overlapped with religious and cosmetic uses. Products derived from faeces were valued for softening and whitening the skin. Urine was distilled for the same purpose. (These practices are not only western, for the application of a cream of nightingale droppings is the first step in the complex process of the geisha's makeup.) The products of a healthy young man had the best reputation for efficacy. In religion, there was the tradition of the impure becoming pure by swallowing the turd of a clerical virgin. Most of this now seems as remote and inexplicable as Swift's Yahoo culture. And in the history of medicine we find it repugnant and, worse, hard to explain; we therefore ignore 'Such gaudy Tulips rais'd from Dung.' Jacques Lacan gave a cosmic explanation. 'La civilisation, c'est le déchet: *cloaca maxima*.' In this model the anal character of civilisation explains everything, including excremental medicine.[41]

Internal use of different varieties of shit was a striking feature of popular medicine. One traditional prescription for curing jaundice required the patient to consume first thing on arising, for a week, five small nanny goat turds in white wine.[42] This concoction may be compared with the *vin de chute*, whose key ingredient was chicken shit, a 'domestic medication' of some popularity in the Berry, and also found in some other places. Its preparation required placing a liter of good white wine under the chicken roost to permit twenty one to twenty five droppings to fall directly into the wine. To recover from the bad effects of a fall, an injured person drank a small glass for several mornings before eating. The product could be kept in storage for emergencies. *Vin de chute* may be cited as an ethnological case of 'common knowledge and empiricism.'[43]

Popular medicine viewed wine as a complement of nutritious food, both essential for good health. Many pithy proverbs expressed this idea. (Two examples. 'Bon vin et bonne chère mettent la médecine en l'air.' And 'un verre de vin vaut cinq francs de médecin.') Some proverbs set up an opposition between food and medicine, sometimes in a crudely amusing way. ('Mieux vaut le devant du cheval du meunier que le cul du médecin.') Proverbial wisdom was not limited to the idea that food and wine help a person avoid sickness; some proverbs gave medicine a bad name or gave 'a negative image of the doctor,' while 'insisting on the benefits of natural medicine. As with beauty, the natural is privileged.'[44] According to one proverb, if people ate cherries, a health-provoking fruit, doctors would have to go around half naked because of a paucity of patients. Without going quite that far, even A. Richerand, one of the most distinguished surgeons and doctors of the early-nineteenth century and certainly no friend of popular medicine, admitted that proverbs about hygiene have a certain value because they are 'the fruit of repeated observations.'[45]

In *Sagesses du corps* (1978) Loux and Richard analysed how health and sickness are encoded in about one third of the body of French proverbs. These proverbs about food and drink dealt with the three key and pleasant life functions of eating, defectation, and sexual relations. There was a popular statement of anatomical homage to the three maternal orifices related to these functions. (Trois trous à ma mère: le trou de morceau, le trou du pet et le trou de la cheville recourbée.) These proverbs can be organized on the basis of 'two big themes: the order of food consumption (rigorous typological distinctions, laws of succession and association, rules of relations between foods) and dietetic equilibrium (quantity and quality of foods, relations between eating and the other body functions).' Physiological functions make it possible to identify two groups of foods. First, there are the foods that rebuild the body, give the body its strength; bread, wine, and meat stand out in this category. Secondly, there are the foods that 'help digestion, that is expel the unhealthy "humors";' these digestion-helpers, such as salad, vegetables, and fruit, help the body get rid of its impurities.[46] In this anthropological analysis there is a considerable overlap between scientific medicine and popular medicine through both the idea of preventing disease and the discourse about the body's needs and functions. Some foods, refractory to the nosographical principle, belong to several categories of analysis.

Wine was particularly privileged as a protean substance. It was, notes Loux, a 'symbolic body-restoring food and as the product of a fruit ('natural herb') played an important role as panacea.' A symbol of blood, wine restored strength to the body. (Un verre de vin rouge dans une vieille panse, c'est comme une poutre neuve dans une grange.) Supplying heat to the body, wine was considered a good preventive medicine against colds. ('Pour les rhumes, il faut le pot de vin.') In Picardie the treatment of colds called for a glass of cider or beer heated by plunging a red hot poker into it. In this wine-scarce area one of the few wine uses was in post-illness anemia, which was treated by giving patients white wine containing onions that had been boiled to a pulp in water with candied sugar added. (More useful Picard advice included recommendations to urinate immediately after being frightened and, more conventional, to spread pigeon shit on the upper lip for a fine moustache.)[47] Since fevers were believed to succumb to heat treatment, wine was also held to cure fevers. A headache being a sign of weakness, wine applied to the head could bring relief. (A mal de tête, cataplasme de vin.) Wine's digestive function was expressed in the gluttonous hope that 'too much food gets drowned in wine.' Wine's purifying properties extended to killing worms and other 'parasites' and even to getting rid of poisons. And the Salernitan *Rule of Health* could be cited in support of most of these medicinal effects of wine. Other foods were given more rebuilding force with wine. So soups with bread and meat, all washed down with wine, were ideal. ('Soupes et vins n'enivrent pas mais réchauffent.') The widespread custom of 'faire chabrot' – adding wine to the remains of the soup thus had a digestive and reconstituting function that glided over into preventive medicine. ('Après la soupe un coup de pur vin préserve d'un écu au médecin.') The seriousness of the prescription, Loux insists, is seen in a lugubrious proverb about failure to follow it leading to death. ('Qui ne boit pas après la soupe approche de son tombeau.')[48]

In some of the oenophilic literature there are certain rules governing the agreement of food and wine. Popular medicine sometimes ignored them, as, for example, in specifying that wine went well with salads and eggs. In popular medicine wine played a catalyzing role in relation to foods. Salad could be harmful especially for the eyes, 'whose limpidity show the clarity of the body's humors.'[49] And salad could produce fevers, presumably the result of illness caused by bacteria. ('Qui vin ne boit après salade est en risque d'être malade.') Though deprived of humoral theory, we can perhaps still see some virtue in this advice on the basis of germ theory. Wine was recommended after eating raw eggs. Protection against the unknown *Salmonella*, perhaps. ('Boire en mangeant un oeuf est un précepte sain/J'échappe en le suivant, au mal, au médecin.' And 'sur les oeufs crus, vin pur.') Followers of the custom of eating peaches macerated in red wine will be happy to know that this is a good practice. ('La pêche aime le bon vin.') Sweet wine is the best wine to drink with this fruit. This seems a matter of taste, but with the pear the drinking of wine was anchored in preventive medicine. The pear had a reputation as a potentially harmful fruit, a curiosity that may be explained by the fact in nature vines and pear trees are not found together. According to this logic, the correspondance not found in nature indicates a danger for the body and has to be corrected. No pear without wine is the rule, even Salernitan. ('La poire est sans le vin un dangereux poison / Que la santé redoute avec juste raison.' And the proverb: 'Après la poire, le vin ou le prêtre.') Cheese being classified as one of the 'heavy foods,' moderate consumption is wise. (The wisdom of Salerno: 'Après la chair, vient le fromage/Qui moins en mange est le plus sage.')

It seems to be a near universal axiom that wine is good for digestion – wine as the catalyzer for most food. There was also a general agreement in popular medicine on the harmful effect of wine without food. Wine growing areas seemed to emphasize the importance of associating wine drinking with eating. More principle than practice, some would argue, but the discourse was unambiguous. ('Boire sans manger est nuisible à la santé.') Excess was condemned, whether in the consumption of wine, cheese, meat, salad, or fruit, whereas moderate consumption was seen as restorative and satisfying for all classes. ('Viande de bouche, restitution de cul.' And a bit cruder: 'son ventre plein, le bourgeois pète, son estomac plein, Jean rote.')[50]

Popular medicine gave an important role to the succession and association of foods, with precise rules for the order in which foods should be eaten. The effects of foods varied with the order in which they were eaten. An extreme example was that wine should be drunk after drinking milk. The explanation of this rule may be an insistence on the precedence of the male element over the female. Associations of this sort were just as important for popular culture as for its elite relative. A more practical explanation was that the wine helps to digest the milk, and so the wine has to come at the end of the food cycle. Salerno warned against consuming these liquids in the wrong order. ('Vin sur lait est souhait / Lait sur vin est venin.') Raw garlic and wine also made a poor couple according to one death-charged argument. ('L'ail cru et le vin rendent la mort sûre.') More curious, in view of the ancient custom of cutting wine with water, was the idea that water and wine do not form a useful alliance in the stomach. Bachelard and popular medicine agreed with the Hippocratic doctors that water is the opposite of wine.[51] ('Eau et vin dans un même estomac/Chat et chien dans le même sac.') Good food, well being, and the happiness of the whole body form a totality.[52] The Hippocratic ideal.

And this *jouissance* of the whole being is related to another powerful idea undergirding popular medicine, namely, that eating well ensures the strength of the tribe. ('La nourriture fait la race.') Perhaps as a result of centuries of exposure to the Catholic dogma of transubstantiation, the French readily accepted 'the symbolic relation of the body with food manifesting itself above all in the homology of wine or meat with the blood.'[53] Color makes the analogy less fanciful than it might otherwise be, and the redness of the blood symbolizes its force. 'Sous sa forme rouge, il [le vin] a pour très vieille hypostase, le sang, le liquide dense et vital.' And 'the beefsteak [accompanied by the national patriotic *frites*] participates in the same sanguine mythology as wine.'[54] Unlike in the United States, white wine thus has a serious mythological disadvantage in a wine culture like France, where it has been associated with weakness, even anemia. ('La faiblesse est marquée par un sang blanc.' And 'se fatiguer, sang de navet.') Being related to blood, red wine can make it stronger; white wine, which is like milk, cannot.[55]

Historically, popular and elite medicines had much in common, with popular medicine heavily in debt to the old elite medicine. Or vice versa, it has been argued in the case of Hippocratic medicine, particularly for phyto or plant therapy.[56] Many of the classics of popular or domestic medicine were written by physicians. Roy Porter has noted the spread of 'rational' domestic medicine through 'printed health manuals, supplanting a traditional, quasi-magical oral health culture with simplified versions of elite medicine.'[57] Among the best known works were Samuel Tissot's *Avis au peuple sur la santé* (1761) and William Buchan's *Domestic Medicine; or the Family Physician* (1769), works translated into major European languages; nineteen large editions, about 80,00 copies, of Buchan's work were sold during his lifetime – he died in 1805. Though he had litttle use for fellow physicians, most of whom he regarded as Latin-spouting dullards, Buchan admired Tissot's *Avis.*[58] Buchan thought that the preservation of health is more important than the cure of disease, important as that may be. In 'diffusing medical knowledge among the people,' one of his aims was 'to improve the art and to banish quackery, but likewise to render medicine more universally useful, by extending its benefits to society.' Buchan gave an important role to wine in domestic medicine; Tissot did not. As late as 1974 part of Buchan's classic (translation of 1789) was republished in France as a cure-yourself volume with the unfortunate title of *Les remèdes de bonnes femmes.*[59] What did this influential classic of popular medicine say about wine therapy?

Buchan's praise of wine in its pure state was more for its potential in preventive medicine than in curing disease, which was more a function of medicinal wines, which contained various items from the *materia medica* recognised as providing effective treatment. It is no criticism of his opinion to say that much of his commentary could have come straight from antiquity. Buchan noted that 'the effects of wine are to raise the pulse, promote perspiration, warm the habit, and exhilirate the spirits.'[60] Being astringent, red wines have the additional power of strengthening the tone of the stomach and intestines, thus helping 'in restraining immoderate secretions.' Thin wines, able to 'pass off by the different emunctories', can 'gently open the body.' So 'the effects of the full-bodied wines' would be 'much more durable than the thinner.' Sweet wines, not being able 'to pass off freely' because of 'a glutinous substance' they contain, 'will heat the body more than an equal amount of any other wine,' provided they are as alcoholic as the others. Buchan praised wine as a cordial medicine or stimulant 'worth all the rest put together.' For wine to provide all these elixir-like properties, it had to be 'sound and good.' No benefit was 'to be expected from the common trash ... often sold by the name of wine,' one of the most falsified products on the market. Americans suspicious of commercial brands were able to make their own wine from recipes easily available in books such as *Dr. Chase's Recipes or Information for Everybody,* though a delicate palate would have found the doctor's wine heavily chaptalized and watered. Complaints about fraudulent wine, which became even more common in the second part of the nineteenth century, continued well into the twentieth century. Adulteration of wine restricted its medical usefulness to the patients able to pay for guaranteed quality.

Wine as a common meeting ground for popular and elite medicine was still evident towards the end of the nineteenth century. The publication of the weekly illustrated *La Médecine populaire* brought together a great deal of the discourse of doctors and of the tried and true practices of popular medicine, including 'Les remèdes des champs'. In 1881 Dr. H. Barella presented to readers the complex composition of wine, explaining how some of the elements – alcohol, tannin, and coloring matter – could generally have a favorable effect on the stomach though actions such as stimulating the digestive functions. The acids – malic, tartric, succinic, carbonic, etc. – were seen as moderating the destructive energy of alcohol in the 'animal economy' and attenuating its effect on the nervous system. Barella believed that the best wines for a sluggish digestion were those rich in tannin and also high in sugar and the natural alcohol produced by the fermentation of the wine. For proof of the efficacy of this medicine he was able to refer to the fact that the hospitals of Paris had been serving the wines of Banyuls and Saint-Raphaël for over thirty years. The authority of Bouchardat stood behind the administration of these wines in treating anemia (including that from chronic gout), chlorosis, intermittant fevers, and illnesses resulting from bad and unbalanced diets; these wines were also given to pregnant women and old people. Run down patients with difficult digestions could benefit particularly from these sweet wines.[61]

Some students of popular medicine talk up their stock by emphasizing the 'recriprocal influences' between elite and popular medicines rather than the 'borrowings of the *remèdes de bonnes femmes* from the old learned doctrines.'[62] So historically one can even identify a sort of collaboration of the two. The doctor used to be called when maternal medicine had failed.[63] In early-nineteenth century Burgundy, the appearance of the doctor signaled that someone was close to death.[64] After plant therapy, simple concoctions or herbal teas, and waters from the appropriate religious sources had been tried, the doctor was called on to try his skills in a difficult situation where three great medical powers of rural culture – Sainte Anne (all diseases), Sainte Catherine (ovarian problems and oversized breasts), and Saint André (impotence) – had all failed.

The knowledge of the therapeutic power of plants, perhaps the chief raison d'être of popular medicine, became less and less important in the nineteenth century because a growing pharmaceutical industry replaced plant preparations of herborist and of family with products that isolated 'most of the active principles of plants to prepare quick acting and better medicines than the plants themselves.'[65] Some French doctors thought that the English were much more knowlegeable than the French in the use of tree and plant medical products.[66] Commentary by some recent French scholars seems to ignore the existence since at least the eighteeenth century 'of what were variously called manufacturing chemists or drug importers and wholesalers,' who sold ingredients to local dispensers for resale to people who diagnosed their own illnesses, according to information in one of numerous medical self help books, and treated themselves.[67] François Magendie's famous *Formulary*, which 'attempted to base the pharmacopoeia on chemically pure drugs ... plant alkaloids such as emetine, quinine, and cinchona.' dated from 1821.[68] (Of course, ingredients and books might not have been available in places deep in the heart of Burgundy in the age of Lamartine.) Veissid argued that 'popular medicine is a branch of medicine that has remained stagnant since the nineteenth century and therefore cannot be so efficacious as living scientific medicine, which ... has not ceased to progress.'[69] One uncompromising defender of the scientific faith even argued that the basis of popular medicine is mainly ethnological, lying outside the domaine of medical science.[70] There remained a therapeutic role for certain plants and herbs, namely that of helping to maintain the organism's equilibrium, a sort of minor and even contested role in modern medicine, though important in human health.

In western culture the functions of items as both food and medicine gradually separated over the past three centuries, and this process did not help the therapeutic status of wine.[71] The existence of common therapeutic practices was evident as late as the eighteenth century – and no doubt there are later examples. One of the big names of late-seventeenth–early-eighteenth century medicine, Philippe Hecquet, praised domestic remedies. Hecquet was able to cite no less an authority than Friedrich Hoffmann, thurifer of scientific medicine, whose work on the *Excellence of Domestic Remedies* was translated into French in 1730. After a love affair with chemical remedies Hoffmann came back to simple things, and Hecquet followed him in emphasizing the use of simple drugs, especially items derived from plants and grains.[72] But the seventeenth and early-eighteenth centuries perhaps provide the last case of this therapeutic sharing in the history of western medicine. The cynic might add the qualification 'until our own time,' when the cost of providing bourgois medical care for the masses has made cheaper therapies and preventive medicine of interest to politicians and doctors. Popular medicine still hopes to be reintegrated into the community that left it outside the pale, and the advocates of cost-cutting efficiencies may grudgingly allow part of the its corpus to achieve respectable status as part of preventive and alternative medicines. And in a certain sense alcohol and wine have always provided a common conceptual meeting ground for different medical worlds.

Notes

1. Quoted in *The New Shorter Oxford English Dictionary*, (Oxford: Oxford University Press, 1996), II: 2292.
2. Charles H. Talbot, 'Folk medicine and history,' in Wayland D. Hand (ed), *American Folk Medicine. A Symposium* (Berkeley, CA: University of California Press, 1976), 10.
3. William George Black, *Folk-Medicine; a chapter in the history of culture* (London: Elliot Stock, 1883). Published for the Folk-Lore Society.
4. See Matthew Ramsey, *Professional and Popular Medicine in France, 1770-1830* (Cambridge: Cambridge University Press, 1988), and the

bibliography in Marcelle Bouteiller, *Médecine populaire d'hier et d'aujourd'hui* (Paris: Maisonneuve et Larose, 1987), 333–55.

5. Bouteiller, *op. cit.* (note 4), 13.
6. Dorothy Porter and Roy Porter, *Patient's Progress. Doctors and Doctoring in Eighteenth-Century England* (Stanford, CA: Stanford University Press, 1989), 192–6.
7. Dr. L. Schlosser, *L'art ancien de guérir* (Paris: Editions France-Empire, 1984), 7–8. He sees the old medicine as a 'médecine de l'homme', which never ignored 'l'homme comme totalité de vie.'
8. A suberb model of this genre of medical history is Ramsey's *Professional and Popular Medicine in France, 1770-1830,* (note 4).
9. Bouteiller, *op. cit.* (note 4), 255–6. Ramsey, 'The Popularization of medicine in France,' in Porter (ed), *The Popularization of Medicine* (London: Routledge, 1992), 105, notes that the split live pigeon was applied to the afflicted part for 18-20 hours to treat pleurisy. Porter and Porter, *op. cit.* (note 6), 194, note that 'In 1771 Dr Richard Brookes advised the application to the head of the split live chicken or pigeon in cases of head pain with delirium. They ask 'was this a medical therapy or a sacrifice?' The answer would appear to be both.
10. Bouteiller, *op. cit.* (note 4), 46.
11. Elizabeth Fee, review in the *Bulletin of the History of Medicine,* 69 (1995), 132–33, of Anne Hardy, *The Epidemic Streets: Infectious Diseases and the Rise of Preventive Medicine, 1856-1900* (Oxford: Clarendon Press, 1993).
12. See T. McKeown and others, 'An interpretation of the modern rise of population in Europe,' *Population Studies,* 27 (1972) and Thomas McKeown, *The Origins of Human Disease* (London: Blackwell, 1988).
13. Jules Romains, *Knock ou le triomphe de la Médecine* (Paris: Gallimard, 1924).
14. Danielle Voldman. 'La médecine en France au début du XXe siècle,' in *La médecine familiale au début du siècle* (Paris: Editions Heures de France), 15. The serious reader will consult W. F. Bynum, *Science and the Practice of Medicine in the Nineteenth Century* (Cambridge: Cambridge University Press, 1994).
15. See the classic chapter on doctors in Theodore Zeldin, *France 1848-1945* (2 vols., Oxford: Oxford University Press, 1973; revised paperback, 1979); for the number of doctors in legislative assemblies, see Jack D. Ellis, *The physician-legislators of France. Medicine and politics in the early Third Republic, 1870-1914* (Cambridge: Cambridge University Press, 1990), 4.
16. This panoramic survey is presented in Bouteiller, *op. cit.* (note 4),

111–114.

17. Schlosser, *op. cit.* (note 7), 7.
18. For the evolution of 'the corpus of popular medical literature' itself, see Ramsey, *op. cit.* (note 9), 122.
19. There were three basic pharmaceutical alcohol preparations prescribed for internal use. The *alcoolature* was obtained from the dissolving action of concentrated alcohol on certain fresh plant substances. The *alcoolat* was obtained by the distillation of alcohol with substances known for their volatile elements – lemon, orange, anis, aloes, etc.; the *alcoolats* were numerous in the old pharmacies. The *alcoolé* was a liquid *préparation officinale* obtained from the dissolving action of the alcohol on one or several bases of medicaments.
20. *La médecine populaire* (1 Nov. 1902), 15, notes that both English and French doctors were prescribing lemon juice after 1844 .
21. Jacques Veissid, *Traité de médecine populaire* (Paris: Société Parisienne d'édition, 1973), 5–7, 16, 123, 142–3, 210, 249, 258.
22. Edward O. Lautmann and others, 'Sexual dysfunction in the United States – Prevalence and predictors,' *Journal of the American Medical Association*, 281 (1999), 537–44.
23. See Arnaud Peri, *Les vins médicinaux* (Paris: Editions Image & Nature, 1997), and Robert van Gulick, *Sexual Life in Ancient China. A Preliminary Survey of Chinese Sex and Society from ca. 1500 B.C. till 1644 A.D.* (Leiden: E. J. Brill, 1961).
24. M. F. K. Fisher, *A Cordiall Water – A Garland of Odd & Old Receipts to Assuage the Ills of Man and Beast* (San Francisco: North Point Press, 1981), 138.
25. Pline l'ancien, *Histoires naturelles. Livre xx: Médecines douces de l'antiquité. La vertu des plantes* (Paris: Arléa, 1995), 68. Translated into French by François Rosso.
26. On Raspail's use of camphor and on camphor generally, see Dora B. Weiner, *Raspail, Scientist and Reformer* (New York: Columbia University Press, 1968), 139–44. On 142 there is a fascinating list of the formulas for the most popular remedies concocted by this 'poor man's doctor,' described by Pierre Mauriac as the 'Don Quijote of medicine.'
27. Adolphe-Benestor Lunel, *Dictionnaire universel de médecine* (Paris: L'auteur, 3 vols., 1861-3), ii, 260, which cites Raspail's *Manuel de médecine populaire* on camphor.
28. Veissid, *op. cit.* (note 21), 5–7.
29. See Sandra Blakeslee, 'Placebos prove so powerful even experts are surprised,' Science Times –The New York Times (Oct. 13, 1998),

D1–4. The placebo effect may not be of any clinical significance: see Asbjorn Hrobjartsson and Peter G. Gotezsche, 'Is the Placebo Powerless? ...', *The New England Journal of Medicine*, 344 (2001), 594–602.

30. Porter and Porter, *op. cit.* (note 6), 195. *The Green Pharmacy* is the title of a book by Dr. Jim Duke. According to *The New York Times* (Oct. 15, 1998), B11, sales of dietary supplements and herbal products in the United States recently totaled $3.6 billion annually, including $200 million for St. John's wort. 'Dr. Duke's Phytochemical and Ethnobotanical Databases' for the Agricultural Research Service are on the web.
31. Françoise Loux, *Pratiques et savoirs populaires dans la société traditionnelle* (Paris: Berger-Levrault, 1979), 154.
32. Loux, *Traditions et soins d'aujourd'hui* (Paris: InterEditions, 1983), 229–230.
33. Françoise Loux, *op. cit.* (note 31), 153–54.
34. Quoted by Loux, *ibid.,* 153–54, from 'Un cahier manuscrit de guérisseur'.
35. These two recipes come from the book *Médecine régionale, mystérieuse et pittoresque* (Niort: Editions Vernaculaires, 1981). Participation et direction littéraire de Jacques Lamare.
36. Black, *op. cit.* (note 3), 161.
37. See Eva C. Keuls, *The Reign of the Phallus. Sexual Politics in Ancient Athens* (New York: Harper, 1985).
38. Captain John C. Bourke (Third Cavalry, U.S.A.), *Scatologic Rites of all Nations. A Dissertation upon the Employment of Excrementitious Remedial Agents in Religion, Therapeutics, Divination, Witchcraft, Love-philters, etc., in all parts of the Globe* (Washington, D.C.: W. H. Lowdermilk, 1891). 'Based upon original notes and personal observation, and upon compilation from over one thousand authorities. Not for general perusal.' Sigmund Freud wrote the preface for the German edition of 1913, published by Ethnologischer Verlag in Leipzig. The French translation, *Les rites scatologiques*, published by Presses Universitaires de France in 1981, contains only thirty one of the original fifty chapters. The French edition was established by the late Dominique Laporte, philosophical expert on excrement and author of *Histoire de la merde* (Paris: Ed. Heures de France, 1978), published by Christian Bourgeois, with the dedication 'Au jeune Flaubert pour la belle explication,' which keeps things nicely medical.
39. Jacques André, *Être médecin à Rome* (Paris: Payot, 1995), 89.
40. Schlosser, *op. cit.* (note 7), 101. *The Oxford Medical Companion*

(Oxford: Oxford University Press, 1994), edited by John Walton and others, 879–80, says of the poem – 'editions vary from several hundred to a few thousand verses' – that 'It is literally a regimen of health and has references to healthy living, diet, liquor, sleep, and remedies of many kinds, including surgical. [One] medical historian ... thought it to be 'the backbone of all practical medical literature up to the time of the Renaisssance'.' For 'Salerno and the impact of translation,' see Vivian Nutton in Lawrence I. Conrad *et al.*, *The Western Medical Tradition 800 BC to AD 1800* (Cambridge: Cambridge University Press, 1995), 139–146.

41. Laporte, *op. cit.* (note 38), 70–97. Laporte draws on the general explanatory scheme used by Bachelard in *La formation de l'esprit scientifique*, which makes an attempt to connect up the digestive essence of the bourgeoisie, medical theories of digestion, and the importance given to excrement in medicine. On 'the excremental vision,' see Norman O. Brown, *Life against Death – The Psychoanalytical Meaning of History* (New York: Vintage Books, 1959), ch. xiii.
42. Loux, *op. cit.* (note 31), 154. M. F. K. Fisher, *op. cit.* (note 24), 46, gives the recipe for breaking a fever, as in measles; the key ingredient is turds of wild jackrabbits dried in the oven and used to make a strong tea to be drunk by the patient every half hour until sweating starts.
43. Bouteiller, *op. cit.* (note 4), 53.
44. Françoise Loux (avec la collaboration de Philippe Richard), *Sagesses du corps. La santé et la maladie dans les proverbes français* (Paris: Maisonneuve et Larose, 1978), 67.
45. See ch. 9 ('De quelques proverbes relatifs à l'hygiène') of A. Richerand, *Des erreurs populaires relatives à la médecine* (Paris: Caille et Ravier, 1812).
46. Loux, *op. cit.* (note 44), 70.
47. René Debrie, 'Contribution à l'étude de la médecine populaire en Picardie,' *Eklitra*, 23 (1976), 2.
48. Loux, *op. cit.* (note 44), 67, 77.
49. *Ibid.*, 73.
50. *Ibid.*, 85–6.
51. Roland Barthes, *Mythologies* (Paris: Seuil, 1957), 76. Barthes noted that the opposition between wine and water is true only mythically (1950s), not so much sociologically, because the old role of water was usurped by milk. Perhaps today, with the revived cult of mineral waters, water has regained some of its old position.
52. Loux, *op. cit.* (note 44), 71–2, 78.

53. *Ibid.*, 78.
54. Barthes, *op. cit.* (note 51), 74–79.
55. Loux, *op. cit.* (note 44), 78.
56. Aline Rousselle argued in the *Annales E. S. C.* back in 1980 that most of the prescriptions in the three books of *Diseases of Women* are so much like a recipe book 'that they derive from a female tradition of home remedies handed down from mother to daughter.' See Helen King, 'Food and Blood in Hippokratic Gynaecology,' in John Wilkins, David Harvey & Mike Dobson (eds), *Food in Antiquity* (Exeter: University of Exeter Press, 1995), 353.
57. Roy Porter, 'The Eighteenth Century,' in Conrad *et al.*, *op. cit.* (note 40), 443–6.
58. The *Dictionary of National Biography*, VII (22 vols, London: Oxford University Press, 1973), 180–1, notes that the first edition of *Domestic medicine* sold for the 'low price of six shillings. In the eighteen edition of *Domestic Medicine; or, a treatise on the prevention and cure of diseases by regimen and simple medicines with an appendix, continuing a dispensatory for the use of private practitioners* (London: J. Smith, 1803) Buchan says that his work has sold about a hundred thousand copies, which presumably includes the translations. See also A. Brierre de Boismont (médecin de l'hôpital des Bons-Hommes , etc.), *Médecine domestique, comprenant les premiers secours à administrer dans les maladies et accidens qui menacent promptement la vie* (Paris: Bibliothèque Populaire, 2d edn, 1833). This book of 104 pages was in the series of the Bibliothèque populaire, which also included Dr. Levasseur's *Pharmacie de la mère....*
59. J. D. Duplanil, *Les remèdes de bonnes femmes, éprouvés à travers les siècles. Tout les secrets des guérisseurs de campagne* (Mandelieu-La Napoule: Editions Intertep, 1974). The translator, Duplanil, was a graduate of Montpellier and the 'médecin honoraire' of the Comte d'Artois. I have looked at the fourth edition of Duplanil's translation, published in 1789: *Médecine domestique, ou traité complet des moyens de se conserver en santé, et de guérir les maladies, par le régime et les remèdes simples: ouvrage mis à la portée de tout le monde*; par G. Buchan, M.D. Another recent work drawing upon Buchan is Georges Vergnes, *La médecine venue du fond des âges. Formules et recettes médico-magiques* (Paris: Laffont, 1979), which notes regional associations with specific folk remedies, many of which included wines .
60. For Buchan's remarks on wine, see 539–41 of the appendix to William Buchan, *op. cit.* (note 58); (London: New Stereotype Edition, n.d.).

61. *La Médecine populaire,* no. 52 (1881), 824–5. Bouchardat's opinion was assumed to be based on his own observations and those of other *maîtres illustres*: Chomel, Rostan, Requin, Grisolles, Trousseau, etc.
62. Bouteiller, *op. cit.* (note 4), 12.
63. Dr Henri Besson, 'Souvenirs d'un jeune médecin d'avant 1914,' in Maximilienne Levet-Gautrat and others, *La médecine familiale au début du siècle* (Paris: Ed. Heures de France, 1978), 29–33.
64. Henri Vincenot, *La vie quotidienne des paysans bourguignons au temps de Lamartine* (Paris: Hachette, 1976), ch. VI, 'Le docteur Bon Temps et ses carnets.' Vincenot also points out the efficacy of 'la pharmacopée bourguigonne ... une étape du savoir médical.' The two staples of pharmacists were camphor, a mild antipruritic in topical preparations and an ingredient of tinctures and oils, and the aloe plant, whose juice supplies a purgative drug.
65. Veissid, *op. cit.* (note 21), 5–7
66. *Nouvelle découverte pour prévenir et guérir diverses maladies sans médicamens* (Paris: Impr. de Chassignon, 1828), par M. Le Barbey, physician and professor of botany.
67. Dr. John C. Gunn, *Domestic Medicine:or Poor Man's Friend, in the House of Affliction, Pain, and Sickness* (2nd edn., Knoxville: F. S. Heiskell, 1832); the work had gone through 213 printings by 1885. R. V. Pierce, M. D., *The People's Common Sense Medical Adviser in Plain English; or, Medicine Simplified* (Buffalo, N.Y.: World's Dispensary, 1875), was in its 14th edn by 1886.
68. Bynum, *op. cit.* (note 14), 119, 164–5. The 6th edn (1827) of the *Formulary for the Preparation and Employment of several new remedies* (London: Underwood, 1928) ... was translated into English in 1828; it had an appendix of the experience of British practitioners with many of the new remedies.
69. Veissid, *op. cit.* (note 21), 5–7.
70. H. V. Valois, preface to Bouteiller, *op. cit.* (note 4), 7–10.
71. For a discussion of plants used as food and medicine, see Virgil J. Vogel, 'American Indian Foods Used as Medicine,' in Hand, *op. cit.* (note 2), 125 ff. Food and medicine are being combined again: see David J. Morrow, 'A medicine chest or a grocery shelf? Debating the merits of 'functional foods',' *The New York Times* (Dec. 12, 1999), section 3.
72. Philippe Hecquet, *La médecine, la chirurgie et la pharmacie des pauvres* (Paris: Clousier, 1742), 3 vols, iii, introduction to the section 'La pharmacie des pauvres.'

2

An Early-Nineteenth Century German–French Model of Wine Therapy

Medicine has always been laden with theories, all fertile in generating different therapeutic discourses. Few theories have generated more squabbling than the views of the radically Bacchic, Scottish physician John Brown (1735-88) on the therapeutic virtues of alcohol. At first examination, the Brunonian system of medicine seems simple and rational, but the fact of the matter is that Brown's texts – even on excitability – have been interpreted according to the situation and interests of readers.[1] Brown's medicine was centred on the excitability or irritability theory, popular in the late-eighteenth century, which classified diseases under sthenia and asthenia according to their over-stimulating (sthenic) and under- or non-stimulating (asthenic) effect on the body. This theory justified the simple treatments of bloodletting, emetics, and cathartics for sthenic conditions and the administration of stimulants, often wine or laudanum (alcoholic tincture of opium), for asthenic diseases.[2]

> Excitement ... the true cause of life, is, within certain boundaries, proportional to the degree of stimulus. The degree of stimulus, when moderate, produces health; in a higher degree it gives occasion to diseases of excessive stimulus; in a lower degree, or excessively weak, it induces those that depend upon a deficiency of stimulus or disability. And, as excitement is the cause both of diseases and perfect health, so that which restores the morbid to the healthy state, is a dimunition of excitement in diseases of excessive stimulus, and an increase of excitement in diseases of debility.[3]

Brown practiced what he preached, even when writing and teaching. He boasted of surviving more than forty hours of literary composition, 'done with dispatch by dining well and drinking a glass of wine every hour.'[4] He needed whisky to face students. Thomas Beddoes describes Brown's countering his languid state by consuming whisky and laudanum: 'before he began his lecture, he would take forty or fifty drops of laudanum in a glass of whisky, repeating the dose four or five times during the lecture. ... He soon waxed warm, and by degrees his imagination was exalted into frenzy.'[5] John Brown and his drunken pedagogy were forgotten by a profession in search of scientific foundations and bourgeois respectability, but the basic principles of his therapy survived.[6]

Brown fancied that with the notion of excitability he had discovered a principle in medicine comparable to Newton's principle of gravity in natural philosophy. If one accepted Newton's axiom that one should not multiply causes, Occam's razor would replace the scalpel. Brown's general theory was solidly rooted in western medicine in a less extreme form. The idea was orthodox enough: deviations from the state of health were to be corrected by debilitating measures in the case of excessive excitement (stenic diseases) and by stimulation in the case of insufficient excitement (asthenic diseases).[7] His emphasis on quantification 'pointed to a therapeutics dependant upon dosage size.'[8] The key thing was that the causes of health and disease were identical in this system.

The influence of Brunonian therapeutics is traditionally explained by a number of factors. First, the use of alcohol and wine in treating diseases had been around since the invention of medicine; this is often forgotten in erudite discussions of the subject.[9] Secondly, the use and abuse of alcohol and opium were well-established features of eighteenth-century medical practice. In the previous century Thomas Sydenham had noted that medicine would be a cripple without opium. 'Opium rampant' was Kramer's description of the European situation in both centuries.[10] Wine continued to be an important item in the doctor's arsenal. William Cullen, Brown's mentor and later enemy, at the University of Edinburgh, prescribed beer, wine, and brandy in appropriate cases. Guenter Risse found that in the 1780s and 1790s more wines and spirits were prescribed at the Edinburgh Infirmary than before.[11] Brown was a man in tune with his times. The eighteenth century saw an increase in the availability of alcoholic beverages, ranging from gin to drinks of higher social status such as champagne, quality red bordeaux and burgundies, cognac, and port. It is probable that the growing social acceptance of alcohol and especially the increasing social distinction of certain varieties of beverages, encouraged doctors to prescribe alcohol and wine more than ever. And it was comforting for the practitioner to know that his alcoholic therapy was solidly 'grounded in conventional forms of doctoring.'[12]

In Edinburgh, as in some German states, Brunonianism served young doctors and reformers as a weapon against the University medical establishment when they proclaimed an alternative medicine of a rigorously scientific nature leading to simple diagnostic procedures and efficacious cures. The optimistic view that Brown's medicine was cheap – in fact, wine therapy could be expensive – opened up the possibility, in principle, of extending the therapeutic privileges of the rich to the poor.[13] On the continent, especially in some Italian and German states, the Brownian doctrine produced resonances different from those in Scotland.[14]

Brown's doctrine had a professional attraction for doctors because of its rejection of the idea of 'the traditional belief in the healing forces of nature' and its consequent empowerment of the doctor as healer.[15] This new therapeutic chutzpah needed a firm foundation, one capable of endowing medicine with as much certainty as the discoveries that were changing natural philosophy in the fast developing sciences of chemistry and physics. As the older medical systems of Hermann Boerhaave and Friedrich Hoffmann cracked and crumbled, many German physicians sought solace in the Brownian system, given philosophical respectability by 'Kant's approval of the Brownian system as the proper framework of vitality and medicine.'[16] A precarious certainty derived from the claim of Brunonianism to provide 'one single cause for vitality – "excitability" – and ... to explain the basis of health and disease on simple quantitative changes of this property....'[17] Not everyone was convinced, even after Schelling incorporated Brunonianism into his *Naturphilosophie*. Jakob Fries pointed out that the Scottish doctrine was unable to:

> supply a legitimate theoretical knowledge of physiology,' which was the later anti-vitalistic achievement of Helmholtz and his emulating successors. For the neo-Kantian Fries only Brown's therapeutic method, which necessarily emphasised drug dosage and could not escape experience, retained some value.[18]

Whatever the positive value of Brown's ideas, many doctors welcomed 'criticism of the tormenting methods of cupping, leeching, and blistering, as well as the endless prescriptions of emetics and purgatives which often contributed to the patient's suffering.'[19] Like Louis XIV, patients came to hate the trinitarian medical repertory of purging, vomiting, and bleeding. Alcoholic beverages and opium seemed pleasant and equally efficacious substitutes. Equally important, the tinkering done by German doctors and the impressive new name of *Erregbarkheitstheorie* given to Brown's doctrine convinced many practitioners that they now had a scientifically-based therapeutics capable of raising their low social status and driving out competing healers, or, according to Broman, even 'inaugurate a revolution in German medicine.'[20]

Andreas Röschlaub, professor at the University of Bamberg, laid the theoretical foundations of German Brunonianism, and Adalbert Friedrich Marcus, director of the Bamberg city hospital provided a firm clinical basis in his *Prüfung des Brownischen System* (1798), which showed the efficacy of the new medicine in the treatment of at least 102 of the 134 patients admitted between April and June of 1798. Marcus keenly appreciated the curative powers of opium, but the Brownian system easily accommodated alcohol and wine as valuable items of *materia medica.*[21]

The first complete professional medical manual on the therapeutic role of wine was probably the treatise published in 1816 by Eduard Loebenstein-Loebel (1779-1819), a Brownian-inspired professor of medicine at the University of Jena and health adviser to the Duke of Weimar.[22] Since there was nothing comparable in French, Daniel Lobstein, Strasbourgeois doctor and accoucheur, quickly did a translation for publication the next year.[23] Very little of what later German doctors say about wine therapy cannot be found in this comprehensive work.[24] This book on wine therapy by a well known professor and literary doctor had considerable success in his native land, much more than it enjoyed in France, which was perhaps medically satiated with the anatomo-clinical method and certainly suffering from the post-Napeolonic surplus of military surgeons, who were unlikely to substitute wine for the knife. Lobstein noted that what had been needed for a long time was a book identifying the origins of wines with their physical and chemical properties, determining precisely their general effects on healthy and on sick people, and giving for each type of wine a detailed therapeutic guide based on the existing state of medical knowledge. (Loebenstein-Loebel made it clear that his book did not discuss the use of wine in the daily diet of healthy people; the book was limited to the use of wine in the treatment of disease.) One of the valuable features of the guide was that it was based on Loebenstein-Loebel's extensive practice, which had permitted him to test all the types of wine about which he had written.

In the development of his wine therapy, in addition to identifying the conditions in which different wines should be used in the sick person's diet, Loebenstein-Loebel pursued the strategy of using different wines according to their individual properties correlated with the specific nature of the disease. The new doctrine scorned doctors who had been unable to attain this therapeutic precision, partly because they had not studied all the ancient and modern texts on the subject. Not least among the virtues of the new approach was the possibility of avoiding prescribing wine where it could do no good or, in the case of certain wines, perhaps some harm.[25] Loebenstein-Loebel emphasised that the wine used in medical treatments had to be pure, non-adulterated, good vintage wines. If taken seriously and rigorously defined, these criteria would have considerably limited the use of wine therapy. To determine the effect of wine on any one person was a complex business depending on the geographical origin and age of the wine, the temperament of the patient – in many people the senses dominated irritability and digestion – and the relations between systems in the organism itself. The doctor had to consider the specific form of the illness, any idiosyncrasy or reaction against wine, and patients' usual consumption habits, especially if they drank several bottles a day.

Loebenstein-Loebel believed wine to be a unique product whose use in medicine could not be compared, as some believed, to that of opium. He reasoned that opium reduces physical movement by acting directly on the central nervous system, including the brain, with a pronounced specific effect on irritability and contractility. With its effects of benumbing, depressing, and weakening the taker, opium could act with good effect only in the case of partial or total 'exaltation of the nervous system': it therefore produced good results in the treatment of insomnia, frenzy, vomiting, and intense pain originating in the nervous system.[26] Erethism required opium and a soporific state required wine. Prudently administered, opium could be useful in treating 'too copious evacuations of the alimentary canal' coupled with disturbances in the lower gut and a 'morbific exaltation' of the senses, especially hearing and sight. Opium could be sparingly used in the case of insomnia with continual anxiety, weak pulse, cold extremities, total lack of appetite, clear urine, and general weakness in the organism. Opium could also be administered in cases of inflammation of the digestive system and secretory organs in the second period of diseases, that is when they threaten to produce gangrene or a scirrhus (hard tumour). Opium was often administered as one of several opium wines, known generically as laudanum. Sydenham's famous laudanum contained 200 grams of opium, 100 grams of saffron, and fifteen grams each of cinnamon and of cloves in 1000 grams of Malaga wine.[27] Neither opium nor wine were to be prescribed when the 'irritable system' (of muscles and nerves) was inflamed. And both opium and wine had to be avoided in brusque, violent inflammation of the nervous and irritable systems. But inflammation was considered a complex condition demanding the care of an experienced and learned doctor: for example, the third period of the evolution of an inflammation of the nervous system absolutely required small doses of the wines of the Rhine and of Würzburg (Frankenwein). Small doses were especially important if there were, among other things, symptoms of spasms accompanied by weakness with a plethora.

Wine, a vivifying medicine, was considered to have an effect opposite to that of opium, increasing the activity and functioning of nerves in the trunk of the body and in the lower stomach while acting in a pleasure-giving and isochronous way on physical movements in the cerebellum and the brain. Wine restored a depressed nervous system, worked magically in lethargy, melancholy, and 'nervous apoplexy.'[28] (The acidity of Rhines, however, made them unsuitable for use in the treatment of apoplexy resulting from general or partial plethora or blockage of the principal ducts.) In the case of nervous apoplexy where patients were weak and had shown previous symptoms, the professor advised the administration every hour of two full soup-spoons of Rhine wine, preferably Johannisberg, Rudesheim, or Hinterhausen. If the patient could not take the wine by mouth, then his head and back had to be washed with a cup or so of wine; expensive wine could still be used.

Wines were classified into different types according to the different effects they had on the organism's systems. The wine administered had to be suited to the system that was malfunctioning as well as to the disease. Loebenstein-Loebel established three categories of wine for medical use. First, acidulous white wines, which acted especially on the depressed irritability and sensibility of the organism. Secondly, French red wines, which were tonic, restorative of the reproductive system and of the sensibility of the neurological system. And third, alcoholic sweet wines, which also acted benignly on sensibility and weakened powers of reproduction. Each region's wine had its own distinguishing characteristics giving it specific medicinal properties. This wine therapy had a clearly stated class basis: the best wines, nearly always expensive, were to be prescribed; if the patients could not afford them, cheaper but still good wines could be administered.

The medical system of Loebenstein-Loebel was firmly anchored in humoral theory, which had long provided the basis of wine therapy. Pliny's *Natural History* (first century A. D.) gave the four basic dogmas on wine: it is a food; it helps digestion; it stimulates the appetite; and it is a psychodynamic agent (not Pliny's language). In the thirteenth century Roger Bacon summed up the humoral theory of wine in a paradigmatic statement. 'Whoever uses wine, properly mixed and at the right time, strengthens the body's natural heat and extends it through the whole system, purges the coleric humors through sweat and urine ... moistens those parts of the body which have become hard through dryness ... and brings on joy and lightness, mitigating melancholy.'[29] Towards the end of the eighteenth century Sir Edward Barry praised Hock wines 'for their salutary and medical qualities.' He found that they 'more equally promote all the excretions than any other wines of the same strength' and 'are more eminently useful for their antiseptic qualities, in all diseases, where the humours are disposed to a putrid state, especially in fevers of that kind.'[30] In Jane Austen's *Sense and Sensibility* the apothecary diagnosed Marianne Dashwood to be afflicted with putrid fever. (For 'the slow or nervous fever,' however, William Buchan had earlier declared that 'almost the only medicine necessary' is wine – a good sound claret – the genuine thing.[31])

According to Loebenstein-Loebel, diseases resulting from 'the degeneration or decomposition of our humors' were not to be treated with opium but with an aromatic white wine. In our day generally only red wine is medically popular, but in the professor's Bacchic therapy of nearly two centuries ago white wines occupied an important position. And no white wines matched the medical benefits of Rhine wines, distinguished more by their bouquet and acidity than their alcoholic content.[32] Through their aroma and acid, these wines acted especially on the nervous system, including the sympathetic nervous system, which regulates the involuntary automatic functions of the body. Loebenstein-Loebel expressed the same opinion as Hoffmann and Barry on German wines. Barry declared that 'no country is at this time [1775] more fertile of various excellent wines than Germany.' [33]

Pure, mature Rhine wines, taken later in the day (*not* in the morning), could be used, often with other medical drugs, to treat about a dozen diseases. In treating 'humid gangrene,' where 'the phenomena of putrefaction predominate,' wine should be used generously with other appropriate medicaments. The top class of the best Rhine wines were recommended for patients suffering from fevers but only after the inflammatory diathesis had passed.[34] In typhus the wine treatment would begin during the last period of the disease, when the body had essentially conquered it. Here Loebenstein-Loebel followed van Helmont in recommending that treatment begin with small doses and then increase in quantity. If the patient could not afford first class Rhine wines, then wines such as those of Marckbrunn, Geisenheim, Mittelheim, and Rothenberg could be prescribed. In nervous or ataxic fevers first quality Rhines would be prescribed after the inflammatory period had passed. In putrid or adynamic fever, when life seems about to end, Rhine wines could be doubly beneficial in strengthening weakened vital forces and in preventing, by their acid and aroma, the decomposition of the humors. In a fever-obsessed age, Hoffmann had followed his medical ancestors in recommending wine in the treatment of putrid fevers, which made the patient ravenous for acids. Wine acted immediately on the nervous system because it contains elements analogous to the 'nervous fluid.' This was also one of the cases in which wines could be helpful when applied externally.

Among the common diseases the doctor encountered, colic, scurvy, and dropsy were identified as responding to Rhine wines. A type of non-inflammatory colic where the faeces resemble laurel berries had to be treated with expensive wines, though some lesser wines such as Mittelheim, Schwartzach, and Erbach would work for poorer patients. Scurvy was ingeniously and broadly defined as an 'asthenic affection of the muscular and lymphatic systems ... with decomposition of the blood.'[35] It responded favourably (for the rich patient) to the alcohol, the aromatic element, and the acid in first class wine. The organism of the poor responded favourably to second class wine.[36] Only Rhine wines were prescribed for diseases of the lymphatic system and use was limited even in these cases. It was important to begin treatment early in the case of dropsy. Rubbing with a hot flannel stimulated the vital properties of the skin and increased the good effects of the wine, which worked less well in idiopathetic oedemas than in symptomatic cases such as those developing after scarlet fever. First class Rhine wines were still an important if sometimes secondary drug in the pharmacopoeia of the post-Enlightenment doctor.

Rhine wines were also prescribed to treat old diseases that have doggedly stayed with us through the centuries: mental troubles, abuse of narcotics, and sexual excess. All mental problems called for Rhine wine, because of their 'marvellous effects on melancholy, tranquil mania, and mental alienation caused by intense sorrow or a violent, unhappy love.' Rhine wines of an inferior quality could be used as aspersions and fomentations for the head. Drugs and sex gave rise to medical problems more difficult to treat.

To fight the baleful effects of opium and other plant narcotic poisons, Loebenstein-Loebel followed in the footsteps of the great doctors (Dioscorides, Paul of Aegina, Fallopius) in recommending that after 'preliminary vomiting' the patient be given heavy doses of acidulous wine at short intervals. He thought it important to use old wines of Johannisberg, Rudesheim, Rothland, and Hinterhausen, which, through their alcoholic and aromatic properties, pleasantly calmed the nervous system while breaking down and eliminating the poisonous narcotic element in the other parts of the organism. Second class Rhine wines also worked, but they had to be at least twenty to twenty-five years old. Loebelstein-Loebel cited an example of a man he had saved by administering large doses of good old Rhine wine after the patient had tried to commit suicide by taking a large dose of opium. Along with induced vomiting and coffee, old Rhines were recommended as the safest and quickest antidotes to opium poisoning.[37]

The enlightened doctor's therapeutic skills must have been tested by patients who, 'weakened by their abuse of the pleasures of love or by onanism,' suffered from dorsal or ischiatic consumption and also lost (unintentionally) seminal fluid. Hippocrates thought that this dangerous combination of ailments afflicted especially young married people and people engaging in excessive sexual activity. 'If you question the patient, he will tell you that ... when he urinates or defecates, he also loses an abundant and liquid sperm; he is sterile; he has nocturnal emissions while dreaming whether he is sleeping with a woman or not.' Other symptoms included weakness, ringing in the ears, and strong fever. When patients presented these symptoms, Hippocrates recommended immediate intervention, including purging. He prescribed various milks, avoidance of sexual relations, no exercise apart from walking, and also moderation in the consumption of wine.[38] The doctor prescribed the wines of Marckbrunn, Laubenheim, Hochheim, Bodenheim, and Nierstein. If the patient was used to drinking these wines, he could get better results by changing to a high quality old wine of Würzburg. And if the patient had digestive problems, neither Rhine or Franconian wines would do. The patient was condemned to the fine, alcoholic red wines of France, although some wines of the Ottoman Empire, essentially of wine-producing regions of the eastern Mediterranean, could also be prescribed because they were reputed to act on the sensibility of the digestive organs and through them to affect the entire organism.[39]

In a later analysis of dessert wines, Loebenstein-Loebel noted the frightful consequences of hideous sexual vices (too frequent emission of semen, too much coition, onanism, and female masturbation), which patients seemed to find pleasant enough to continue for years. Once his patient's virtue had been restored, he prescribed top-quality ('première goutte') Tokay, but in small doses so as not to give further stimulation to the patient's imagination and sex organs. In addition to the usual precautions with these patients, it was necessary to see if wine drinking produced temporary congestions or penile erections. The doctor did not forget that the the patients already suffered from too much of a good thing.

Because of the aromatic and especially the acidic qualities of Rhine wines, Loebenstein-Loebel regarded them as unsuitable in many diseases, especially those related to the digestive and blood-vascular systems. So spasms, weakness, and indurations and hard tumours in the digestive system, as well as idiopathic and symptomatic diarrhoea, colic, and iliac passion (ileus), were not treated with Rhines. But in 1838 a doctor in Cologne published a case history of a woman aged sixty seven suffering from a dreadful case of ileus whom he cured by the administration of a soup spoon of champagne every half hour: after four hours of this treatment she had a copious bowel movement.[40] Perhaps the acidity was countered by the carbon dioxide. Rhine wines were not used when the patient was being given mercurial oxides, for the wine's acid would further irritate the stomach. Nor were sufferers from heartburn to drink these wines. And they were to be avoided in all acute and chronic chest diseases because the acid would excessively irritate inflamed or suppurating lungs and aggravate diseases such as asthma. All acute inflammations and inflammation of the peripheral nervous system, including 'rheumatism and gout' required avoidance of Rhine wines.[41] So did haemorrhaging of any kind and all heart problems, especially those related to the lesser or pulmonary circulation. Loebenstein-Loebel's final prohibitions fell within the urological empire: Rhine wines should not be used for patients suffering from kidney stones, inflammation of the urinary tract, and gonorrhea; nor should they be used by women afflicted with *les fleurs blanches* or the whites.[42] In many of these diseases, the prescribed wine was burgundy or bordeaux.

Loebenstein-Loebel did not consider other German wines (Franconia, Mosel, the Palatinate or Pfalz) to be without medical virtues; he particularly had a good word for the wines of Franconia, though the wines of both Franconia and Mosel were not to be used in cases in which Rhine wines were contra-indicated.[43] In old *Frankenwein,* acid takes second place to sugar, aroma, and alcohol, thus enabling it to be useful in influencing the digestive functions, especially when the digestion seems stalled and the stomach sensitive. Wines of Leisten and Stein were used to treat 'putrid or nervous' dysentery, which also responded to burgundy if there were no inflammation. Arnica, which Stahl called the quinine of the poor, was probably used by patients who could not afford wine.[44] *Frankenwein* was considered particularly effective in treating recently developed non-feverish rheumatism manifesting itself between the skin and muscles of the extremities. Often in these cases, pain would start somewhere in the lower gut and run down the spermatic cord into the testicles, which could become red, tender, and swollen. The anguished male could be consoled with alcoholic wines of Franconia and the Palatinate, the preferred ones being from Roth, Neustadt, Ettinghofen, and Forster.

In the early-nineteenth century the framing of fever as a disease was nearly as complex as it had been in the era of Cullen (1710-90).[45] Loebenstein-Loebel used the hoary categories of hectic, continued, and essential fevers.[46] Horn's well known handbook of practical medicine of 1803 recommended with Brownian enthusiasm the early use of wine in treating fevers.[47] For a category designated as slow hectic fever, Loebenstein-Loebel found that old wines of Stein and Leisten were best; in the case of a great loss of weight, the patient drank several glasses of wine daily, but the pleasure was lessened by the addition of egg yolk corrupted by a little nutmeg. The same wines worked for essential fever, even if the fever occurred after the large evacuations typical in women who go through too long a period of wet-nursing; they worked also after too frequent losses of seminal fluid and in cases of gonorrhea. Fever was still viewed pretty much as 'a finalised reaction of the organism defending itself against a pathogenic attack or substance ... a sign not of the disease, but of the resistance to the disease. ... Fever is an excretory movement, purificatory in intention....'[48] Wine helped drive out the disease.

Older Franconian wines were used to treat amaurosis, loss of sight from disease of the optic nerve.[49] Schmucken used Rhine wines to which he added 60 to 100 crushed woodlice. (The woodlouse, like the armadillo, 'formerly played a considerable role in the medical art'; they were used to produce diuretic, appetite-stimulating, and anti-scrofulous effects in the organism. Galen recommended them to relieve abdominal obstructions.[50]) Loebenstein-Loebel, who could lay claim to a certain expertise in ophthalmology, preferred the wine of Stein or Leisten with added tartrate , a salt or ester of tartaric acid, which could be obtained from the tartar (potassium hydrogentartrate) deposits in wine vats or barrels.[51] In France the woodlice wine was included in some standard works but recognised as effective only if it contained potassium nitrate or saltpetre, which occurs naturally as nitre, or another substance having a special action on the urinary tract[52]. Poor people, unable to afford the old Franconian wines, could use the wines of the Mosel or the Palatinate. The dose was generous: one or two goblets with a meal and a glass in the afternoon at about four or five o'clock; the amount could be increased according to the patient's experience with wine. German wines had to be used in special cases of idiopathic amaurosis, such as that caused by a particular weakness of the optic nerve, without an excess of blood. The pure wines of Burgundy were much preferable for symptomatic amaurosis and in many other cases, including those where the digestive organs were affected at the same time.

Loebenstein-Loebel found that Rhine wines and the wines of Burgundy and Bordeaux were the most medically useful. Wines of the Hapsburg empire did not have much of a therapeutic role. Austrian wines had little use in medicine because of their low alcohol and low level of sugar. He admitted that at Whippach in the Carniole there was a wine called 'creator of children,' which was the best he could do for Austria. Hungarian wines were excellent and therapeutically indispensable – in Hungary. Both Hoffmann and Barry had a high opinion of Hungarian wines, especially Tokay and St. George Auspruch. Loebenstein-Loebel was not so keen on them. The best whites did not travel well and the reds were comparable to middle-range burgundies rather than the mythical bull's blood. Still, some Hungarian wines were useful in treating hysterical, weak women who had had miscarriages and in treating hypochrondiacs. And Tokay *première goutte* retained its role in lubricating the passage from deviation to normality in sexual behaviour. But the Hapsburg Empire provided a minor harvest compared to the therapeutic riches of French vineyards.

France had a long-established reputation as the country best able to maintain quality in producing, preserving, and exporting wine. All three capabilities were important for doctors, and the last was especially important for those practising outside France.[53] In spite of having been involved in a long quarrel over its therapeutic virtues versus those of champagne, burgundy was a favourite of the medical profession for both drinking and prescribing. It was a wine of distinction. Loebenstein-Loebel noted that Frederick the Great preferred it above all other wines; the father he hated loved champagne. He might also have identified the rich, Corton-loving Voltaire as an excellent reference for burgundy and noted that Diderot once followed the advice of Madame d'Epinay to cure a terrible head cold with copious amounts of burgundy. He got well in one day, after eating and drinking for eleven hours.[54] Burgundy had the reputation of producing the best table wines. German doctors seem to have considered burgundy as the most salubrious of wines. (French medical opinion divided along regional lines and would probably have given bordeaux this honour.) Hoffmann, however, seemed unenthusiastic about burgundy because its higher sulphur content made it stupefy the patient more than Rhine wine. Loebenstein-Loebel attributed a curious remark to Chaptal that burgundy is the least acid of French wines. This would have been a useful piece of medical knowledge if true. No matter. Other qualities made burgundy a great medical wine, at least up to its fourth year, after which, Loebenstein-Loebel noted, its qualities declined. Earlier doctors had treated rich people, including Burgundian rulers, by prescribing old burgundy because of its valuable medicinal properties. Some Normans may have done as well on cider vinegar.

Because of its abundant sugar content, balanced by the right proportion of alcohol, a good burgundy was believed to act energetically on the sensibility of the digestive organs. An extra benefit, available only within the medical system subscribed to by Loebenstein-Loebel, was that pure burgundy from a good year countered the degeneration of the humors and the blood. Burgundy was believed to influence the whole organism, with the highly desirable result of strengthening it. In treating certain illnesses doctors could not do without it, and Loebenstein-Loebel used it with the greatest success in a whole range of diseases. Like physicians since antiquity, he showed his faith in his knowledge and healing skill by speaking mostly of curing patients. We have no reason not to believe him.

Loebenstein-Loebel got good results in prescribing burgundy for external and internal use in the treatment of 'goutty diseases' not accompanied by inflammation or high fever, especially when the head was affected or even when goutty feet produced, by metastasis, foci in the intestines, the brain, or the urinary tract. In combination with other medicinal drugs, burgundy could produce surprising effects when drunk even up to six months after the illness. Between three and six goblets were prescribed with meals. Between meals the patient was comforted with a strong infusion of thyme and burgundy. The wines recommended were Volnay, Beaune, Chassagne, Nuits, Chambertin, Pommard, and Montrachet. Beer and *eau-de-vie* were forbidden, and so was white Meursault. White Chambertin was acceptable for a goutty person with no digestive problems even if he was perhaps bulging with haemorrhoids. Although Barry appreciated the perfumed and balmy Nuis (Côte de

Nuits), he declared Chambertin to be 'generally preferred to any other wine in Burgundy, as it is said to contain all the good qualities of the other wines, without any of their faults, and on that account is sold as dear as any wine in Burgundy.' Also in Barry's medical repertory was Chassagne, 'one of the noblest wines in the world,' preserved by its saline acid principle for three to four years, after which its 'tartness begins to wear off, and a more balsamic softness succeeds it.'[55] Less inclined to wax eloquent over the aesthetic properties of burgundy, Loebenstein-Loebel noted that all non-inflammatory digestive diseases responded to it. Even a poisoned patient could be given burgundy with egg yolk and nutmeg. And for digestive problems there was also the possibility of adding burgundy to the German drink Bischoff, which was made from unripe oranges. Loebenstein-Loebel also gave burgundy a role in treating various types of fevers. After this impressive prologue on diseases treatable with burgundy, the *Traité* goes on to deal with the diseases in which burgundy could be particularly useful.

One group of these diseases had a dermatological common denominator. For a patient with a scrofulous condition the doctor prescribed up to a daily bottle of second class burgundy. Children got three to six coffee spoonfuls. No wine surpassed burgundy in the treatment of venereal diseases, once formally part of the dermatological empire. Patients weakened by the disease were furthered destroyed by the cure, mercurous oxides, one of whose results was to put the digestive organs in a state of atonia. In this situation no wine was better than burgundy to aid the curative action of mercury and direct it towards the skin. Burgundy could also help in the treatment of inveterate gonorrhea accompanied by an ulcerated urinary tract and in the treatment of extraordinarily weak patients. The dose was limited to one half bottle a day. By giving them a disease grouping of their own with a different dose (one half to one bottle daily according to the case), Loebenstein-Loebel indicated the importance of mercury poisoning and other illnesses caused by mercury, which often totally changed the mass of humors. When the metal produced tumours and eruptions, burgundy was the 'sovereign remedy,' independent of the phosphoric acid, quinine, and sulphur combined with musk and orange rinds given to the patient, who also benefited from baths of hops, sulphur, and juniper wood. (Known for improving digestion, hops were widely used in nineteenth-century Paris hospitals.) Rich patients filled their prescriptions with Romanée, Chambertin, Volnay, Chassagne, Beaune, and Nuits, while poorer patients consoled themselves with wines such as Auray, Monthelie, and Mercurey. If any of these measures caused bladder troubles, which old people might have even without medical help, these wines would produce excellent effects, even when other wines could not be tolerated and other red wines caused pains during urination. Burgundy was seen as a friend of the genito-urinary system.

Burgundy was accepted as a valuable tool in treating two specifically female diseases. In cases of chronic leucorrhoea, whether the discharge originated in the uterus or the vagina, whether the disease was symptomatic or idiopathic, and whether the cause was venereal or not, first and second class burgundies were in the doctor's bag of tricks. But they were drunk only after the first period of inflammation had passed. Up to three goblets could be drunk at *dîner* (lunch). Wine must have been a welcome change from the ordinary drink of salep mixed with burgundy and water. (Salep refers to a drink made with the bulbs of orchis, whose shape was more inspiring than the taste of the drink.) Wine was believed to stimulate and strengthen the lymphatic system, correcting the changes that the lymph underwent in illness. Being sensitive, an infected lymphatic system required that wine be given prudently. The practice of humoral medicine was a complex business.

Complexity was compounded with delicacy in the treatment of young anaemic females, whose greenish complexion explains the use of the term chlorosis to describe their iron deficiency. Loebenstein-Loebel listed some of the problems with which the doctor had to deal in this category of patient: diminished irritability (the ability of excitable tissue such as nerve and muscle to respond to stimuli); altered blood and lymph; disturbance of intellectual functions; weakness of digestive organs accompanied by a disturbed appetite and a desire to eat odd things – earth, charcoal, and rinds, for example. Next to ferruginous medicines, nothing was better than red burgundies for curing this disease.[56] Sometimes it was necessary to prescribe a burgundy fortified with iron from a small sack of iron filings that had been suspended for eight days in a recorked bottle. A patient drank two or three glasses daily if there was no sign of nervous irritability, which required the dose to be cut in half or even a quarter at the beginning of treatment. Second and third class burgundies were recommended: Auray, Monthelie, and Mercurey in the second class; and wines from Châlons, Torny, Chénas, and the Mâconnais, etc. in the third class. Some wines of the southwest were also prescribed: Château Margaux, Cahors, Grand Constant, and even the côtes, and any others that were not too heavy.

Chlorosis used to be given the more exciting if misleading label of 'erotic fever.' Bad food was regarded as one of the causes of this type of burning libido. But the physician's gaze also found the etiology of chlorisis in sexual perversion: tribadism or female homosexuality and onanism (meaning masturbation, not *coitus interruptus*).[57] Naturally, the females had to renounce these vices before wine produced any effects; without a moral decision, no cure was possible. Once safely protected by the laws of modesty, the patient could be treated with the wine of burgundy combined with iron-fortified medicines, quinine, aromatics, and quassia.[58] The patient was not be permitted to enjoy the sensuous stimulation of good pure burgundy. The wine was assumed to work independently of the required proper diet and exercise in fresh air. This program did not work if the patient had been suffering from the disease for a long time, or if there was organic disease in the liver, the spleen, or the lungs.

Doctors assumed that burgundy helps the body when water gets where it should not, as in hydrocephalus, for example. In the case of pleural effusion, the accumulation of fluid within the pleural cavity, especially in old people with healthy lungs and heart, red burgundy was the recommended wine at lunch. But in case of accompanying obstruction in the lower gut or of constipation, fine white burgundies or old Rhine wine were substituted.

In his discussion of the use of burgundies combined with other remedies in treating haemorrhages, Loebenstein-Loebel noted his successes. Women exhausted by too many pregnancies could benefit from burgundy in more ways than one: it could be injected into the uterus. He preferred red burgundies to other French red wines because 'the latter are too heavy and too stimulating, acting with too much violence on the sanguine system, which could have unfortunate consequences.' French wines, especially burgundy, were not to be used in treating haemoptysis or coughing-up of blood. The doctor needed to know nearly a dozen conditions governing the use of burgundy when a patient was haemorrhaging, and though the doctor might have used a checklist to be sure that his patient was included in the category of case benefiting from burgundy, only wise judgment and intuition acquired by practice could enable the doctor to make the best decision in such a case.[59] But no doctor needed to doubt that burgundies were especially good in convalescence after certain haemorrhages.

The other French wine Loebenstein-Loebel dealt with in considerable detail was red bordeaux. His comments on the wines of the Languedoc were not generally friendly, though he admitted that if properly developed the best of these wines were just below the good wines of Bordeaux. Of course it was impossible to specify precisely the effects of all French wines because doctors, including Loebenstein-Loebel, had not observed their actions on patients. So the analysis had to be limited to the most important French wines, a category that serendipitiously corresponded to the wines he had used in his own practice. Barry had limited his recommendation to the wines of the Graves, both red and white. Though the Graves were excellent, Barry was not keen on their medical uses because of the difficulty of getting a pure bordeaux as a result of the adulteration and mixing with Spanish wines that went on in Great Britain and Ireland. (He might also have condemned the master mixers of Bordeaux.) Small wonder, he said, that port was 'preferred to the French claret.'[60]

In moderate doses the effect of bordeaux on the organism seems similar to that of burgundy.[61] So it seemed reasonable to Loebenstein-loebel that bordeaux and burgundy could often be prescribed for patients suffering from the same diseases. Bordeaux had a reputation for acting quicker and producing a more exhalted effect in the vascular system because it was, he thought, more alcoholic than burgundy. (Loebenstein-Loebel lived in the pre-Chaptalian age of winemaking.) The proper dose of bordeaux warmed the body and acted on the mental faculties: good humour and gaiety replaced sadness and melancholy; hypochrondiacs forgot their sicknesses. Red bordeaux also had its uses in treating headache, migraine, and even in treating the uncomplicated atrophy or emaciation of children.[62] High quality bordeaux, especially Château Margaux and first and second quality médocs were recommended for a languid digestion because they act as a tonic on the digestive organs, spreading their effect to the brain and the vascular system. On the basis of the general theory of a miasmatic or environmental etiology of disease, Loebenstein-Loebel argued that the power of wine to promote transpiration, and secretions and excretions in general, made it valuable in dissipating several morbific miasmas, which themselves arose from diseases.

Loebenstein-Loebel recommended French red wine in his capacity as a patient as well as a doctor. After experimenting on himself, he found the pure and alcoholic reds of France much better than white wines for treating goutty diseases. Having inherited gout from his father, he first decided to follow conventional wisdom in drinking the wines of Würzburg with meals. But he decided to drink only bordeaux and burgundy on finding that they left him less affected with gout and its accompanying stomach troubles than did white wines. (Because of the incompatibilty of beer with wine for a goutty person, beer had to be cut from the diet.)

A patient's occupation determined the kind of wine that the doctor prescribed. The sedentary life called for Châteaux Margaux and Haut Brion and the fine médocs because they were considered less heavy than other wines of the southwest, including St. Julien. For persons who worked outdoors the doctor recommended the wines of Libourne (St. Emilion) and even of Roussillon. In fact all red wines were supposed to give quicker and better results in the organism when patients spent lots of time outdoors, whether active or not. Many of the diseases in which bordeaux was the preferred wine, complementing other medicines, were related to digestion and the dual category of gynaecological-sexual problems.

Doctors accepted bordeaux as the ideal simulant for restarting flow in stalled female fluid systems. Lochias could be set flowing again if they had stopped because of weakness of the uterus or of the body itself. Loebenstein-Loebel considered the problem of the cessation of menses associated with a bad state of health in which the patient suffered from headaches, vertigo, heaviness in limbs, pains near the anus and the sexual organs, with a discharge or the 'whites,' poor digestion, and inflated and tender breasts as well as a swollen and hard lower belly. The doctor had to be sure that there were no physical obstructions in the patient's vagina or defects in the womb before proceeding with wine therapy. But there was no doubt in Loebenstein-Loebel's mind that she would greatly benefit from drinking the wine of the Médoc (or, more generally, the southwest) prepared with an iron supplement: Château Margaux and Haut Brion for the rich patient and cheaper wines for the poor, who could benefit just as well from a pure Côtes du Rhône of good vintage – Châteauneuf and Tavel would do nicely. Loebenstein-Loebel had also used successfully if prudently the fine wines of Roussillon in treating suffering women, including those in a state of general atonia if they did not have any organic lung or liver defects, which would work against a cure.

As in the treatment of chlorosis, so in the case of amenorrhea resulting from an organism weakened by moral or physical causes, moral vices such as masturbation and lesbianism had to be taken care of before treatment could be definitively efficacious in bringing back the menses. The opposite problem of excessive bleeding during menses was amenable to a similar treatment. In all female fluid-flow problems, where the red wines of France along with other standard remedies were clearly indicated, the patient could benefit from a cinnamon-mint-balm-haematite concoction, produced by simmering the ingredients on the fire for twenty four hours. Though van Swieten had prescribed it with success, any patient who gagged on this liquid had to be given other medications and Château Margaux. With excessive or too frequent menses the only recommended wines, given with other suitable medicaments, were the *corsé* or rich and full wines of the Médoc (first class), Cahors, Châteaux Margaux and Haut Brion, and Grand Constant, beginning with small doses at long intervals; the wines used to treat amenorrhea were too heavy in this case. Dysmenorrhea or painful menstruation was not included as a medical condition worthy of the médocs.

Loebenstein-Loebel found that the wines of Châteaux Margaux and Haut Brion, along with the first and second quality Médoc wines and Cahors wines, were particularly good for the treatment of 'nervous phthisis' in the absence of an organic defect, if, rather than ravaged by alcohol, the nervous system was weakened by emotion through sorrow, unhappy loves, onanism, or an excessive indulgence in sexual pleasures. Dessert wines could also be given to some patients, perhaps to those who would be shocked by the idea of drinking dry French wine and to whom sweet wine would seem medicinal. Some other patients might be sad, melancholic, with diarrhoea alternating with stomach pains and a lack of appetite. The red wines of France, described in this context as 'fins et légers' rather than *corsés*, administered in small doses, could be 'extremely salutary.' But the doctor had to remember that it was necessary to supplement the wines with 'a moral and physical treatment' to restore the health of the patient.[63]

Civilisation produces a lot of heartburn and doctors have not been remiss in coming up with remedies. The Greek-derived word cardiolgy can be used to dignify this potentially serious nuisance, which is 'associated with reflux of some of the acid contents of the stomach back into the lower end of the oesophagus' or gullet.[64] (About ten per cent of contemporary Americans suffer from this potentially serious complaint, now called gastroesophageal reflux disease.[65]) Loebenstein-Loebel found that in this affliction the stomach nerves could be acting up with the viscera in a state of atonia, or the stomach could be overloaded with glairs or with acids. Then Château Margaux, first and second quality wines of the Médoc, and wines of the côtes, Gaillac, and Cahors should be prescribed. For poorer patients, lesser wines such as Tavel and

Châteauneuf. Madeira was also effective. A successful cure depended on the patient's completely giving up acid foods and beer. Thirst was quenched with watered and sugared red wine. The professor found in his practice that when no other medication could conquer this often stubborn complaint, the fine wines of France succeeded.

There were two French white wines that had a significant role in Lobenstein-Loebel's therapeutic scheme: white bordeaux and champagne. The most famous white wines of Bordeaux earned a place of honour in the therapeutic repertory because they were believed to help the circulation of the blood with less of an effect on the lymphatic system than that of red bordeaux.

Old white wines of the Graves used to be recognised as quite useful in treating 'nervous hypochondria,' that 'morbid state of depression for which there is no real cause,' according to the *Concise Oxford Dictionary*[66]. Armed with a long list of digestive and nerve-related symptoms, Loebenstein-Loebel had no problem with its etiology. The lifestyles of some people contributed to this disease: excessive scholarly or professional activity (as in the case of the male literary hypochondriacs of Georgian England), too many cares and worries, and extreme weakness produced by onanism or an immoderate amount of coition. If a patient was in a particularly serious state, with failure of memory, vertigo, and light shaking of limbs, which indicated a need for an alcoholic and sweet wine, then some of the following whites could have a salutary effect: old Barsac, Castillon, Sainte-Foi, Loupiac, and Sainte-Croix-du-Mont. No beer or red wine allowed. The professor, finding old Barsac to be particularly beneficial, did not hesitate to advise his patients to drink two or three glasses daily with their meals and to quench their thirst with a drink of three parts water and one part Barsac. These white wines would not work without a proper diet and outdoor exercise. The patient's lifestyle might have to be changed in order to produce a cure. All properly Hippocratic.

White wines of the southwest, including those of the Graves, if not too sulphured, were used in the treatment of 'nervous hysteria,' but only in the absence of physical problems such as intestinal troubles. These wines could not be used if deprivation of coition caused the hysteria. A patient with no aversion to wine who has recovered from a hysterical attack could be given the wines of Poudensac, Citran, Entre-Deux-Mers, Graves (fine), Barsac, as well as Tursan. The 'old and authentic' Jurançon was also acceptable. Patients began with three or four half goblets a day and could also quench their thirst with a mixture of two-thirds water and one-third wine.

Loebenstein-Loebel found Bordeaux whites useful, along with other traditional medical drugs, in treating a mixed bag of other ailments, most of which seem to have little in common: Werlhof's disease, Millars' asthma, chronic gout, jaundice, and oedema of the womb, whether in the Fallopian tubes or the womb itself.[67]

For oedema of the womb Loebenstein-Loebel found one particular concoction very effective. One or two roots of the plant bryony and two ounces of absinth were macerated in a bottle of Haut-Barsac for eight days, after which time the patient drank one half goblet at ten a.m. and another half goblet at four p.m. After eight days the dose rose to two goblets. Any other appropriate medicines were given concurrently and the 'lower belly' was washed with Haut-Barsac. The patient had to stick to the proper diet.

In the case of jaundice without inflammation, the patient could take, instead of bordeaux, small doses of one of several wines, including Jurançon, the good wines of Bayonne, and even those of the Dauphiné. Loebenstein-Loebel had much success in adding calamus and absinth to the wines. Beer and acid food and drink were strictly forbidden.

Werlhof's disease or purpura haemorrhagica, now called idiopathic thrombocytopenic purpura, could be treated with small doses of white wine if general weakness or constipation made it imprudent to give French red wine. A very weak patient drank up to three glasses of Barsac or Graves daily and quenched his thirst with a decoction of malt mixed with one of these wines. The doctor had found that an extremely useful medicine in this case was a couple of slices of an orange in a pint of cool water added to a quarter pint of Haut-Barsac or Bergerac. Old Rhine wine was used to sponge down the patient when he was not sweating. All 'white wines of Bordeaux and Bayonne,' if old and authentic, could be given in Werlhof's disease unless there was 'a sthenic fever,' which indicated a condition of too much excitability (reaction to external stimuli) excluding the use of wine. All this wine often produced a cure. Otherwise, the doctor could administer a decoction of husks of nuts, quinine, sulphuric ether, and teinture of oranges.

So the white wines of the southwest filled several gaps in wine therapy better than any other wines and made it possible to take advantage of the recognised medicinal properties of French wines when the nature of the disease made it impossible or at least imprudent to use the great French reds.

Loebenstein-Loebel assigned champagne (*vin mousseux*), preferably *oeil de perdrix*, a modest role in his therapeutic scheme, far less of a role than many Champenois doctors gave it. Champagne was regarded as an excellent wine for the digestion because of its sugar and carbon dioxide. Giving off its own special bouquet, this wine 'decomposes the acidities in the primary ducts or canals, it gives tone to the organs, and brings back calm and gaiety to patients who are sad and hypochondiac.'[68] One of the chief medical uses of champagne was to cure vomiting. In the case of idiopathic vomiting resulting from a nervous stomach but without scirrhus or inflammation, small doses were spread out and gradually increased in amount and frequency. The symptomatic vomiting experienced by pregnant women was controlled by some consumption and also by external application. Champagne was used to give some pain relief to non-plethoric sufferers from kidney stones if they did not have a predisposition to inflammation. Even patients with gravel had their pain reduced and copious urine produced by heavy doses of champagne – one glass five times daily, and the dose could even be increased to three glasses at a time. Heavy medication.

In his discussion of the treatment of chronic gout, Loebenstein-Loebel used the case history of one of his patients, a fifty-year old man who had alternate attacks of gout and kidney stones every three years. With the noon meal the patient was given three glasses of champagne but only one glass with the evening meal. He drank no beer or other wine. His ordinary drink was concentrated *uva ursi*. He walked one hour before the meal and two hours after. After three months the doctor switched the patient to burgundy and still required him to drink *uva ursi*. Loebenstein-Loebel declared him cured of both illnesses.

Loebenstein-Loebel included the wines of Spain, Portugal, and Italy in one chapter, which indicates that he did not use them as much as German and French wines. Yet several of these wines, especially madeira and port, were important in his therapeutic repertory. The wines had a reputation for acting primarily on the lymphatic system and on the skin. They were good for helping patients gain weight. They exerted a secondary action on the stomach and on the total organism by producing a certain well-being. They seemed to act more directly on the nerves of the spinal column than on the brain because they did not at all produce as agreeable an excitation or stimulus as French wines and old Rhine wine (few wines do.) These wines had a clear therapeutic specificity, with the effects of the wines differing from one another, some acting strongly on irritability and others on sensibility. As usual, the doctor's remarks were limited to the personal observations he had made in treating patients.

Loebenstein-Loebel gave little attention to Italian wines. The sweet, heavy wines could be given in teaspoon doses to weak invalid children, with Lacryma Christi prescribed for the sick children of rich parents. He cited two cases. An eight-year old boy with whooping cough who had this wine prescribed was also sponged down with a strong infusion of orange leaves and musk. A six-year girl with diarrhoea who refused to take medication was inveigled into treatment by a little Lachryma Christi del Vesuvio, still a famous wine in the early-nineteenth century. Like Hoffmann, Barry had said some favourable things about the potential of Italian wines. The problem was that there were 'seldom any good Italian wines imported' into the U. K. Good chianti (called Florence) used to be imported, but by the 1770s 'only a sort of *gros rouge* in flasks was imported to be used to make artificial claret and burgundy, and to give lightness and spirit to heavy vapid port.'[69] Neither German nor English medicine made much use of Italian wines.

The therapeutic empire of dessert wines extended to children's diseases: whooping cough, scarlet fever, and measles, especially asthenic measles. After his six-year-old daughter, who had whooping cough, failed to respond to conventional treatment, Loebenstein-Loebel began the treatment used in the critical moments of a patient's life. This meant applying sinapis (mustard) to the calves of the legs, the inside of the thighs, and the lower belly, with the patient also taking every two hours a teaspoon of a mixture of quinine and the herb serpentaria or snake root (both soaked in boiling water for half an hour), to which were then added a scruple of phosphoric acid and a half once of orange-peel syrup. He alternated this concoction with a teaspoon of 'the most exquisite and oldest madeira.' He rubbed the girl's chest and between the shoulders with an ointment made from althaea, cajuput oil, camomile oil, and musc. After a few days, a different decoction was administered every two hours: quinine mixed with phosphoric acid and orange syrup. The child drank madeira with meals.[70] And she recovered.

Loebenstein-Loebel used madeira and malaga in 'treating the most dangerous diseases.'[71] Madeira was not wrongly associated with old age; it was the wine for people suffering from senile marasmus or for people wasting away. But it enjoyed other therapeutic virtues and was used in the period of convalescence from intermittent and malignant fevers, as well as in cases of heartburn not caused by saburra (foul granular matter in the stomach), heavy and spasmodic vomiting without complications, certain types of asthma, and both acute and chronic goutty affections. In the case of skin diseases such as scabies (itch, mange) and eczema two to three glasses of madeira or malaga were prescribed during meals. Other remedies were important in treating these skin diseases: scabies required cleaning the skin with malt baths and drinking a strong, concentrated decoction of sarsaparilla; stubborn eczema required baths with malt and juniper. These wines recharged the 'principe vital'; they change the cacochymia of the body's fluids. Sometimes Loebenstein-Loebel cured scabies using no medicine other than wine.

Haemorrhoids came under the regime of madeira: two to three glasses of madeira a day could be prescribed; indeed up to a full bottle was allowed for this widespread, generally minor form of agony. Ordinary Tokay was an acceptable substitute. The wine, recommended with easily digested food, worked better for patients who exercised outdoors. Of course the wine was prescribed in the case of haemorrhoids of several specific etiologies: those resulting from weakening factors like drastic purgatives, those coming from sad passions, or from excessive mental tension. Then there were haemorrhoids stemming from onanism and those that sprang from 'the excesses of the pleasures of love.'[72] Sexual activity outside conventional social guidelines was dangerous. (Towards the end of the century, the classic treatise on dietetics by Munk and Ewald, professors at the University of Berlin, advised people with piles to drink Mosel, a good bitter beer, tea, and cocoa.[73])

Loebenstein-Loebel gave port wine a modest place in his therapeutic repertory. Like William Buchan, he used it as the vehicle for medical products in creating medicinal wines.[74] Port was used in the treatment of vertigo, paralysis of nervous origin, all problems of the digestive organs (heartburn, spasmodic vomiting, and diarrhoea after digestion), life-threatening eruptive fevers, and gout that internalised in the humors (a category constructed of all the metastatic diseases). In the case of this feverish threat to life, the most powerful remedies also had to be used: musk, phosphorus, camphor, volatile oils, and ethers. For vertigo, rubbing with sulphuric ether was recommended along with the taking of a concentrated decoction of quinine, teinture of valerian, and cinnamon. Treatment of the nervous paralysis called for rubbing of the sacrum with alcohol several times a day; then for eight to ten days the patient took two glasses of a filtered medicinal wine consisting of a bottle of port to which had been added crushed mustard, cinnamon bark, and roots of galingale and of valerian. After presenting this admirable model of specificity in fitting port and botanicals to diseases, Loebenstein-Loebel ended his work with a flourish of authority by quoting, with more enthusiasm than accuracy, from the 'immortal work' of Thomas Sydenham on the use of wine in treating disease.[75]

Wine still had an important role in German medicine at mid-century which continued well into the second half of the nineteenth century. There were 211 prescriptions based on wine in the *Pharmacopöea universalis* (1846). The therapeutic canon established by some well known medical texts gave wine a role in the treatment of a great variety of diseases, but wine was especially valued in treating states of depression, fevers, conditions of general weakness, including loss of appetite, and heart and circulation problems and in promoting convalescence. Perhaps we see here the influence of the notoriously fluid German diagnosis of *Herzinsuffizienz.*[76] Wine had retained much of its therapeutic versatility, though it got pretty much limited to being recommended for purposes of strengthening and stimulating the body and promoting convalescence. Towards the end of the century new therapies usurped the functions of wine. Wine therapy was also burdened by the fact that the dangers of alcoholism had long cast a shadow over the therapeutic use of any form of alcohol. With many new items in their therapeutic arsenal, doctors in 1898 could take seriously the declaration of Robert Koppe that alcohol therapy was one of the great errors in the history of medicine; wine therapy could hardly be regarded as radically different. An anti-alcoholic age had dawned in medicine. The Nazi regime vigorously promoted an anti-alcoholic ideology. Sarrazin's survey of the German medical scene in the twentieth century regretted finding no evidence of anything such as the medical pro-wine movement starting in Bordeaux in the 1930s, which attempted to resurrect *Weintherapie.*[77]

Notes

1. Christopher Lawrence, 'Cullen, Brown and the poverty of essentialism,' in W. F. Bynum and Roy Porter (eds), *Brunonianism in Britain and Europe, supplement no. 8 to Medical History* (1988), 1–21.
2. Sthenic (*sthenos*, strength) means with morbid increase of vital action, especially of the heart and arteries. See W. F. Bynum, *Science and the Practice of Medicine in the nineteenth century* (Cambridge: Cambridge University Press, 1994), 17, and Erwin H. Ackerknecht, *A Short History of Medicine* (rev. edn, Baltimore: The Johns Hopkins University Press, 1982), 129.
3. John Brown, *The Elements of Medicine* (2 vols., London: J. Johnson 1795), vol. i, 14-15. Brown was a student of William Cullen's at Edinburgh but took his degree at St Andrews. Ackerknecht, *op. cit.*

(note 2), 129, notes that Cullen's medical system was founded 'on the assumption that the basic phenomenon of life and disease is a "nervous force".'

4. Brown, *op. cit.* (note 3), 19, paragraph xxxi, note f.
5. Thomas Beddoes, M.D., introduction to Brown, *ibid.*, I, lxxxvii.
6. Bynum, *op. cit.* (note 2), 17, notes that Brown's system, which 'never made much headway' in Britain, 'found many willing disciples' in Germany and Italy.
7. For precise details, see Günther B. Risse, 'The Brownian System of Medicine: Its Theoretical and Practical Implications,' *Clio Medica*, v (Amsterdam: B. M. Israel, 1970), 45–51.
8. Roy Porter, *The Greatest Benefit to Mankind. A Medical History of Humanity* (London: HarperCollins, 1997), 262.
9. Risse, 'Brunonian therapeutics: new wine in old bottles?,' in Bynum and Porter (eds), *op. cit.* (note 1), 46. Risse does not forget it.
10. *Ibid.*, 47, with reference to J. C. Kramer in note 8.
11. *Ibid.*, 51. Michael Barfoot, 'Brunonianism under the bed: an alternative to university medicine in Edinburgh in the 1780s,' in Bynum and Porter, *op. cit.* (note 1), 22–45, says that there was 'no visible impact [of Brown's doctrine] except perhaps in the Infirmary, where more stimulants were used in the 1790s' (39).
12. Risse, 'Brunonian therapeutics,' *ibid.*, 48–9.
13. Barfoot, 'Brunonianism under the bed: an alternative to University medicine,' *ibid.*, 36–9. Risse, 'Brunonian therapeutics,' in *ibid.*, 52, notes that the Edinburgh Infirmary took action to control expenses on alcoholic beverages in the 1790s.
14. On Pisa and Bamberg, see Risse, 'Brunonian therapeutics, *ibid.*, 54–62, and 'Kant, Schelling, and the early search for a philosophical "science" of medicine in Germany,' *Journal of the History of Medicine* (April 1972), 149–51.
15. See Risse, 'Brunonian therapeutics,' in Bynum and Porter, *op. cit.* (note 1), 61.
16. Risse, 'Kant, Schelling,' *Journal of the History of Medicine* (1972), 146.
17. *Ibid.*
18. Frederick Gregory, 'Regulative therapeutics in the German romantic era: the contribution of Jakob Fries (1773-1843),' *Clio Medica* (Amsterdam: B. M. Israel, 1983), 179–89.
19. Risse, 'Brunonian therapeutics,' in Bynum and Porter, *op. cit.* (note 1), 59–60.
20. Nelly Tsouyopoulos, 'The influence of John Brown's ideas in Germany,' in *ibid.*, 63–74, and Thomas H. Broman, *The*

transformation of German academic medicine 1750-1820 (Cambridge: Cambridge University Press, 1996), 144 .

21. Broman, *ibid.*, ch. 5, 'Breaking the shackles of history: The Brunonian revolution in Germany.'
22. Eduard Leopold Loebenstein-Loebel, *Die Anwendung und Wirkung der Weine in lebensgefährlichen Krankheiten, und deren Verfälschungen; nach eignen Ansichten und Erfahrungen* (Leipzig: Brockhaus, 1816).
23. Ed. Loebenstein-Loebel, *Traité sur l'usage et les effets des vins dans les maladies dangereuses et mortelles, et sur la falsification de cette boisson.* (Strasbourg: Levrault, 1817). Traduit de l'allemand par J. Fr. Daniel Lobstein (Docteur en médecine de la Faculté de Paris, Correspondant de la Société latine et de la Société minéralogique de Jena, etc. Ancien médecin aux hôpitaux militaires et aux armées françaises, etc.). There is a two-page dedication of the translation to Jean-Jacques Leroux, a survivor from the faculty of medicine in Paris in the ancien régime; Leroux became professeur de clinique interne and dean of the new faculty.
24. An excellent survey of German wine therapy in the nineteenth century has been provided by Hans Christian Sarrazin, *Der Wein in der Therapie des 19. Jahrhunderts* ('Inaugural-Dissertation zur Erlangung des Doctorwürde der Hohen Medizinischen Fakultät der Johannes Gutenberg Universität Mainz,' 1952).
25. 'C'est ainsi que Hippocrate, Galien, Coelius Aurelianus, Borellus, Helmont, etc. ... indiquent le vin dans les fièvres inflammatoires et intermittentes.' Loebenstein-Loebel, *op. cit.* (note 23), 4.
26. *Le petit Littré* defines the medical meaning of exaltation as an 'augmentation démesurée de l'action d'un organe ou d'un système d'organes.'
27. There were also tinctures of opium: simple and camphorated (*élixir parégorique*). According to *La médecine populaire*, no. 19 (27 Jan. 1881), 291, opium concoctions were used in combatting vomiting; both wines and tinctures were given as drops in sugared water. And the laudanum could be added to an enema.
28. The *Concise Oxford Dictionary* defines apoplexy as a 'malady arresting powers of sense and motion, usu. caused by effusion of blood or serum in the brain.' *The Oxford Medical Companion* (OMC hereinafter) calls it 'a stroke,' and goes on to give the deadly details: 'a sudden impairment of brain function due to haemorrhage from, or obstruction of, cerebral blood vessels.' The term is also applied to vascular catastrophes in other organs (e.g., pituitary apoplexy, ovarian apoplexy).
29. Cited in Christopher Hoolihan, 'Wine and Regimen from

Hippocrates to the Renaissance,' *Caduceus*, 9 (1993), 7–8.

30. Sir Edward Barry (Fellow of the Royal College of Physicians, and of the Royal Society), *Observations historical, critical, and medical on the wines of the Ancients. And the analogy between them and modern wines. With general observations on the principles and qualities of water, and in particular those of Bath* (London: T. Cadell, 1775), 447.
31. Willliam Buchan, *Domestic Medicine. A Treatise on the Prevention and Cure of Disease, by Regimen and Simple Medicines* (London: J. Smith, 1769; A new stereotype edn, London, n.d.), 181.
32. Frank Schoonmaker, *The Wine of Germany* (Revised by Peter M. F. Sichel; London: Faber and Faber, 1983), 27, notes that 'the Mosel and Rhine wines ... [are] so light in alcohol [8-10%?] that many of them could not be classified as wine if they were produced in California,' where a mind-numbing 14% (and more) is not unusual.
33. Barry, *op. cit.* (note 30), 444.
34. T*he Oxford English Dictionary* defines diathesis as 'a permanent (hereditary or acquired) condition of the body which renders it liable to certain special diseases or affections; a constitutional predisposition or tendency.' *Le Garnier Delamare - Dictionnaire des termes de médecine* (Paris: Maloine, 1992, 23d edn) notes that the word has fallen into disuse since great morbid processes such as tuberculosis, syphilis, and arthritis have been identified.
35. Still in a pre-vitamin age, Littré defined scurvy (*le scorbut*) as an 'affection générale non fébrile, qui a pour caractère un affaiblissement notable de l'énergie musculaire et qui est accompagnée fréquemment d'une altération plus ou moins prononcée des gençives.'
36. Michael Foehr's Berlin dissertation (1835) found Mosel wine effective in treating scurvy. In 1866 Franz Meurer found Saar wine and Mosel wine to be useful. See Sarrazin, *op. cit.* (note 24), 33.
37. The physiological properties attributed to coffee, a European craze after the middle of the seventeenth century, are noted by Wolfgang Schivelbusch, *Tastes of Paradise: A Social History of Spices, Stimulants, and Intoxicants* (New York: Vintage Books, 1993), 19. Recognised as a panacea it is 'good for colic, ...fortifies the liver and the gall bladder, brings relief in cases of dropsy, purifies the blood ....'
38. Hippocrate, *Maladies*, x (Paris: Les Belles Lettres, 1983), 188. Translation by Jacques Jouanna.
39. Loebenstein-Loebel, *op. cit.* (note 23), ch. ix, 117–123, 'De la nature des vins de Turquie.' Discussed in this fluid category were wines of Syria, Bulgaria, Tripoli, the Greek islands, and Cyprus, among others. Greek wines were particularly recommended. Vins cuits were

not recommended.

40. The case history, supplied by Dr. Ulrich of Cologne, was presented as 'another case of ileus cured by the wine of the Champagne,' in *Journal des connaissances médicales pratiques et de pharmacologie,* vi (1838-39), 150; it was reprinted from *Casper's Wochenschrift fuer die gesammte Heilkunde.* Ileus is a painful, frequently fatal, internal obstruction, especially in the ileum (portion of the small intestine).
41. Lobstein used the term 'système végétatif,' which may be an early version of what is called the 'système neurovégétatif' - 'ensemble des structures nerveuses qui contrôlent les grandes fonctions involontaires (la vie végétative): circulation, sécrétion, excrétion,' etc. See *Le Nouveau Petit Robert* (Paris: Dictionnaires Le Robert, 1993).
42. Leucorrhea (leukorrhea) – the whites – is a mucous discharge, sometimes purulent, from the vagina. In the nineteenth century the French referred to *la leucorrhée as les fleurs blanches*; now it is the more pedestrian *les pertes blanches.*
43. The therapeutic powers of *Moselwein* were defended by Karl Graff in several works, including *Der Moselweinals Getränk und Heilmittel* (Bonn: A. Marcus, 1821). He found it effective in the prevention of urinary calculus as well as in the treatment of haemorrhoids, cholera, and numerous other diseases, including gout.
44. *Le Petit Littré* notes that the plant arnica 'a été préconconisée comme stimulante et éminemment fébrifuge (Stahl l'appelait le quinquina des pauvres), et quelquefois aussi comme une panacée contre tous les accidents des chutes (*panacea lapsorum*).' Quinine is a febrifuge alkaloid derived from the bark of the quinquina tree.
45. For an excellent discussion of fevers and especially of Cullen on fevers, see W. F. Bynum, *op. cit.* (note 2), 21–23 (see the index for a listing of the different kinds of fevers). Roy Porter, *op. cit.* (note 8), 402, also makes some enlightening remarks on 'the ceaseless surge of fevers' in the nineteenth century. And there are even some clear statements on the eighteenth-century concept of fever in chapter 10 ('Crisis in Fevers') of Michel Foucault, *The Birth of the Clinic: An Archaeology of Medical Perception* (New York: Vintage Books, 1995).

46 The Concise English Dictionary defines hectic fever as 'that which accompanies consumption and similar diseases, attended with flushed cheeks and hot skin.' An essential fever would have no 'striking local manifestations,' as Bynum, *op. cit.* (note 2), 46, put it in discussing Broussais; Bynum also notes (22) that 'Cullen's main division was between the intermittent and the continued fevers.'

47. Ernst Horn, *Handbuch des praktischen Arzneimittellehre für Ärzte und Wundärzte* (Berlin: Oehmigke der Jüngese, 1803). Sarrazin, *op.*

cit. (note 24), 36, notes that F. G. Voigtel's four volume *Vollständiges System der Arzneimittellehre* (edited by C. G. Kühn, Leipzig, 1816-17) was even more in favour of *Weintherapie* than Horn.

48. Foucault, *op. cit.* (note 45), 178–9.
49. *Le petit Littré*'s nineteenth-century definition of amaurosis was 'a blindness caused by the paralysis of the retina and the optic nerve'. In the 1860s, Ernest Hart, ophthalmic surgeon to St. Mary's Hospital, used the ophthalmoscope to distinguish many diseases referred to as amaurosis. See Hart, 'On some of the diseases constituting the condition commonly called amaurosis,' *Lancet*, ii (1864), 566; Hart had given a lecture to the Harveian Society on Nov. 5, 1863. The OMC defines it as 'blindness from other than local ocular causes.' Tay-Sachs disease, afflicting mainly Ashkenazi Jews (middle and northern Europe), used to be called amaurotic family idiocy. This fatal infantile form of cerebral sphingolipidosis causes, among other things, blindness, and produces a characteristic 'cherry-red spot on each retina.'
50. *La Médecine populaire* (1 Nov. 1902), 283-4. Dr. A. Larbalétrier, author of the article, recognised that certain chemicals, which were medically useful, had been found in wood lice, but he thought that the value of the lice had been much exaggerated. '...On a beaucoup exaggéré leurs propriétés médicales. Cependant ils ont pu rendre quelques services à cause des chlorhydrates et des azoates de potasse et de chaux que l'analyse chimique y a découverts.'
51. See Loebenstein-Loebel, *Grundriss des Semiologie des Auges für Aerzte* (Jena: Cröker, 1817).
52. J.-L. Alibert, *Nouveaux élémens de thérapeutique et de matière médicale* ... (Paris: Béchet jeune, 1826; 3 vols, 5th edn), iii, 202.
53. 'Nul pays, dit l'ingénieur Servière, n'offre des dispositions aussi bien entendues pour produire, conserver et expédier les vins ....' Quoted by Loebenstein-Loebel, op. cit. (note 23), at the beginning of chapter 5. Joseph Servière wrote several books on the wine business; see e.g., *Der theoretische und praktische Kellermeister* ... (Frankfurt am Main: Gebhard and Korber, 1811).
54. Diderot's letter to Sophie Volland, cited in François Lapraz, *Beaujolaiseries – Histoires et petits histoires du Beaujolais* (Lyon: Editions du Merle, 1979), 168. Diderot classifed Brouilly and the côte de Brouilly as burgundies in this cure, which was certified by Dr. Louis, the surgeon Barry, and Madame Diderot.
55. Barry, *op. cit.* (note 30), 428, 433.
56. Bynum, *op. cit.* (note 2), 6, notes that though most 'eighteenth-century remedies were botanical ... preparations of mercury,

antimony, phosphorus, arsenic, and iron were also popular.'

57. Modern French [*le nouveau petit Robert*] retains la tribade for female homosexual but drops the euphonic la tribaderie. It seems that this word comes from the Greek for lewd woman through the verb to rub. The *Concise English Dictionary* defines tribadism as 'unnatural vice between women.'
58. Quassia is a bitter medicinal decoction made from the bark of the quassia or other trees of South America, especially Surinam.
59. Loebenstein-Loebel, *op. cit.* (note 23) 56–57.
60. Barry, *op. cit.* (note 30), 422, 436, 439.
61. There were five medical conditions that precluded consumption of red bordeaux: constipation, atrabiliousness or black bile affliction, inflammation, liver attack, and consumption.
62. Sir William Wilthy Gull (1816-90) gave a medical description of the condition anorexia nervosa, the 'slimmer's disease,' in 1868.
63. Pituitous phthisis, whose name indicates the secretion of phlegm or mucous, required restricting the patient to the moderate consumption of pure first and second quality médocs, which had to be free of added *eau-de-vie,* with the midday meal.
64. OMC, 365. The French seem to take the pain seriously, or perhaps because it afflicts digestion it seems serious: 'une douleur très vive qui se fait senti à l'épigastre, vers l'orifice supérieure de l'estomac' (*Le petit Littré*). *Le nouveau petit Robert,* drops 'vive,' which is reserved for la gastralgie - 'une vive douleur.'
65. Jane E. Brody, 'Personal Health,' *The New York Times* (25 September 1996), B6.
66. Sydenham believed in 'a hysteria-like syndrome in males ... hypochondriasis.' Mark S. Micale, *Approaching Hysteria. Disease and Its Interpretations* (Princeton, NJ: Princeton University Press, 1995), 22.
67. In Werlhof's disease 'there are spontaneous haemorrhages into the skin and mucous membranes and many other tissues and organs. This is now known to be caused by a diminution of platelets (thrombocytes) in the blood.' OMC, 1001. An oedema is the 'swelling of tissue through increase of its (chiefly intercellular) fluid content, due to passage of extra amounts of water out from capillaries, e.g. in inflammation.' M. Abercrombie *et al, The Penguin Dictionary of Biology* (Harmondsworth: Penguin, 1980, seventh edn.), 209.
68. Loebenstein-Loebel, *op. cit.* (note 23), 61.
69. Barry, *op. cit.* (note 30), 442.
70. Loebenstein-Loebel, *op. cit.* (note 23), 157.

71. Malaga, from Andalusia, is a blended sweet wine similar to Marsala; its production is falling because it has declined seriously in quality and lost its raison d'être. Madeira is from Portugal's Atlantic islands; it was of higher quality and more famous in the early-nineteenth century; it is comparable to port and cream sherry; malsmey is the best of the madeiras.
72. Loebenstein-Loebel, *op. cit.* (note 23), 142.
73. I. Munk et C. A. Ewald, *Traité de diététique, à l'usage des médecins, chefs d'Administration, directeurs d'hôpitaux, de prisons, de pensionnats, etc.* (1886; 3d edn, 1897; Paris and Brussels: Carré et Naud, 1897), 531. Translated by J. F. Heymans and P. Masoin.
74. William Buchan, *Domestic Medicine*, appendix, 540, gives the recipe for an anthelmintic wine: red wine containing rhubarb and worm-seed.He was quite keen on the virtues of medicinal wine in treating 'debility of stomach and intestines.' He used wines as the vehicle for antimony, ipecacuanha, Peruvian bark, cardamum seeds, orange peels, etc.
75. Loebenstein-Loebel, *op. cit.* (note 23), 112–6, cites Sydenham, *Praxis med. experiment.* (Lipsiae: T. Fritsch, 1711). Dr. John Swan translated and prepared an edition of *The Entire Works of Dr. Thomas Sydenham* (London: E. Cave, 1742). The index has twelve references to wine.
76. See Lynn Payer, *Medicine and Culture* (London: Penguin Books, 1988), chapter on 'West Germany: the lingering influences of romanticism'.
77. Sarrazin, *op. cit.* (note 24), 49–52.

PART II

A REMARKABLE NINETEENTH CENTURY MEDICINE

3

Alcohol Therapy

The role of alcohol as panacea was given an impressive statement by Arnau de Villanova (1235-1313), physician to kings and popes. In time, medical literature came to make a simple distinction between the external and internal use of alcohol, mixed in various proportions with other substances and applied or administered according to time-tested directions, although experiments were sometimes tried by an adventurous few.[1] The operation in 1686 on Louis XIV's anal fistula, then called *la grande opération*, must be history's most famous proctological event. Post-operatory care included soothing the royal rectum by the application of compresses soaked with red wine in which absinth, pomegranate rinds, roses of Provins, and myrtle leaves had been boiled.[2] For subjects unable to afford or unwilling to be cured by surgery, another procedure for treating a fistula was to clean the affected area with a concoction including turpentine, egg yolk, honey, water and spirit of wine. This mixture was also injected into the rectum to strengthen the affected area. In the nineteenth century alcohol or glycerine combined with other substances were applied to the ailing anus.

Until the beginning of the nineteenth century, the substance distilled from wine was the only organic body possessing the properties associated with alcohol, especially its ability to combine directly with acids and produce ethers.[3] Beginning in the 1830s, a group of chemists, Dumas in particular, radically changed the structure and content of scientific knowledge about alcohol. In 1835 Dumas and Péligrot showed that wood or methyl alcohol is really one type of a series of bodies with the same general properties. Berthelot, Wurtz, Cannizzaro, and others established the basis of the final classification of alcohols into the five classes of primary, secondary, tertiary, phenols and mixed-function. One of Berthelot's 'earliest triumphs was the synthesis of alcohol.' Berthelot also introduced the concept and name of polyatomic alcohols in his research on glycerine and gave alcohol the modern chemical definition of 'neutral compounds made up of carbon, hydrogen, and oxygen....'[4] By the 1850s the doctor serious about alcohol had to learn a lot of new chemistry, including the novelties of isomerism and synthesis of organic compounds.

At mid-nineteenth century, no alcohol seemed more valuable in medicine than glycerine, a trihydric alcohol discovered by Scheele in 1779 and worked on by Chevreul and especially Berthelot.[5] Pasteur discovered its presence in wine. Trials in the U.S. and the U.K. with this alcohol produced encouraging medical results. In 1854, the year in which the Académie de médecine heard a report on the medical uses of glycerine, hospitals in Paris used only twenty five kilos of it. By 1862 these hospitals were using 1500 kilos of glycerine a year. Its use as an excipient had become clear. Before long it was used to dress wounds and to treat fissures in nipples as well as to treat skin and eye diseases. Charles Robin popularised its use in the microscopic study of tissues. Perhaps most important in explaining this increase was the success that Jean-Nicolas Demarquay had in using glycerine to fight an epidemic of hospital gangrene, followed by his subsequent research and experimenting on the subject.[6]

By the 1860s alcohol had acquired an impressive list of uses in standard medical literature, including applications in surgery. Alcohol was an ingredient in a mixture applied topically to treat hypertrophy of the breasts; it was used as a cooling agent for burns – hot wine alcohol was also used by some doctors; it was mixed with chloroform to promote the healing of anal fissures; and camphorated alcohol was used to clean wounds and control infections. Pure alcohol could be gargled to cure a sore throat in three hours. Diluted with water, alcohol was injected into the appropriate genital tracts to treat leucorrhea and drainage from gonorrhoea. The venereologist Philippe Ricord reported good results in treating gonorrhoea with injections of fifty grams of an astringent wine (red) and 100 grams of distilled rosewater; he got better results with 150 grams of red wine and one gram of pure tannin – two grams in cases of vaginal injections.[7] Alcohol was injected into the testicles to cure hydrocele. One standard nineteenth-century procedure was to evacuate the liquid from the testicle before injecting about five grams of pure alcohol into the *tunica vaginalis.* A. F. Richard treated fourteen cases of hydrocele by injecting into the drained vaginal tunic five grams of cold alcohol at thirty six degrees Baumé and leaving it there. Thirteen of the patients could return to work immediately.[8]

Alcohol was the recommended treatment for bleeding after childbirth: several enemas of four ounces of port with twenty drops of laudanum every twenty minutes. Some texts recommended that because of its anti-bleeding property, alcohol should be injected into the uterus to stop the haemorrhaging.[9] An infusion of red roses in wine could also be injected for leucorrhea as well as for uterine bleeding. Compresses with hot alcohol could stop excessive menstrual bleeding. Historically, menorrhagia must have been a serious medical problem. Books on social history sometimes refer to women in childbirth dying of bleeding because of the physiological effects of a diet poor in vitamins and minerals. Anorexia as well as amenorrhea are known historical entities, but excessive menstrual bleeding seems to be an ignored topic. In the medical literature, however, female bleeding of various types was taken seriously. French doctors, influenced by English medical practice, were aware that they were also emulating a popular practice in treating difficult menstruation by having the patient drink 'une dose assez forte de punch' to end the affliction.[10] Some practitioners used Bordeaux wine, which presumably produced a more pleasant state of inebriation but was equally efficacious. One treatment recommended for life-threatening menstrual bleeding was to give the patient half a bottle of Marsala: a cure followed drunkenness. Béhier used this treatment several times with a patient who had a large uterine fibroid tumour causing bleeding during menstruation. Alcohol was perceived by both physician and patient as an effective agent of healing.

Traditionally used internally to cure illnesses or to act as the vehicle for carrying other substances into the system, alcohol was a tonic as well as a medicament. The possibility of a patient's abuse of alcohol put the doctor in an iatrogenic quandary from which he could escape only by severely limiting the amount given and carefully regulating the doses. Some doctors continued to be afraid of turning people into addicts though the medical use of alcohol. The spread of the 'doctrines of Broussais,' which insisted on a universal diagnosis of all illness in terms of gastroenteritis-inflammation to be treated by the panacea of therapeutic bleeding, militated against the internal use of alcohol and various alcoholic drinks.[11] To what extent it is hard to say. The patients of Broussais (and of his numerous acolytes) who were suspected of suffering from irritated organs were condemned to a diet of chicken bouillon or gummy water. R. T. H. Laennec saved a part of French medical practice for wine by using the popular method of administering various alcoholic drinks, including doses of hot wine and thirty to forty grams of eau-de-vie in an infusion of violets. Trousseau's highly successful *Traité de thérapeutique* (1836) also gave alcohol and wine important roles in medical practice.[12]

One of the advantages of alcohol was that it could be administered in various ways: pleasantly as a medicament to be swallowed, unpleasantly through a feeding tube put into the stomach, or by an enema. Alcohol is rapidly absorbed by the wall of the large intestine. François Aran, a doctor at the Saint-Antoine hospital who did work on diseases of the uterus and the heart, recommended the wine enema in 1855 as a tonic and general stimulant in treating chlorosis, dyspepsia, pulmonary tuberculosis, and convalescence from serious illnesses. Some doctors reported quick success during World War I in treating typhus with intestinal wine enemas. The amount injected into a purged rectum was 150 to 200 grams of good quality wine cut with water. Some doctors added bouillon with the fat removed and a few drops of Sydenham's laudanum (tincture of opium). If 250 to 330 grams were required, it was preferable to give the enema in two stages within twenty four hours. Children and women might require modification of the therapy. In the 1880s Jules Simon treated infant cholera by a bath in warm red wine. The proper stimulation of impressionable women could be obtained with an injection of 150 grams.[13]

Alcohol was used as an antidote to arsenical poisoning until replaced in the second half of the century by remedies such as sesquioxides of iron. In the 1860s bites by poisonous snakes could still be treated in a fashion similar to that of treating bee stings, that is by having the victim take large doses of alcohol, including wines and champagne; the wine or whisky was laced with ammonia, spirits of turpentine, or a little strychnine. Getting drunk to treat bee stings was still good therapy in some circles in the 1930s. Alain Cuénot recommended that the patient be given repeated small doses of a wine with an alcohol level of fourteen to sixteen per cent in order to maintain a state of drunkenness for several hours. Experiments had shown, the argument went, that wine alcohol raises body temperature, thus countering the temperature-lowering effect of the venom. The exciting effect of the alcohol counters the depressing effect of the venom on the nervous system. In the blood the alcohol resists the chemical reactions brought on by the poison. And finally the alcohol in passing off through the lungs, the skin, and the kidneys, promotes the exit of the poison. Once again a popular and cheap medication had found a complete and logical scientific explanation of its action.[14]

Among nineteenth-century diseases on which old remedies could be tried, the most frightening was cholera, which swept through western European cities in five pandemics; as late as 1892 it left about 10,000 dead in Hamburg. Before this 'new plague' was brought under control by public health measures, 'many treatments were tried; nothing worked.'[15] Alcohol was a frequently prescribed remedy.

Magendie prescribed it during the vintage cholera year of 1832, when about 2.3 per cent of the population of Paris died – 18,402 is one impressively precise figure, shockingly high when compared to London's 7000 deaths.[16] Cholera had a mortality of about fifty per cent; 3560 people died during the Liverpool epidemic of 1866. The situation was similar in Paris. In the eleventh arrondissement, which used to include the Luxembourg quarter, cholera killed 1200 out of a population of 50,636 in three months of 1832, mostly those under five years old and older people. Proportionately, more women than men died. Though wearing a flannel belly band might have been as good as anything, doctors carried out their duties by aggressively treating patients. When cholera patients arrived at the hospital Magendie had them rubbed down repeatedly with a mixture consisting of equal parts of camphorated alcohol, ammonia, and turpentine oil. Among the stimulating drinks given were strong punch and hot, sugared wine laced with alcohol and cinnamon. Hot enemas and stimulating infusions, some with camphor or opium, accompanied what were often the sufferer's last rites. From 28 March to 23 August 1832 Magendie treated 594 cholera patients: 374 were cured; twelve were sent off to other hospital rooms to convalesce; 208 died, but thirty eight of this group had come to the hospital as hopelessly ill. Magendie lamented that it was hard to avoid a mortality of one third of cholera patients.[17] As John Snow found out in London, alcohol gave protection against cholera only if one drank it instead of water; this was the case of the London brewery workers who drank free beer.[18]

In 1865 an editorial in *Lancet* declared that there were 'few things more remarkable in the recent history of medicine than the extent to which alcohol has been introduced, and the importance which has been attached to it in the treatment of disease.'[19] John Harley Warner consecrated this development as 'a revolution ... in British medical practice, between the early-1830s and the 1850s. Therapeutics largely underwent a reversal from the practice of depletion using bloodletting and purgatives to stimulation with alcohol and nourishment; the brandy bottle replaced the lancet.'[20] Why therapeutics changed is usually explained as the transformation of the concept of disease from an overstimulating type requiring depletive practices to an enfeebling type requiring stimulation and nutriments.[21]

Warner found that 'in the 1860s many British physicians utilised the new physiological research on alcohol to restructure fundamentally the current theories of alcohol's therapeutic action' in acute diseases.[22] He identified three major alcoholic theories that succeeded one another between the 1850s and the 1870s. First, alcohol is a food: originating in the late-1850s, the major axiom of this theory was Todd's belief, based on Liebig's nutritional physiology, that alcohol is a non-nitrogenous, respiration-supporting aliment and an assimilable nervous stimulant. Secondly, the diametrically opposed theory that alcohol is totally eliminated from the body: after 1859, the spread of the so-called total elimination theory left alcohol as an unassimilable stimulant, but Todd's defenders succeeded in emasculating the total elimination theory by the end of the 1860s. Thirdly, the belief that alcohol lowers body temperature led to the conversion of doctors excited by fever theory, and in the late-1860s laboratory and clinical evidence confirming this idea led to justification of the use of alcohol as an antipyretic in certain cases.[23]

Yet it difficult to accept the judgment that, in the decades after the debates of the 1860s, changes in physiological teachings led to changes in therapeutic theory but not in the clinical use of alcohol. There is lots of evidence of alcohol's being rejected in clinical practice and replaced by other therapeutic agents in the second half of the nineteenth century. The claim that 'alcohol remained a fashionable and widely prescribed therapeutic agent through the end of the nineteenth century' should not lead us into forgetting the critics of alcohol therapy and the doctors who rejected it.[24]

Medical explanation was sometimes based explicitly on scientific research, but science was also the source of a current of hostility to alcohol and wine as dangers to health. The learned hygienist Jean Champouillon, expert on mineral waters and thermal cures, had called the attention of the Académie des sciences to the rapid rotting of the corpses of drunkards and alcoholics. In *Le démon alcool* Prosper Desprine, a doctor in Marseille, celebrated the spread of phylloxera because it was destroying French vineyards.[25] By the late-1860s Bordeaux's Académie de médecine had become so alarmed by contradictory theories circulating in the medical profession on wine drinking that it chose 'the physiological and therapeutic action of alcohol' as the subject for the prize awarded in its annual competition. Four memoirs were submitted to the Bordeaux academy. A work by Angel Marvaud, professor at the 'Ecole de médecine militaire du Val-du-Grâce' (Paris), won the gold medal in this *concours* (1869-70).[26]

As the *chef de service* in a big hospital during the seige of Paris by the Prussians, Marvaud was able to experiment on 500 sick people, eighty of whom had typhoid fever, 300 smallpox, and twenty five scarlet fever; other groups had measles, pneumonia, and other diseases. Marvaud did not contest the general idea of the clinical usefulness of alcoholic preparations. Disagreeing with the common view that alcohol is a source of heat and calories, he nevertheless came to a conclusion that must have comforted the Bordeaux academy. He found alcohol to be an energetic depressant of temperature, and so recommended its use to lower fevers and to prevent patients from wasting away. Marvaud also endorsed the use of alcohol as a stimulant of the nervous system. With the backing of a vast clinical apparatus, Marvaud supported a positive physiological function for alcohol, showed its usefulness in public health, and retained its role in the diet of the worker.

Much work that was more experimental than clinical gave less solace than Marvaud's to alcohol therapists but still permitted them to retain an uneasy faith in wine alcohol. Dujardin-Beaumetz and Audigé were inspired by the fact that the physiological study of alcohol had acquired its socio-medical importance because of the increasing abuse of alcoholic drinks as well as the role of alcohol in therapeutic medicine as a powerful and energetic medication and in toxicology. 'Whether considered as food, medication, or poison, alcohol's interest to medicine is clear.' A set of experiments they carried out in Paul Bert's laboratory at the Sorbonne convinced these two doctors of the existence of a general law. 'In a natural series of similar bodies, the most active are those containing the greatest number of atoms,' and from this they concluded that the toxic properties in the series of alcohols produced by fermentation followed in a mathematical way their atomic composition. (Both doctors were students of Wurtz, a great defender of atomic theory in chemistry and a professor in the Paris faculty of medicine.) So the higher its atomic number, the more toxic the alcohol. The practical lesson here was that all alcohols other than ethanol were unfit for human consumption. Amyl and butyl alcohols were found to be especially toxic. It was fortunate that the principal alcohol in wine is ethanol.[27]

Touting the advantages of experimental physiology over chemical analysis, which inconveniently found no difference between ethanol produced from grapes and that produced from the sugars and starches of other products, Dujardin-Beaumetz and Audigé ploughed on to study the toxic properties of 'commercial alcohols.' Many dogs received sub-cutaneous injections of these alcohols, got drunk, and died. These canine sacrifices enabled the doctors to confirm the discovery of Isidore Pierre, a faculty chemist in Caen, that eaux-de-vie made from grains and sugarbeet contain amyl, butyl, and propyl alcohols, all toxic. Wine drinkers were reminded of how lucky they were that wine alcohol is the least poisonous of all the alcohols because it is made up nearly exclusively of ethanol, the least toxic of the series.[28] Given the toxicity of most medicaments, the results of this research were more relevant for drinkers than for patients.

Representatives of respectable medical science promoted the moderate use of alcohol in the treatment of diseases throughout much of the nineteenth century. Todd's advocacy of alcohol as a 'specific power,' indeed, nearly a panacea, became so widespread in London practice by the 1860s that *Lancet* observed that alcohol had made 'Dr. Todd as famous as vaccination [had] made Jenner, or chloroform Simpson.'[29] Across the channel he was regarded as a 'chef d'école' who had given 'considerable development to the new ideas' on alcohol as the chief remedy in treating acute fevers. Todd held that acute diseases depressed vital power and wasted or disintegrated tissue, and saw the accompanying inflammation as 'a process of deranged nutrition,' which 'drew nutriments from the blood for the formation of morbid products like pus.' Believing that the vital power of the body cured disease, Todd could do little except prescribe alcohol for stimulation of the nervous system, thus 'strengthening vital force,' and food to keep the patient alive until 'nature provided a cure.'[30]

W. T. Gairdner pointed out that the practice of using alcoholic stimulants had been widespread in the profession long before Todd 'adopted the routine.' Todd was 'rather the expositor of a general tendency in medicine than the deviser of anything really new and striking in theory in this matter....' Gairdner's teacher, Alison, had taught a moderate version of the doctrine as early as 1826; his pupils, Robert Graves and William Stokes, had spread the gospel in Ireland. This doctrine 'had a powerful influence in breaking up the bad old routine of depletion in [treating] typhus fever, which was almost universal in the earlier part' of the nineteenth century.[31] Todd thus appears in this account as the genial practitioner of and propagandist for the alcoholic paradigm. Why did Todd get so much credit and blame for following an old therapeutic practice? Perhaps, as Warner notes, because he gave it a solid scientific basis, providing 'the 'scientific physician' with a clearly articulated theoretical justification for the use of alcohol, firmly grounded in the doctrines of contemporary physiology.'[32]

Medical discourse about fevers still contained a considerable residue of the eighteenth-century idea that fever 'was a disease itself' rather than 'a sign of underlying disease.'[33] But doctors talked about typhus fever with diagnostic certainty. Gairdner optimistically declared that 'typhus fever, as marked by the eruption, is a remarkably well-defined disease, in which, with proper securities against error, there is likely to be but little difference between the diagnosis of one well-informed hospital physician and another.'[34] W. W. Gerhard had distinguished typhus fever from typhoid fever in 1837, but one finds them paired as diseases throughout medical literature in the nineteenth century, and the fact that they share several common features may partly explain the diagnostic conflation. Current literature identifies the causal organism in typhoid as one of the *Salmonella* bacteria and that of typhus as a species of very small intracellular bacteria (*Rickettsia Prowazekis*), transmitted by arthropod vectors. Transmitted by lice, typhus was the plague of armies, prisons, ships, hospitals, and other insalubrious institutions. Typhus mortality can vary between under five per cent in children under fifteen and about forty six per cent in people over fifty. Charles Murchison (1830-79) and colleagues estimated it at about eighteen per cent. The untreated typhoid mortality can be up to twenty five per cent of infected persons. In 1882 Paris endured a five-month outbreak in which 2300 people died.[35]

A more sober medical historiography has given Todd some credit as a pioneer in laying down 'definite principles for the treatment of specially serious cases of fever, such as influenza and rheumatic fever, besides inflammations associated with exhaustion in which life was in jeopardy.' He is usually given the chief credit for the development of alcohol therapy. On the basis of his observation of patients Todd 'proved' that the best type of treatment was 'a steady administering of alcoholic stimulants at short intervals, day and night, while the danger lasted.' This treatment maintained the patient's strength and shortened the period of convalescence. In the case of delirium due to exhaustion and an abnormal condition of the blood, Todd often gave acetate of ammonia as 'a frequent adjunct to his alcoholic treatment' and 'most commonly added chloric ether, and not infrequently quinine to his plan of treatment,' which, unlike bleeding and lowering remedies, brought relief from the illness.[36] This shotgun approach in therapy made it difficult to be certain that alcohol played a role in the patient's recovery. What is certain is that Todd prescribed alcohol freely, without questioning its possible role in producing a high mortality rate among the patients at King's College Hospital. 'Dr. Todd ... thought nothing of prescribing half an ounce, or even an ounce of brandy every hour in case of fever.' Even conservative medical minds eventually wondered if there were a correlation between alcohol consumption and the high death rate (twenty five per cent) in the cases of typhus treated by Todd.[37]

Todd accepted the 'chemical theory [*à la* Liebig] that alcohol is transformed within the system' into carbon dioxide and water, thereby producing heat. The authoritative voice of the Parisian professor of hygiene, Apollinaire Bouchardat, supported Liebig's claim that alcohol is a food that helps respiration (*un aliment respiratoire*). This was one answer to the question of whether alcohol is destroyed in the organism with none expelled through activities such as breathing and urinating. Bouchardat and Sandras tried to establish the intravascular transformations of alcohol, and in their experiment, which used dogs, cocks, and ducks, they recognised (or thought they did) the presence of acetic acid. Some doctors were sceptical.[38]

The medical reputation of alcohol appeared to have been given a hard blow in 1860, when three French medical men, Lallemand, Perrin, and Duroy, published their experimentally-based work showing that alcohol is not a food and, worse, that it has bad effects on the brain, the liver, and the kidneys. Béhier recognised the revolutionary implication of this research by modifying profoundly his view of the physiological role attributed to alcohol, including alcoholic drinks. The work denied the doctrine of intravascular combustion. Both French and English researchers soon exposed the weakness and errors of the heretical teachings of Lallemand, Perrin, and Duroy, thus enabling the pro-alcohol camp to continue believing in the scientific basis of their therapy.[39] Perrin did not change his mind, or at least he he declared, after reviewing the work of his critics, that 'alcohol possesses none of the properties found in a food substance.'[40] Doctors are no better than scientists at changing their minds, and both groups never lack good theories and experiments on which to base their practices. In any case, though Perrin rejected the idea that alcohol is a food, he still recognised the therapeutical value of moderate doses as a stimulating and comforting agent.[41]

In 1861 Todd's principles of treatment were reduced to the following set of axioms and prescriptions by Edward Smith, assistant-physician to the Brompton hospital for consumption and diseases of the chest. Alcohol acts primarily on the nervous system: beneficially in increasing the generation of nervous power, without producing a smell of alcohol on the breath; or injuriously, in the case of too large a dose, by adversely affecting 'the nutrition of nerve matter' and producing a perceptible breath odour. Alcohol does not produce a 'true secondary depression of the vital powers,' except for too large doses, which upset the digestive process. 'Alcohol does not cause inflammation of the lungs, heart, or liver' or inflammation or congestion of the brain, though the brain is affected by 'poisoning of the nerve-cell and nerve fibre.' Alcohol, 'carefully taken,' has a positive effect on the cardiovascular system: it 'upholds the calorifying process,' thus preventing 'oxidation of the nervous and other tissues,' and 'strengthens the action of the heart, and reduces the frequency of the pulse.' (Todd had insisted on the need for adhering precisely to his prescription of dose and frequency: a dose of two drachms to two ounces of alcohol, repeated as often as food was given.) Food and alcohol have 'the same intention – *viz.*, to save the tissues from oxidation.' So in the patient's recovery from disease, alcohols 'uphold nervous force, and supply the most assimilable material for combustion. They calm the nervous system, and avert delirium.' In cases of coma and delirium from excess of alcohol, more alcohol should be given. Though it is dangerous to withdraw alcohol from the patient, there are cases in which it should not be given; their signs would be 'referable to deranged digestion – as flatus, eructations, sicknesses, and dry tongue and mouth.' Another case for withholding the panacea would be 'the smell in the breath, which indicates that the alcohol is passing off unchanged.' Smith summarised Todd's system as 'the belief that alcohol increases nerve-nutrition, strengthens the heart's action, lessens the rapidity of the circulation, shields the tissues from oxidation, and produces heat.'[42]

Smith based his views on the work done by Lallemand, Perrin, and Duroy. His repetition of their experiments confirmed the 'chemical theory' that moderate doses of alcohol pass through the body unchanged – usually called the 'total elimination theory.' So he rejected Todd's more orthodox view that alcohol is transformed in the system, for 'the arguments [Todd] used ... [were] not sufficient to establish his theory of the action of alcohols, or to warrant his peculiar plan of administering them.' Smith was not interested in discussing specific diseases in which alcohol could be used but rather in 'its true action, and ... the general conditions of the system to which it is fitted.' Since the 'same conditions exist in some stage of many diseases ... it is better to confine ... attention to the separate indications for its use, than to regard the whole phenomena of a disease as a unity, to be treated on a uniform plan. The indications being given, it will be easy to specify the diseases and stages of diseases to which its action is suitable.' So much of Todd's specific medicine had no evidence supporting it – e.g., the idea that hydrocarbons and particularly alcohol 'have an especial affinity for the nervous system.' Todd's practice rested 'only upon the ground of his personal authority.' A matter of great importance in the practice of medicine. Smith thought it was time to move the debate over the use of alcohol in the treatment of disease to a discussion of 'its merits on scientific grounds, and to remove it from the domain of hypothesis and empiricism.' So he reproduced the French experiments, adding experiments on himself and another person to determine the effects of alcohol in moderate quantity on the heart, brain, cerebro-spinal tract, respiratory tract, and the sympathetic system. After establishing the experimental fact that alcohol passed from the system by way of the breath in some people, by the skin in people who perspired freely, and by the kidneys in people who were big pissers, Smith was ready to give a scientific summary of alcohol's specific modes of action.[43]

Like doctors since antiquity, Smith was impressed by alcohol's reinforcing action on the heart and the resulting 'fulness [of the bloodvessels as a result of the tendency of alcohol to accumulate fluid] and freeness of the circulation,' with the blood being 'carried to the remote parts and to the surface.' Increasing the force of the circulation prevented or removed 'the tendency to local congestion of organs as the lungs and the liver,' and improved 'the whole nutritive and vital powers of the body.' Among 'the common and general actions of alcohol,' Smith included a second group of effects beginning with a lessening action on the skin, 'whereby the loss of heat is reduced, the urgent necessity for food and vital transformation is lessened, and the sensation of warmth is increased.' In the same category of effects can be included the local action as stimulant upon the stomach and alimentary canal with an increase of vascular action. Since Smith rejected the idea that the body consumes alcohol, he had to accommodate a conflict between the notion that alcohol generally interferes with the production of heat, required by his general theory, and the accepted clinical fact that alcohol does produce increased warmth when the patient consumes it. His ingenious supposition of a 'general temporary increase in the vital actions' provided a solution of the paradox.[44]

Smith believed that alcohol hinders alimentation, with retention of water and consequent lessening of the excretion of urea as a result of 'the diminution in the excretion of urine by the kidneys.' It is clear that Smith believed that alcohol has tremendous lessening powers: it lessens muscular power, it lessens nervous power, as shown by the muscles and the mind, it lessens vital action. The power of alcohol 'to lessen the salivary secretion' had 'to impede the due digestion of starch,' and this added to Smith's gloomy view of its effect on the digestive process. Fortunately for drinkers, Smith found that there are 'other important elements in ales, wines, and spirits having a different and independent action; so old wines directly lessen vital action, and ales directly promote transformation of food.' Aromas of wines have a 'conservative effect ... fitted for the cases of excessive nervous actions, in which to reduce the action would conduce to health.' New wine also had its use, particularly in the treatment of fever. 'The newer wines, containing little aroma and more spirit than old wines, have a better action.' A quotation from Aretaeus summed up these uses of wine and showed the learning of the doctor.[45]

By 1864, the *Lancet* was expressing grave concern over the excessive use of alcoholic stimulants, especially in London. 'There has been an unseemly extremeness in the doctrines of leading members of the profession of late years, represented by a lingering faith in bleeding on the one hand, and a newly acquired belief in brandy on the other. ... We have long had a most disagreeable fear that the lavish prescription of alcoholic stimulants ... would one day be discovered to be a great medical error, only less than the opposite system which preceeded it. It has been pushed amongst all classes of patients – rich and poor, women and children; in acute cases, in hospitals and in private practice....' Money that could have been used to send convalescent patients to the seaside or to paid overdue bills was being 'squandered over bottles of wine.' And there was the moral effect that this 'fashion of the faculty' had on the public. Of course, these considerations of 'mere cost or morals in a life-and-death situation' were 'essentially secondary.' The important question was if there were 'any physiological or therapeutical facts' proving that the big drink had 'a saving or curative effect in fever, not to be got in any other way.' A paper in the *Lancet* by W. T. Gairdner seriously questioned the efficacy of the excessive treatment; further, it aired the suspicion that 'alcohol tends 'to poison the blood'.' So one could 'doubt whether, the blood being already poisoned, as it is in fever, alcohol is likely to contribute anything to its purification.' The situation seemed ripe for the question put by Sir Robert Peel, quoting a saying in the north: 'Did he die by the doctor, or did he come by his death fairly?'[46]

Early in 1864, the *Lancet* published Gairdner's 'very important clinical paper' on the use of alcoholic stimulants in typhus fever.[47] Gairdner was 'regarded as one of the most promising' of his 'generation of physicians in Scotland'; formerly with the Edinburgh Infirmary and then the Glasgow Infirmary, he was an authority on 'vitality and disease in large cities and on a large scale.' His paper therefore attracted considerable attention and perhaps even had some influence in the medical community. *Lancet* pontificated that it was 'upon such men as Dr. Gardiner' that devolved 'the duty of mediating between the extreme views of the past and the, perhaps, equally extreme views of the present.' Convinced that the truth lay in 'neither extreme, but somewhere in the middle,' the journal looked to moderate sceptics like Gairdner to restore 'the credit of medical practice.'[48]

In the Glasgow Fever Hospital, where typhus 'constituted by far the largest proportion of all the fevers treated,' Gairdner enjoyed advantages other than a large diseased population to study. It was possible to get a 'tolerably accurate estimate both of the usual mortality of typhus fever, and of the amount of stimulants usually administered.' And his medical practices pretty much agreed with those of his colleagues, thus avoiding clashes that might vitiate the study. In fact, practice in Glasgow and Edinburgh, and probably Scotland generally, avoided the tendency to excess in prescribing stimulants that was characteristic of doctors in London and probably many parts of England.[49] Between November 1862 and December 1863 Gairdner had 595 cases of typhus admitted under his care. Each case was 'the subject of a special diagnosis.' The aggregrate mortality was seventy one, about twelve per cent, though for two months it rose to nineteen per cent because of the 'graver character of the cases admitted.' In epidemics the mortality rate could rise to about twenty five per cent: in the Edinburgh epidemic of 1847-8 the rate was 20.6 to 24.72 per cent. Over a period of fourteen and one-half years, Charles Murchison had found for all ages an average rate of mortality of 20.89 per cent, but the 'larger proportion of old and destitute persons' admitted to the London Fever Hospital was, Gairdner recognised, partly responsible for the high rate. It was still better than the rate of twenty-five per cent at King's College Hospital under Todd, who also had a high rate, possibly seventeen per cent, for young people, compared to a rate of 6.2 per cent at the London Fever Hospital over a ten year period. Out of Gairdner's 189 young typhus patients, only one died, a child aged six, 'admitted moribund.' Gairdner explained that his great success in treating fevers resulted from his general practice of 'supporting the strength,' which might require a moderate dose of stimulant for some adult patients but never for young patients. Nine-tenths of his patients required no stimulants at all. *Lancet* found it more striking that the ten per cent of his cases getting 'a good allowance of stimulants were the identical ten per cent which died.'[50]

Gairdner emphasised that his practice had nothing in common with 'the depletion and starvation school of physicians,' who completely avoided the use of stimulants in treating fevers because they 'excite the circulation.' That school's system for countering febrile excitement worked 'by depressing remedies, and by starvation or extreme restriction of the diet.' Gairdner belonged to another school of physic, which believed that 'to the young, in typhus, and very probably in most other fevers, stimulants are not less than actively poisonous and destructive, unless administered with the most extreme caution, and in the most special and critical circumstances.' In general, alcohol poisons the system, 'by loading the blood with material which is inconvertible into blood or material, and which interferes with the vital changes necessary to preserve the balance of waste and supply.' Since 'all routine methods of administration tend to abuse,' each patient needs individually tailored medical care. Gairdner's excellent therapeutic results justified the *Lancet*'s favourable endorsement of his practices.[51]

Initially it did not seem that the quarrel over the usefulness of the alcoholic treatment of disease could be settled by statistical studies. Charles Murchison's comparative study of Todd's treatment of typhus and typhoid fever at King's College Hospital and cases treated at the London Fever Hospital, where alcohol was used, not abused, ignited an inconclusive squabble in the *Lancet* in the 1860s. Murchison used alcohol more in cases of typhus than typhoid fever. Unlike cholera, typhus had what Bynum calls a class-specific image.[52] With a death rate some pessimists put as high as twenty-five per cent of an untreated population, doctors were inspired to take risks, but Murchison resisted the temptation to follow the enthusiastic prescribers. He limited doses to six to eight ounces of brandy daily, given only after the tenth or twelfth day and rarely in cases of relapse – sixteen ounces in twenty four hours would have been exceptional.[53] Murchison was in the good moderate or even abstaining company of Alexander Tweedie, Robert D. Lyons, and Gairdner, as well as the better known Bright and Addison. Recognising the dangers of alcoholic medicine, even Francis Anstie, the English hero of the pro-alcohol group, took a moderate position in the debates.

Writers had noted that a sick person could ingest doses of alcohol that would poison a well person, but more and more doctors came to warn about the danger of making sick people sicker with large doses of alcohol. A striking example of Brown's 'therapeutic alcoholism' was reported by Hugh Norris in 1878. Nine years before, Norris had attended a patient suffering from 'a severe attack of pleuro-pneumonia, which left considerable condensation in both lungs, and consequent extreme prostration of the vital powers. For this he took, under medical supervision, one ordinary bottle of brandy, one bottle of champagne, and one bottle of old port wine *daily for nine months*, at the expiration of such time he began to reduce this amount of stimulant.' This account was corroborated by the patient's wife. Norris also accepted the account because the patient, his friend, was a minister of the gospel. The patient, then in 'fair health,' a 'small, attenuated man of fifty two or fifty three years' was still 'active in profession.'[54] This accounts conforms to other medical accounts of some sick people able to consume with no visible ill effects amounts of alcohol that would kill healthy people.

Heavy doses of alcohol were standard treatment for intermittent fever; if quinine could not be administered, the malarial patient could always be treated by alcohol alone. Other febrile diseases were reported to succumb, at least sometimes, to the ingestion of prescribed doses of alcohol. Doctors worried about the method of administration and dosage. And some doctors did experiments that showed the pro-alcohol group to be wrong in their theories, or at least to have considerably exaggerated the success of alcohol cures. In his treatise on continued fevers Murchison rejected the excesses of Todd's alcoholic medicine.[55] The etiology of disease and therapy were just as much subjects of disagreement and debate in the nineteenth century as they are today, perhaps even more.

Anti-alcoholic therapy received a solid boost when *Lancet* published the results obtained by Samuel Wilks in treating without stimulants twelve cases of typhus and typhoid fever at Guy's Hospital.[56] His results backed up those reported earlier by Gairdner and those obtained in the 121 cases of fever treated by Chambers with a mortality rate of only two and one-half per cent. Both Gairdner and Chambers emphasised 'the essential point of supporting the patient, not by stimulants, but by nourishing food.'[57] In some of his twelve cases, Wilks administered some wine and in one serious case turpentine fomentations and brandy. Given in capsules or in emulsion, turpentine used to have a wide range of medical uses ranging from increasing the flow of urine to checking the growth of bacteria in the lungs. It was also added to enemas to help expel gas.[58] One of Wilks' twelve patients died, chiefly as a result of an abscess, it seems. So medical treatment for fevers had returned to 'the old practice of the hospital ... laid down by Drs. Bright, Addison, and Barlow.... The teaching of these professors was to the effect that a large number of cases ran their course without any treatment than careful watching and feeding; that they required no other medicine than a simple saline; but that some needed a stimulant during the progress of the disease, and others required it from the commencement.'[59] The answers to the questions of when and how much could only be determined by the experienced practitioner.

In treating febrile patients Wilks enthusiastically encouraged them to consume plenty of milk, still identified well into the twentieth century as the best form of nutriment in the treatment of typhus.[60] One of the traditional treatments for rich people with typhoid fever was 'three or four cups of beef-tea daily, some jelly, eight or ten ounces of brandy, five or six glasses of champagne, and medicine containing five grains of ammonia every four hours.' Wilks pointed out that the victim would die of starvation. And he could not help feeling 'almost overcome with regret' seeing his 'hospital patients doing well and ... the young people in a rich man's house literally dying of *starvation and stimulation*.' Like most of the medical profession, Wilks followed Robert Graves's law of 'feed a fever.' The problem was how to provide nutrition when 'the condition of the alimentary canal precludes the use of solid food.' Wilks' miracle food was milk, four or five pints daily. And Wilks was able to advertise that his 'success with fever' was consequently 'much greater than heretofore.'[61]

Todd had also claimed that he obtained respectable results in treating pneumonia, limiting the death rate to one-ninth of the patients treated even though most arrived in dreadful condition. It was estimated that two-thirds of the patients would die if treated with stibious or antimonious tartar, and only one-eight of them would die with other treatments. Wilks impatiently dismissed the brandy treatment on the basis of his own clinical experience and, above all, because of the results reported by John Hughes Bennett at the Royal Infirmary in Edinburgh.[62] 'What the need of this [the brandy treatment] can be with Professor Hughes Bennett's statistics before us, I do not comprehend.'[63] Bennett was skilled at curing patients through the restorative treatment, which did nevertheless involve the administration of moderate amounts of port wine.[64]

Contemporaries regarded Bennett's treatment of pneumonia and phthisis (pulmonary tuberculosis) as his most valuable therapeutic work. These diseases were considered as important in themselves and representative of two great classes of disease, acute and chronic. His German-influenced prescription for the patient suffering from phthisis was fresh air and cod liver oil; the oil was also a classic remedy among Scottish fishermen.[65] *Lancet* gave him an excessive eulogy on his death in 1875. 'Dr. Bennett, more than any other man, has contributed to reform the treatment of them [the two diseases], and to overthrow the view which has ruled medical men for centuries. ... He reduced the mortality of uncomplicated pneumonia to *nil*; he demonstrated not only the dispensableness, but the injuriousness, of the antiphlogistic treatment. ... Other physicians were working in the same direction even before Bennett. But he devised a treatment of his own which has given most brilliant results, and he adhered to it and to the pathological views on which it was based ... to establish its truth, and so largely revolutionise[d] the practice of medicine in acute diseases....'[66]

Pneumonia provided a therapeutic battleground for rival theories and treatments. The restorative treatment called for strong beef-tea (sometimes laced with port wine), eggs, steak, and rice pudding. A patient could have six ounces of port wine prescribed daily. The restorative repertory also included the administration of colchicum and antimonial wines, solution of acetate of ammonia, and salines, among other chemicals. So mainly through the vehicle of port wine, alcohol retained a minor role in the restorative treatment of pneumonia; Bennett advocated it as a substitute for the 'recently inculcated' venesection or bloodletting, an old palliative practice that produced the best effects, according to 'systematic writers,' when carried out on the very day of the attack. Bennett found that large warm poultices applied to the painful sides gave more relief than bloodletting and possibly served 'to assist the transformation of the exudation in the lung, and facilitate recovery. ... Beef tea and wine were, however, assiduously administered.' The treatment of pneumonia at the Royal Infirmary offers an unusual view into the therapeutic powers and limits of nineteenth-century medicine. Bennett was able to use the annual number of cases treated between 1839 and 1864 to show the evolution of treatment and the great improvement in mortality or cure rate achieved by the restorative treatment. Bennett identified the period before 1848 with an antiphlogistic practice, which produced more than one death in every two and a half cases. In the second period, 1848 to 1856, when Bennett was able as clinical professor to introduce a restorative practice, the death rate fell to less than one in four and a half cases. In the third triumphant period, beginning in 1856-7, 'when the bloodletting controversy began which fixed so strongly the attention of medical men on the restorative treatment of pneumonia,' the death rate dropped further to one in seven and three quarter cases, about thirteen per cent. Bennett boasted that 'these figures speak for themselves.'[67] (The present mortality for pneumonia is thirty per cent without treatment and five per cent with antibiotic therapy.)

When doctors think about the history of medicine, they sometimes flounder around in search of a theory that will give a more solid scientific basis to their practice along with better therapeutic results – the two results sometimes coincide. *Lancet* thought that a solid theory had been found by 1865.

> One great discovery has been made of late years - that there is a method in diseased processes; that there is a good 'nisus' in the worst of them; that when disease overtakes the body, it finds the body not unprepared to meet it, and make the best of it, but with many provisions for conducting it to a kindly and harmless issue; and that the height of medical wisdom is to recognise these provisions, to place the body in the best natural circumstances, and gently assist all the natural processes of cure.[68]

The word *nisus* is reminiscent of the idea of 'life force' or *nisus formativus* developed by the anatomist-physiologist J. F. Blumenbach (1752-1840), but it also is reminiscent of the ancient doctrine of the *vis medicatrix naturae* or 'self healing tendencies of the body.'[69] The spectre of vitalism may even be lurking in the shadow of this latinism.

This latest theory rejected the 'old medicine,' which 'erred in treating disease and nature too roughly,' and the 'new treatment by alcohol,' whose excess 'was scarcely less 'perturbing' than the old one.' A case study illustrated the danger of the alcohol treatment. 'Thirty-six ounces of brandy in twenty-four hours to a girl fourteen years old, with fever and a diseased heart, was apt to be a disease of itself....' The alcohol put a strain on the heart, the excreting organs, and the brain.The effect on the brain was believed to be unfortunate because in the new model of medicine recovery depended to a considerable extent on the brain's efficiency. *Lancet* was happy to 'receive intimation ... that the days of this fashion are numbered, and that a more moderate, a more physiological method of treating disease is destined to replace it.'[70]

Trying to explain the excessive English enthusiasm for the therapeutic use of alcohol and the reaction against it, the French doctor Paul Gingeot fell back on the convenient idea of its being a new therapeutic fashion whose excesses in one direction led ineluctably to an excessive reaction against it. It made some sense to argue that doctors believed, like many people, in the tonic or strength-giving proprieties of beer, wine, and spirits; it made more sense to say that doctor and patient were in agreement on the prescription of a stimulant than to say that the doctor was pandering to public taste.[71] Culture creates the treatment if not the disease. *Lancet* also sniffed at the vagueness and simplicity of the popular concept of debility or weakness, which in 'defying the definition of the physiologist and the analysis of the chemist,' provided a 'great recommendation' for the theory to doctors, 'busy men who have not much time to spend over the choice of their theories.' In 1865 *Lancet* noted that it had long expressed doubt concerning the double theory that all diseases are but 'different forms of this universal disease of weakness' and that 'alcohol in some form or other is the panacea for it.'[72] Gingeot believed that perhaps the major problem was the therapy's lack of a solid foundation, either clinical or experimental, which meant that its administration was based solely on arbitrary theoretical ideas.[73]

Nineteenth-century English ideas on treating diseases influenced many French doctors. The older pro-alcohol group in France, including Pinel and Laennec, and most of the French medical community, restricted the administration of alcohol to the treatment of fevers, especially typhus. Wine and *eau-de-vie* were used in cases of typhoid and the adynamic pneumonia that prostrated old people. French doctors generally prescribed small repeated doses of strong alcohol. Although he condemned the prescription of excessive doses, Charles Murchison was often cited in favour of this therapeutic strategy. L.-F.-J. Béhier's 'conférence de clinique médicale' of 1864 made the alcoholic treatment, in its largest sense, an important issue. In 1864 Béhier became professor of internal pathology at the faculty of medicine in Paris before soon switching to the chair of *clinique médicale* at the Hôtel-Dieu. He supposedly gained some notoriety by introducing into French practice the English method of administering alcohol in cases of pneumonia. Bréhier emphasised that in the case of older people (66-77 years) the eau-de-vie had to be given with a light hand and accompanied by bouillons, potages, and other light food.[74] (The age range for these patients was probably not unusual among Bréhier's well-off clients: the great clinician was Guizot's favourite doctor as well as the physician of other ministers and of the Maison du roi Louis-Philippe.)

Paul Gingeot, who had interned under Béhier, noted that his

patron had prescribed wine in the case of acute diseases before the pro-wine articles by William Stokes came out in *The Dublin Journal of Medical Science* in 1839. Bréhier prescribed *eau-de-vie* in amounts varying between 80 and 300 grams with 80-120 grams of edulcorated water – 'la potion de Todd' – in doses of one spoonful every two hours. Like Todd, he found that alcohol stopped delirium, slowed down the pulse and breathing, and caused an abundant perspiration, and that the patient recovered strength 'without the slightest sign of drunkenness.'[75] After Hyde-Salter (Charing-Cross Hospital) reported in *Lancet* (14 Nov. 1863) that large doses of alcohol stopped asthma attacks, Bréhier tested the claim by successfully treating a member of his own family: a small glass of rum did the trick. Bréhier was proud of keeping up with the latest work done in pathological anatomy and in chemistry. An aging Trousseau found that it was easier to denounce the chemical invasion of medicine than to try to understand the chemistry. Bréhier enthusiastically took over the somewhat disused English custom of giving sub-cutaneous injections to become the 'grand maître des piqûres' who could end the pain of the elite promptly with a needle.[76] Although wine and *eaux-de-vie* had been part of French medical practice for ages and was justified on the grounds of clinical experience and the opinions of the greatest medical authorities since antiquity, alcohol therapy in order to be scientific needed the patina of English science as the guarantee of certainty and efficacy. In administering doses of alcohol according to the rules of English science, the doctor avoided the stigmata of popular medicine and folk remedies based on wine.

The lively discussions following the publication of research on alcoholic therapy indicated that the 'alcohol question' was very much alive in the medical world after the 1860s. Gingeot, well aware that Bréhier's therapy was based on Todd's teachings, believed that the French movement for the study of the physiological and therapeutic properties of alcohol had originated in England. This was as unsurprising for Gingeot as for Béhier because England was perceived as a country in which alcoholic drink had too large a role in the diet. French doctors envied the situation of doctors in Britain, where the medical use of alcohol was helped by a long history of consumption of fermented drinks in all social classes. It is not clear how French consumption produced a different situation in France, but by eliminating wine from figures on the consumption of alcohol the French were able to claim that the English drank more than they did. With the approval of Dr. Simon, his 'nouveau chef,' Gingeot was able to carry out on children an experimental alcoholic treatment whose effects he already knew for adults and old people. A drinkable *esprit-de-vin* used to be given to children suffering from worms, which were expected to leave their drunken host. Although he followed Murchison in doubting some of Todd's more optimistic ideas – for example, that alcohol was able to effect special repairs of nervous tissue – Gingeot thought that after the death of Todd an excessive reaction had set in against the use of alcohol therapy.

Abuses there had been, but total discrediting of the treatment was not justified. And given the nature of modern therapy it was not possible to banish alcohol from medicine. Why not? Gingeot's answer surprises us. No longer a matter of inspiration without serious links to scientific knowledge, therapy had become scientific. Gingeot argued that the idea of the physiological effects of alcohol had given the liquid an important place in the doctor's arsenal. So there was no point in arguing that alcohol was frequently useless in treating acute diseases or that it had been misused in chronic affections, which was true but incapable of damaging the body of achieved results. Gingeot could still assert in 1867 that the new method had proved itself theoretically and practically. Even if new imperfections of the alcoholic therapy were discovered, this would be a reason for further research, not a reason for rejecting it. One a treatment had entered into general practice, the fact that it was not totally successful, or even if limited in success, was no reason for dropping it from the medical arsenal.[77]

Even in its heyday there were troubles with alcoholic therapy. A major problem was that there was no evidence that alcohol could 'antagonise' a disease in the way that quinine antagonised malarial fever, mercury antagonised syphilis, or, more doubtful, alkalis antagonised rheumatic fever.[78] Nor was it long before distinguished doctors challenged this new medicine by citing experimentally-based statistics showing that diseases like typhus could be treated successfully without any stimulants at all. Eventually most doctors came to recognise that many cases of fever could be treated without alcohol. Todd's giving up to thirty ounces of brandy daily to a young patient was hard to justify, especially since it was believed that young people rarely died of fever. Once the major weapon in the treatment of cholera, alcohol came to be regarded as dangerous and was replaced by 'caustic alkalis,' including a hot disinfecting enema of potassium salts several times a day. Theoretical and therapeutic opinion showed some signs of slowing turning away from alcohol, though with some of the replacement therapies the patient was not necessarily better off.

The practice of administering stimulants had, according to its opponents, remarkable survival powers. A valuable drug in the medical arsenal, alcohol was also widely accepted as a food and an antiseptic. In 1867 Wilks felt obliged to deliver a clinical lecture on the 'indiscriminate use of alcoholic stimulants in disease,' which was published in *Lancet*.[79] Wilks believed that 'the most important question in therapeutics ... [was] the value of alcohol in disease.' He was alarmed at the abuse of an item that should have been on the list of drugs and administered with the same caution as other articles in the *Pharmacopoeia*. 'Alcohol ... although an excitant, is a sedative to the nervous system – is, in fact, an anaesthetic.' A drinker feels better after a glass or two of grog like 'the Turk who feels better for his opium.' To give brandy to all patients was quack medicine, 'as much a universal remedy as revalenta, chlorodyne, Morrison's pills.' A doctor should 'always seriously [consider] the advisability of alcoholic treatment before [having] recourse to it.' Wilks noted that he had obtained good results after discontinuing the use of stimulants in a case of bronchitis.

Reflecting on the success of his non-alcoholic treatment of a sixty-year old patient, Wilks found remarkable 'how slight a scientific basis is founded for the treatment of pneumonia.' Not many years before, 'the antiphlogistic method was adopted, including bleeding, antimony, calomel, etc.; then came the 'let alone' method'; and then 'the brandy treatment.' Wilks thought that the antiphlogistic treatment saved more patients than the brandy treatment. Although generally agreeing with Wilks, *Lancet* noted that he rather overrated 'the careless and excessive use of stimulants by the profession now.' It was getting easier to round up a group of distinguished medical men who either totally opposed the therapeutic use of alcohol or allowed it only in moderation while avoiding giving it 'in the early stages of the disease, in which circumstances you are apt to get the injurious and narcotic effects of alcohol.'[80]

The therapeutic use of alcohol did not lack defenders. As some doctors pointed out, alcohol still had the undeniable virtues that had led the profession to incorporate it into the practice of medicine in the first place. Since these valuable properties were increasingly forgotten in the quarrels over its effectiveness in treating specific diseases, Robert Barnes thought it necessary to defend its three virtues.[81] Barnes was convinced that doctors and nurses who had tended cases of fever would 'be able to bear testimony to the stimulating and the *sustaining* powers of alcohol.' As a result of 'close clinical observation,' Barnes concluded that alcohol 'is to a certain extent *a substitute for food*, by sustaining the powers of life under circumstances where the call for food is urgent and obvious, but cannot be supplied. One proof of this lies in the extraordinary tolerance of alcohol with which we are familiar during fever.' The third virtue of alcohol, which Barnes believed to be as important as the other two but neglected in the debates, was its antiseptic property in fever caused by zymotic diseases.[82] Alcohol countered both the specific poison produced by the fever and the poisoning process 'resulting from perverted nutrition and impeded excretion.' So 'under alcohol the secretions in fever improve [and] the diarrhoeal stools become less offensive.' Once this antiseptic principle justifying the use of alcohol was accepted, other substances could be administered as an internal medicine by those opposed to the universal use of alcohol. Barnes himself had 'encouraging success' in treating cholera with carbolic acid. Mordey Douglas had three cholera patients drink a solution of ammonia in hot water and administered enemas of a dilute solution of permanganate of potash. Most patients would probably have preferred sipping brandy and port wine to drinking ammonia and having a solution of potassium salts 'thrown up the bowel two or three times during the day, as hot as the patients would bear it.'[83] But in the professional world the preferences of the patient may be sacrificed to the dictates of scientific medicine, which discovers by experiment on animal and patient the best treatment for disease.

Some doctors were eager to end a debate exposing the fragility of the scientific basis of their practice. Douglas hoped that the highly visible work done by Francis Anstie would 'give a fresh impetus to the study of the action of alcohol in disease, and that its ... empirical prescription ... [would] soon be replaced by scientific data.'[84] Anstie was sure by 1868 that new research had 'made it necessary that the theory of stimulation in febrile diseases should be reconsidered, from its very foundation.'[85]

In the 1870s arguments for and against the therapeutic use of alcohol were based on the latest medical understanding of the mechanism by which alcohol worked in the organism, especially in the blood, the fluid tissue of life. And the effect of alcohol on temperature had become of great concern to doctors. With the 'systematic use of medical thermometry,' physicians could emulate measurement-mad scientists, though the medical 'preoccupation [was] with the destructive effects of heat in the febrile patient and a search for means of therapeutically lowering temperature.'[86] Fever was classified as a killer which destroyed 'life by the rapid exhaustion of the nutritive properties of the blood.' Alcohol came to be used as a medicament to lower body temperature and prevent the wasting of tissue. Barnes explained how alcohol worked as an antiseptic in zymotic disease that used up of 'the vital properties of the blood.' The idea that disease consumes items in the blood is what might be expected in a fermentation model of disease: the process is analogous to the yeast's 'consumption' of sugar to produce alcohol and carbon dioxide. But zymotic diseases posed another danger to the patient by producing poison. 'First, there is the specific poison of the fever, multiplying itself; secondly, there is the empoisoning process, resulting from perverted nutrition and impeded excretion.' Although he had no quantitative data, Barnes believed that the alcohol rapidly entered and mixed with the blood, where, in an undecomposed state, it slowed up 'the double process of empoisonment.'[87] With the idea of an antiseptic capable of countering poison produced by diseases that act analogously to fermentation, the medical profession was not a great conceptual leap away from the model of the germ theory of disease.

Mordey Douglas assumed the operation of much the same mechanism to explain the action of alcohol and, except in the case of high fever, to argue against its therapeutic use. There was general agreement that the eventual decomposition of alcohol in the blood produced heat, but this was part of a paradox, for alcohol also lowered temperature for some time 'by appropriating the oxygen of the blood,' thus lessening 'the combustion of better fuel' and retarding 'tissue-change.' In the 1860s and beyond, the limited medical grammar of the digestive process could only handle a vague discourse about tissue's being replaced by nitrogenised food or azotised substances in the blood.[88] The argument was that what is injurious to the body in health is 'of value in the severe state of fever. The fever-poison, by quickly acting upon the azotised substances, causes the high temperature, rapid emaciation, and nervous exhaustion. Alcohol, by taking up the oxygen, keeps the fermenting poison at bay, and thus lowers the temperature, prevents the rapid destruction of tissue, and consequent shock to the nervous system.' Douglas believed that as the temperature of the patient approaches 'the normal standard,' alcohol should be decreased or discontinued because it causes 'an increase of imperfectly oxidised bodies in the system,' thereby retarding the convalescence.[89] Late-eighteenth century chemical theory, with its elevation of oxygen 'to the principle of a general explanatory 'principle',' seemed to have become part of the medical model of fever.[90] And the concept of oxidation, so important in the Pasteurian model of the evolution of wine, had become an axiom on which to base the treatment of fever. Whatever sense or nonsense we can make of the discourse, it enabled the nineteenth-century doctor to acquire a veneer of certainty by using the language of chemistry. Bichat's dream fulfilled again.[91]

Unlike Barnes, Douglas rejected the idea that alcohol would ever be shown to be of use in treating the zymotic diseases. Douglas analysed how alcohol would work in a patient striken with cholera, a disease in which 'alcohol used to be looked upon as the sheet-anchor, but ... [then] generally [came to be] regarded as an intensifier of the collapse.' The problem was again the assumed affinity of alcohol for the oxygen in the blood, whose capacity for oxygenation was probably already reduced by the disease. Lessening the amount of oxygen in the blood would lower the temperature of an already chilly patient. Worse, 'the retarded oxidation of tissue would favour capillary congestion, and ultimately stagnation of the blood.' Alcohol would retard 'the interchanges between the blood in the capillaries and the tissues.' (Current wisdom is that alcohol promotes peripheral vasodilation.) Why then did doctors nearly universally accept alcohol as a stimulant? Douglas thought that this erroneous conclusion had been arrived at because the 'increased action of the heart and throbbing of the large arteries' were considered 'as always synonymous with accelerated circulation.' The action of the heart, 'the principal agent in the circulation of the arteries,' did not extend to the capillaries, which were subject to another force, the *vis a fronte.* The increased activity of the alcohol-stimulated heart could not counter this congestion of the capillaries. Since 'in cholera it appears desirable not to retard, but to favour oxidation,' Douglas followed chemical logic in prescribing 'caustic alkalies to promote that change.' And although we sometimes cannot follow the scientific reasoning of these doctors, ignorant of how cholera introduced poison into the intestines or of the existence of electrolytes, we should keep in mind that often their therapies 'worked' for reasons that would require an entirely new type of scientific explanation.[92]

Lancet greeted the new year in 1870 with a confident statement on the achievement of 'some real progress toward the establishment of satisfactory principles' in 'professional opinion upon the question of alcoholic stimulation in disease.'[93] To generate the maximum of confidence a treatment had to be based on experiment. And this was the point at which the alcohol treatment had arrived by 1870: a solid body of therapeutic knowledge resting on experimental results. True, authorities still differed on the value of the alcoholic treatment, which involved 'a good deal of extreme and irrational practice, both in the direction of excessive stimulation, and of the opposite fault of an unreasonable fear of the remedy.' But with the establishment of 'the outlines of a greatly improved knowledge, both of the therapeutic powers and the capacity for mischief which alcohol possesses,' optimists hoped that this schism would soon end.

Any decision to use the alcohol treatment was supposed to be governed by the general classification of the disease treated, whether it was acute or chronic. A whiff of the nosographical imperative still hung lightly in the air. In the treatment of 'acute diseases attended by febrile phenomena,' there were three things or facts that were 'reasonably plain' certainties. First, if alcohol acted well, it did so 'as an antiphlogistic stimulant': it lowered high temperature, reduced a fast pulse, and, 'while raising nervous power,' calmed the disturbances of the nervous system accompanying and possibly caused by 'the elevated temperature of the blood in pyrexia [fever].' Second, not all patients benefited from alcohol. Young people and previously robust patients did best without it, others could take daily only three ounces of wine, which would be for them 'fully the physiological and therapeutical equivalent of twenty-four ounces given to another and smaller class of patients.' The physician had to experiment cautiously with the patient in order to discover the right dose because no generalised prescription was possible.[94] 'The third settled fact' was that alcohol often produces its best effects 'in cases with very high temperature and flushed face.' These were the cases in which 'alcohol was formerly thought (on purely theoretical grounds) to be most dangerous.' But there could be no justification for pouring 'large quantities of stimulants into a fever patient' just because he is pale and has a weak pulse. And so ended in 1870 the list of the medical certainties in acute diseases.

There were also a couple of probabilities the physician could gamble with. First, it was probable that the antiseptic property of alcohol gave it 'part of its influence in fevers' by destroying 'the activity of certain bodies ... by means of which the *contagium* sets up the febrile disturbance within the blood.' Since there was no consensus on germ theory, the bodies could be called 'organisms, or not,' as pleased the reader. In inflammation, it was believed that alcohol probably stimulated the sympathetic nervous system, contracted the arterioles, and partly interfered 'with the migration of blood-corpuscles through the vascular walls, as [Carl] Binz and his pupils' had shown that quinine could also do. Alcohol has different effects on different people depending on the amount of alcohol they are capable of absorbing: different people oxidise alcohol at different rates. As soon as the alcohol mingles with the blood, there is an antiseptic effect with an influence on the 'migrative tendency of the corpuscles,' though the 'subsequent progress of oxidation' determined 'the *general* effect on the patient' for 'good or bad.' In the treatment of acute diseases, one thing was accepted as certain: if signs of narcotism – that is paralysis of the nervous system – were produced, the alcohol was doing harm, and had to be immediately diminished or stopped.[95]

In contrast to the happy state of affairs in the treatment of acute diseases, there was 'much less of intelligent progress in medical opinion' on chronic diseases. *Lancet* 'regretted that a large number of practitioners [persisted] in acting on the assumption that in non-febrile diseases the amount of alcohol to be administered ought to be measured by the degree of debility, merely as such.' This practice had a 'direct and mischievous corollary,' the growing prescription of a 'lavish profusion' of stimulants in 'numerous *nervous* afflictions to which weakly persons (more especially women) are prone.' *Lancet* condemned 'unthinking and illogical' doctors for have driven 'hundreds of neuralgic, hysteric, and epileptic patients ... into drunkenness or lunacy, or both.' This 'grave scandal and mischief' required an immediate reform. The writer justified this virtuous outburst as the duty of medical journalists, though the condemnation was limited to the 'prescription of alcohol for *debility, merely as such*.' *Lancet* men, though 'no bigots against alcohol,' also declared that they were 'heartily sick of the unthinking abuse which has been lavished on what it is the fashion to call 'indiscriminate stimulation in acute diseases'.'[96] Of course a sustained reading of *Lancet* in the 1870s shows that there was still some confusion on the therapeutic status of the alcohol treatment. The confusion lay deep in the medical profession itself. Yet an evolution had taken place in medical opinion on the subject of alcohol. Whereas it used to be unusual to find opposition to the treatment, by the late-1870s the reverse was true.

In 1875 *Lancet* could still be impressed enough with the therapeutic power of alcohol to report the details of a striking case of a patient's recovery from rheumatic fever and carditis in which alcohol was freely used in the treatment.[97] On January 25, 1875, University College hospital in London admitted under the care of Wilson Fox a twenty-three year old married woman with an impressive case history. She 'had suffered from an attack of rheumatic fever in infancy, and thirteen weeks prior to her admission from inflammation of the kidneys.' She had delivered two months before admission. Two weeks before admission she had an attack of rheumatic fever after catching cold, with all the joints being successively affected; she also had bronchitis and 'expectorated much yellow phlegm.' (When there were later 'occasional returns of joint pains and fever,' she was given 'a mixture containing five grains of iodide of potassium and five grains of iodide of iron, three times a day.' A side effect of this standard treatment was that after a fortnight 'a crop of purpura came out on the legs and feet, lasting three days.') On the day after admission her condition was serious but not hopeless: she was slightly cyanotic and anaemic, experiencing chest pains with 'sonorous and sibilant râles, and breathing rapidly, rising to '52 in the minute' the next day. The heart's apex-beat was not well defined ... and there was a soft, long presystolic murmur audible at the fifth interspace one inch inside the nipple.' Weak pulse and high temperature were also noted. Aggressive treatment had to begin at once.

The treatment of this patient was 'a good illustration of the advantages to be derived from the free and unsparing administration of alcohol in cases of carditis.' On January 26 she was given as much beef-tea and milk as she could take and her dose of brandy brought up to one ounce every two hours. Two days later her stimulant was changed to 'a mixture of rectified spirit and water – two pints of the former to one pint of water, flavoured with one ounce and a half of tincture of orange-peel.' The dose, increased to half an ounce every half hour, was 'given with champagne or milk as the patient ... [could] take it.' By the fifth day the patient, having gotten worse, even refused to drink brandy. Then she took a turn for the better, recovering enough to take brandy and milk. Custard, eggs, and Brand's essence of meat were added to the diet. After more than a month in the hospital she recovered enough to get up for a short time. The case was complicated by her recurrent attacks of rheumatic fever and an attack of dry pleurisy. But by April 30 the patient was well enough to be sent off to Eastbourne.

Fox's comments on the case make clear the medical reasons for his use of the alcohol treatment. Though the patient had no pericarditis and little endocarditis, there was 'evident carditis, with a retarded pulse (60).' Fox accepted the traditional therapeutic belief that 'the remedy in such cases' is alcohol, with 'everything else in the way of medicine' being discontinued. Alcohol being a stimulant to the heart, it should be given, Fox maintained, 'when the pulse is very rapid and feeble, or very weak, intermittent, and retarded.' Digitalis, valuable in treating patients with the first type of pulse is too dangerous because it is so effective in reducing the pulse. In the case of a woman patient with carditis, Fox believed in giving alcohol 'with unsparing hand till regularity of pulse is produced.' Death in such cases could come from exhaustion, syncope, apnoea, and thrombosis in the heart. 'So long as the heart contracts efficiently so as to empty its cavities thrombosis will not occur' because no 'stagnant blood' is left between the columnae carneae to give rise to clots. Within this system of medical thought, alcohol was one of the essential tools with which the doctor fought off death.

Although the debate on alcohol dribbled on into the last quarter of the nineteenth century, an important stage in closure was reached by 1870, when Parkes and Wollowicz gave an epoch-making paper at the Royal Society.[98] The results of their experiments on the effects of alcohol on the healthy human subject contradicted those obtained by previous researchers. A review of the pamphlet in *Lancet* took the optimistic view that the conclusions should be accepted because of the great care and trouble taken by the experimenters and the extreme sensitivity of their instruments. Part of the reason for the disagreements obtained in different experiments might have resulted from the use of ethyl alcohol mixed with water and of brandy; so researchers using beer or wine, which contain different substances in addition to alcohol, might have gotten different experimental results.

In one sense, the great importance of this piece of physiological research was 'the remarkably negative character of the results.' It had been confirmed that 'moderate doses of alcohol do not hinder the oxidation-processes, which are the true life of the healthy body....'[99] The main points of interest for the practicing physician concerned the effects of alcohol on the vital functions of the diseased body. The research had also given 'confirmation of the maxim that alcohol, given in small and in large daily quantities respectively ... has widely different effects upon the system.' More than two ounces of alcohol produced symptoms of narcosis; a small amount stimulated the appetite, but more than two ounces depressed it, with large amounts nearly destroying it. Alcohol stimulated the action of the heart but excessively so in the person given a high dose; it was also able to cause an improper increase in capillary circulation. 'It did not seem to impede primary digestion.' Neither alcohol nor brandy lessened temperature, even during an attack of ephemeral fever. Since neither normal nor 'moderately narcotic' doses of alcohol affected the amount of free acidity or of phosphoric acid in the urine, the researchers concluded that the nervous system was not affected.

Parkes and Wollowicz believed it improbable that 'alcohol in quantities that can be properly used in diet has any effect' on 'the metamorphosis of nitrogenous tissues' or on 'animal heat.' It also seemed 'unlikely (in the face of the chemical results) that it [alcohol] can enable the body to perform more work on less food, though by quickening a failing heart it may enable work to be done that could not be so. It may then act like the spur in the side of a horse, eliciting force, though not supplying it.' The researchers coyly concluded that though the experiments recognised the great practical use of alcohol in rousing a failing appetite, exciting a feeble heart, and accelerating a languid capillary circulation,' it would be out of place in the paper to extend their remarks to medical practice, except to succumb to to the temptation of saying that doctors should exercise moderation and caution in prescribing alcohol.[100] The further the research was from the practice of medicine, the more authority it had in its recommendations.

As the end of the 1870s drew near, medical discussion was shifting from the role of alcohol in therapy to an issue we are still arguing about, namely the effect of moderate drinking on health. Two sets of 'evil effects [were recognised as] permanent, and ... these ... [were] related to diminished nutrition and to excessive stimulation.' It had not been determined 'how much the molecular and fatty degeneration of highly organised tissues, such as muscle, nerve, and secreting cells, are due to overaction.' An editorial writer for *Lancet* thought it not improbable that 'part at least ... [was] consequent upon deranged glycogenesis, due to frequent irregular stimulation of the liver, though, perhaps, more to direct action upon the tissues themselves.' (Claude Bernard had discovered in 1848 that the liver releases glucose and, in 1857, that it also forms glycogen, the 'animal starch.' By the time his *Leçons sur le diabète et la glycogenèse animale* appeared in 1877, medical speculation on the therapeutic implications of liver processes was becoming common though the knowledge remained necessarily difficult to apply in treating patients.[101]) Stimulation was still a popular concept in medical explanation of disease but had become more specific in etiology than before. 'Excessive stimulation ... appears to be the chief agent in the production of sclerotic changes though how far this ... is aided by vaso-motor paralysis ... is uncertain.' Moderate consumption, however, was still viewed by *Lancet* as safe and even beneficial. It was seen as fallacious to argue that the degeneration of tissue caused by an excessive amount of alcohol would also be produced by a moderate amount over a long period. The argument that moderate consumption produces a slow decay of organs assumes that the body is 'only a machine, forgetting that it ... is a machine ... constantly renewing itself. Such mechanical and chemical pathology loses sight of one of the most essential factors in animal life.'[102]

Doctors were coming to have a keen analytical understanding of the complex action of alcohol on the organism. One should say alcohols. *Lancet* had proclaimed in 1864 that 'the modern Prometheus ... is the organic chemist.'[103] Although doctors had not yet learned enough about alcohols to talk like chemists, Sir Benjamin Ward Richardson (1826-96), in a lecture to the Hunterian Society in April 1878, referred to the 'heavier alcohols, the butylic and amylic.'[104] He noted their distinct effect of causing a 'tremor of the muscles, a condition resembling delirium tremens, which condition seems to be peculiar to their action, and to separate them from the methylic and ethylic alcohols and from ether in respect to physiological action.'[105]

Richardson thought it important for the doctor who administers alcohol to keep in mind the four stages or degrees of its action. In the first stage vascular and nervous excitement is prominent; in the second 'there is some slight failure of power, muscular, nervous, and mental;' in the third 'there is great failure of these powers, with reduction of temperature;' in the fourth stage, 'there is complete narcosis, with great reduction of temperature.' Richardson believed that it had been shown 'on a sufficiently large scale to admit of a fair argument, that disease, using the term in its widest sense, can be treated without the use of alcohol.' But he also recognised that alcohol could retain its place in the physician's arsenal along with drugs such as opium and chloral but only 'if he knows how to use it properly – if, that is to say, its true physiological action and its true therapeutical application be understood.' Alcohol did not mean wine, beer, stout, or spirits; it meant pure alcohol, which Richardson tested for three years in his medical practice, prescribing it 'as he would any other remedial agent.' Thus 'alcohol comes ... into its true therapeutical position ... [as] an antispasmodic ... a paralyzer of organic muscular fibre ... [and] beyond the first stage of its action ... a reducer of animal temperature.'[106]

Alcohol was no longer needed 'to induce the third or fourth degree of narcotism' in order to make operations painless. Better relaxants of muscle fibre existed to reduce a dislocation or to produce relaxation 'in instances of spasm, such as asthma, colic, tetanus, or angina pectoris': for example, chloroform, ether, and nitrite of amyl.[107] Alcohol, 'administered in its purest form,' could 'serve now and then as an adjuvant.' Nor was alcohol acceptable any longer as a febrifuge. Reducing fever by making a sick person drunk was now believed to accelerate the motion of the heart, induce delirium, trouble the digestion, and, as an after-effect, produce depression. No defender of alcohol invented the palatable category of side-effects for these results.

In the end Richardson found that there remained a few situations in which alcohol still stood out as a remedy. First, in certain kinds of heart trouble, such as weakness, irregularity – perhaps we would refer to arrhythmias, 'fatty change of the structure,' and 'granular degeneration, ... the skilful administration of alcohol' could sometimes be of benefit if the effect of the remedy remained in the first stage of vascular and nervous excitement. The alcohol had still to be 'combined with some other antispasmodic, – usually with nitrite of amyl, which in doses of two to five minims in half a fluid ounce of alcohol,' made 'an excellent combination.' In the emergency treatment of 'resistance to the passage of the blood' in cases of shock – we might say vasospasm or coronary vasoconstriction, Richardson admitted that 'alcohol stands out as a remedy.' It was not recognised so useful, however, in treating a sudden haemorrhaging. True, alcohol enabled 'the feeble heart to recommence work,' but as 'a relaxer of vascular tension,' it opened 'the way to secondary loss of blood' in the vessels and presented therefore 'a danger beyond its advantage.'[108]

Even in its justification of the moderate use of alcohol in treating some acute diseases, *Lancet* increasingly found itself in a defensive position, as was made clear in a report early in 1877 that the medical staff of the Dorset County Hospital had decided, whenever possible, to do without alcoholic stimulants as medicine. The annual wine and spirits bill was reduced from £143 to £43. *Lancet* defended alcohol as a medicine and as a food, though the second claim was becoming increasingly difficult to uphold. What worried *Lancet* was that the growing movement in favour of non-alcoholic treatment in large towns – London even had a 'so-called Temperance Hospital' – would spread to the treatment of acute diseases and therefore double mortality in such cases. The reasoning was that 'the results in a provincial hospital, such as that at Dorchester, cannot be applied to hospitals in large towns.' *Lancet* accepted as axiomatic the existence of a clear rural-urban difference. 'It is the common conclusion of those who have had opportunities of comparing the treatment of the sick in rural districts and in London, that the sick poor in the country neither need nor bear the amount of stimulation which in London is indispensable in the treatment of severe acute diseases.'[109]

We may find this urban-rural division a strange idea, and so did some contemporary doctors. Norman Kerr thought that a nearly non-alcoholic medicine would reduce mortality. His 'not inconsiderable experience in the treatment of the sick poor both in city and country practice' had led him to conclude that excluding alcohol from ordinary practice would considerably reduce mortality in 'severe acute diseases from what it was 'under the alcoholic *régime*.' Kerr believed that the Dorset Country Hospital should have been commended for 'reducing the cost of intoxicating liquors ... with no detriment to the sick.' No doctor should forget that 'alcohol is a powerful drug, and ought to be administered with as great caution as any other poisonous remedy.'[110]

Alcohol no longer played a major role in the therapeutic discourse of medicine. It was not yet reduced to a few lines in medical books but the mighty remedy had fallen rapidly from its perch of therapeutic domination.[111] In *Lancet* of the 1880s it was difficult to find anyone willing to risk a defence of the alcohol treatment. Typical articles dealt with doubts and dangers. In a paper on the transformation of alcohol and on the formation of alcohol and urea in the living body, given in 1882 to the Cambridge Philosophical Society, Latham observed that no one had been 'able to detect the ordinary products of the oxidation of ethylic alcohol in the body.' The question was what became of it? And was it food, physic, or poison?[112] The medical view seemed to have shifted heavily in the direction of seeing alcohol chiefly as a sometimes useful poison.

Even if a doctor accepted the therapeutic value of alcohol, he could not automatically use it in appropriate situations. It was argued, for example, that there is a danger in giving eight ounces of alcohol to a hospital patient who is an abstainer. The patient could die as a result of the shock to his system, unhabituated to any alcohol, let alone the large amount given in some standard treatments. With other remedies available, some doctors thought it unwise to take an additional risk in treating patients.

Although they hardly needed heavier artillery, the anti-alcohol doctors had their fire-power considerably increased in 1883 by a report of the Harveian Society on 'the mortality referable to alcohol.' *Lancet* presented the report as 'a very serious indictment ... against alcohol.' After examining 10,000 cases of death, a committee of the Harveian Society found a much higher death rate 'among intemperate persons' than 'that generally prevailing among adults.' In diseases of the liver and chylopoietic viscera the death rate was four times higher. But with the exception of pneumonia and pleurisy, lung diseases carried off 'a smaller proportion of persons given to excess in alcohol than of the general population.' The explanation of this anomaly was a further indictment of alcohol: liver, kidney, and brain diseases killed the heavy drinkers before diseases such as phthisis and bronchitis could. It was just a 'displacement of the mortality from the more common [respiratory] diseases,' which accounted for thirty five per cent of the whole adult mortality. It seemed that 'much of the suspicion with which alcohol' was by then 'regarded by the intelligent classes' was 'due to medical teaching and ... medical example.'[113] And *Lancet* might have added that this suspicion also reflected a reversal of medical opinion in one generation.

It could be debated whether this shift in therapies was the result of internal changes in medicine itself or the result of external events. But such a debate would probably be as unenlightening as a similar one was in the history of science. An explanation of the shift in therapies was given in 1889 by an army doctor, A. G. Bartley. Here is his account of this change of paradigms, as we used to say in Kuhnian times.

> In the 1860s it was common to treat delirium tremens ('alcoholic poisoning') by giving stimulants and opium. It is no longer the case. I always avoided the use of alcohol in my medical practice. Aitken's *Practice of Physic*, which was and still is the chief authority in the medical service, forbids alcohol and prescribes food in all possible ways.[114] We now see an unmistakable diminution of the consumption of alcoholic liquors in hospitals. This is probably due in great measure to the greater temperance of the general community – a change in fashion rather than a reform of practise. It was said long ago that the evils wrought by a theory have never in history discredited the theory; and certainly this would seem to be true in the practise of medicine. The melancholy history of the use of calomel [mercurous chloride used as a purgative] and opium in India is a saddening illustration. A few men here and there question the theory, and gain adherents chiefly among the young. The older men are not so much converted. They die out, and by-and-by the world awakes and exclaims how foolish the last generation was.[115]

Notes

1. On the topic of alcohol in medicine there is a remarkable article by Louis-Félix-Jules Béhier, 'Alcool (thérapeutique)' in the *Dictionnaire encyclopédique des sciences médicales*, vol. ii (Paris: P. Asselin, 1865), 592–611. See also H. Triboulet et Félix Mathieu, *L'alcool et*

l'alcoolisme (Carré et Naud, 1900). For the history of American use of alcohol and wine up to 1860, see Sarah E. Williams, 'The Use of Beverage Alcohol as Medicine, 1790-1860,' *Journal of Studies on Alcohol*, 41 (1980), 543–566.

2. The *Journal de la santé du roi Louis XIV de l'année 1647 à l'année 1711*, written by Vallot, d'Aquin and Fagon (1862), 401. Various concoctions prepared for the king's ills are listed on 416–30. E.g., vin de quinqina, pour le roi, 1686 (d'Aquin): écorce de racines de quina pulvérisée; faites infuser dans le vin de Bourgogne.
3. Triboulet et Mathieu, *op. cit.* (note 1), 3.
4. Sources for this information on the history of the chemistry are *La grande encyclopédie*, ii, 34–52; Satish C. Kapoor, 'Dumas,' in C.C. Gillispie (ed), *Dictionary of Scientific Biography* – hereinafter *DSB* (New York: Scribner, 1970-80), iv, 242–8; and M. P. Crosland, 'Berthelot,' *DSB*, ii: 63–72.
5. Clifford A. Hampel and Gessner G. Hawley, *The Encylopedia of Chemistry* (New York: Van Nostrand, 1973, 3d edn), 1580, point out that 'the term 'glycerol' is generally used for the pure chemical compound, whereas glycerine (or glycerin) commonly refers to commercial materials of whatever grade or purity. All three names are often used without distinction.' Nitroglycerine (glycerol trinitrate) is an ester of great medical importance, used in the treatment of angina pectoris; like amyl nitrite, it is a smooth muscle relaxant and peripheral vasodilator.
6. Louis Hébert, *Des alcools employés en médecine* (3d edn, Paris: F. Savy, 1863), 61–4.
7. Jean-François-Napoléon Dougnac, *Le vin au points de vue physico-chimique, physiologique, hygiénique et thérapeutique* (Bordeaux: Delmas, 1933; 2d edn, 1935), 275, and Bréhier, *op. cit.* (note 1), 595. Béhier reports on the success of Chapelle in Angoulême in treating fourteen cases of anal fissure by brushing the lesion with a mixture of fifty grams of alcohol with ten grams of chloroform; Dr. Tournié got similar results with six cures reported; so Trousseau's lack of success with one case at the Hôtel-Dieu looked like an anomaly.
8. A. Trousseau and H. Pidoux, *Traité de thérapeutique et de matière médicale,* vol. ii (1836), 801, and Béhier, *op. cit.* (note 1), 597.
9. Béhier, *loc. cit* (note 1), 598, and *L'Union médicale,* vii (1860), 566.
10. John Brown, *The Elements of Medicine* (2 vols., London, 3d edn, 1795; translated into French in 1805); John Thomas Ingleby, *A Practical Treatise on Uterine Hemorrhage in connection with pregnancy and parturition* (London: Longman, 1832); Robert Bentley Todd: *The Cyclopaedia of Anatomy and Physiology* (5 vols., London:

Longman, 1836-52); *Clinical Lectures on Certain Acute Diseases* (London: Churchill, 1860). Some French sources point out that well before the advent of Todd's alcoholic therapy, Louis, Laennec, and Chomel in France used alcohol in treating diseases. Bréhier, 'Alcool,' 598, refers specifically to the English influence (including Ingleby's work) on the internal use of alcohol in controlling hemorraghing.

11. On Broussais (1772-1838) see Pierre Huard's article in DSB, vol. ii, 507-09; Jean Héritier, *Le sève de l'homme de l'âge d'or de la saignée aux débuts de l'hématologie* (Paris: Denoël, 1987), 91; and Jean-François Braunstein, *Broussais et le matérialisme* (1988).
12. Trousseau and Pidoux, *Traite thérapeutique et de matière médicale* vol. i. Trousseau was then an Agrégé à la faculté de médecine de Paris and Pidoux a Professeur particulier de thérapeutique. Constantin Paul was added as a collaborator for the 9th edn.
13. Dougnac, *op. cit.* (note 7), 240-1.
14. *Bulletin de l'organisation internationale du vin* (hereinafter *BIV*), no. 75 (août 1934), 99, citing as its source *Je sais tout* for July. Until the recent use of fomepizole (sold under the brand name Antizol), the standard medical treatment for ethyl glycol poisoning was to get the patient drunk. 'Antidote for pretty poison is found but at big price,' *The New York Times*, (23 March 1999), D6, reporting on an article in *The New England Journal of Medicine*, also of 18 March 1999.
15. For a description of death by cholera, see Roy Porter, *The Greatest Benefit to Mankind. A Medical History of Humanity* (New York: HarperCollins, 1997), 403. Cholera is 'an epidemic diarrhoeal disease characterized by devasting intestinal loss of fluid and electrolytes, the replacement of which constitutes the vital element of treatment.' The '*Vibrio cholerae* or comma bacillus elaborates an enterotoxin which promotes the secretion of electrolytes in the bowel lumen.' See John Walton and others (eds), *The Oxford Medical Companion* – hereinafter OMC (Oxford: Oxford University Press, 1994), 136–7.
16. In 1849 nearly 20,000 died from cholera in Paris. See Catherine J. Kudlick, *Cholera in Post-Revolutionary Paris. A Cultural History* (Berkeley, CA: University of California Press, 1996), 1–2. Dr. B. Lunel, *Vade-mecum des pharmaciens* (2d edn, Paris: L'auteur, 1864), 97, cites the following governmental figures for cholera deaths in France: 1832 – 102,735; 1849 – 110,110; 1854 – 145,531.
17. M. F. Magendie, *Leçons sur le choléra-morbus faites au Collège de France* (Paris: Méquignon-Marvis, 1832).
18. W. F. Bynum, *Science and the Practice of Medicine in the Nineteenth Century* (Cambridge: Cambridge University Press, 1994), 79.

19. *Lancet* (Feb. 11, 1865), 153.
20. John Harley Warner, 'Physiological theory and therapeutic explanation in the 1860s: The British debate on the medical use of alcohol,' *Bulletin of the History of Medicine*, 54 (1980), 236.
21. *Ibid.*, 236–7, note 4.
22. *Ibid.*, 235.
23. *Ibid.*, 235–6, 256–7.
24. *Ibid.*, 256; see also note 85.
25. Prosper Despine, *Le démon alcool. Ses effets désastreux sur le moral, sur l'intelligence et sur le physique. Moyens d'y porter remède* (Paris: F. Savy, 1871), a salvo of forty seven pages. Between 1858 and 1871 the number of outlets for alcohol (cafés, *débits de liqueurs* and *débits de vins*) in Marseille increased from 647 to 1585.
26. Angel Marvaud, *L'alcool. Son action physiologique, son utilité et ses applications en hygiène et en thérapeutique* (Paris: V. Rozier, 1872), a volume in the Librairie de la médecine, de la chirurgie et de la pharmacie militaire.
27. MM. les docteurs Dujardin-Beaumetz (médecin des hôpitaux) et Audigé (lauréat de la faculté de médecine), *Recherches expérimentales sur les alcools par fermentation*, extract of the *Bulletins et Mémoires de la Société de Thérapeutique* (1875).
28. Les docteurs Dujardin-Beaumetz (médecin de l'Hôpital Saint-Antoine) et Audigé, *Recherches expérimentales sur la puissance toxique des alcools* (Paris: E. Donnaud, 1879).
29. 'The alcoholic treatment of disease,' *Lancet* (11 Feb. 1865), 153. Todd (1809-1860) was appointed in 1836 to the new chair of physiology and general morbid anatomy in King's College. See entry on Robert Bentley Todd in the *Dictionary of National Biography*, (Oxford: Oxford University Press, 1971) lvi, 433.
30. Warner, *loc. cit.* (note 20), 241. Warner points out how Todd's theory of alcoholic action 'drew heavily on the principles of nutritional physiology' of Justus Liebig.
31. W. T. Gairdner, M.D. (physician to the Royal Infirmary, and professor of practice of physic in the University, Glasgow), 'Facts and conclusions as to the use of alcoholic stimulants in typhus fever,' *Lancet* (1864), 291.
32. Warner, *loc. cit.* (note 20), 244.
33. 'In 1790, 'fever' was a common diagnostic tag, accounting for almost a quarter of the mortality between 1774 and 1793 in some London parishes.' Bynum, *op. cit.* (note 18), 21–22.
34. Gairdner, *Lancet* (1864), 291.
35. Jack D. Ellis, *The physician-legislators of France. Medicine and politics*

in the early Third Republic, 1870-1914 (Cambridge: Cambridge University Press, 1990), 192.

36. 'Todd,' *Dictionary of National Biography*, op. cit. (note 29), lvi, 433, and Paul Gingeot, *Essai sur l'emploi thérapeutique de l'alcool chez les enfants et, en général, sur le rôle de cet agent dans le traitement des maladies aiguës fébriles* (Paris: A. Delahaye, 1867), 13.
37. *Lancet* (1864), 358.
38. Edward Smith, M.D., LL.B., F.R.S., 'On the mode of action of alcohol in the treatment of disease,' *Lancet* (1861), 212; Béhier, *op. cit.* (note 1), 578–83; Warner, *loc. cit.* (note 20), 242, note 23; Bouchardat and Sandras, 'De la digestion des boissons alcooliques et de leur rôle dans la nutrition,' *Archives générales de médecine* (1846), supplément, 233–44.
39. L. Lallemand, M. Perrin et J.-L.-P. Duroy, *Du rôle de l'alcool et des anesthésiques dans l'organisme. Recherches expérimentales,* (Paris: F. Chamerot, 1860), an expanded version of their article in *Union médicale* in 1859. See Warner, *loc. cit.* (note 20), 245, note 32. For an account of the experiments refuting the 'total elimination theory' and counter-experiments, see Warner, *loc cit.*, 250–3. Edmond Baudot's article 'De l'alcool; de sa destruction dans l'organisme' in the *Union médicale* in 1863 noted that the trio's method, using Masing's reagent, was totally unsuited to that kind of research. With another method, using the alcoholometer, Baudot found that twenty out of twenty two times alcohol was not eliminated by the kidneys. Baudot, 'De l'alcool, de sa destruction dans l'organisme,' *Union médicale,* 2nd series, xx (1863), 273, 357, 374, 390; xxi (1864), 40. On Massing's method, see Warner, *loc. cit.*, 245, note 33.
40. Béhier, *op. cit.* (note 1), 584.
41. Maurice Perrin (1826-89), a military doctor known in surgery and opthalmology, became director of the Ecole du Val-de-Grâce and president of the academy of medicine.
42. Edward Smith, *Lancet* (1861), 212.
43. Smith, *Lancet* (1861), 80, 212, and Warner, *loc. cit.* (note 20), 244–9.
44. Smith, *Lancet* (1861), 134.
45. *Ibid.*, 134, 213.
46. *Lancet* (1864), 357-8. The saying is quoted in the issue of June 25, 1864, 731.
47. W. T. Gairdner, M.D., 'Alcoholic stimulants in typhus fever,' *Lancet* (1864), 291–4; editorial commentary, 357–8.
48. *Lancet* (1864), 357–8.
49. Gairdner, *loc. cit.* (note 47), 291.

50. *Lancet*, (1864), 358.
51. Gairdner, *loc. cit.* (note 47), 294.
52. Bynum, *op. cit.* (note 18), 76. *Lancet* (Nov. 16, 1867), 608–09, says that the death rate in typhus cases was calculated at 1/10. During the period 1862-66 in Liverpool of the 7669 people who died of typus 7143 were classified as the 'weekly-wage class.'
53. Gingeot, *op. cit.* (note 36), 13.
54. Letter from Hugh Norris, printed under the heading of 'therapeutic alcoholism' in *Lancet* (May 4, 1878), 186. Nancy Mitford, in *The Pursuit of Love* (1945), 225–6, recounts her 'uncle's lapses into insobriety,' which 'had no vice about them; they were purely therapeutic. The fact is he was following a new régime for perfect health, much in vogue at that time, he assured us, on the Continent.'
55. Charles Murchison, *A Treatise of the Continued Fevers of Great Britain* (London: Parker and Brown, 1862; 3d edn, 1884; German translation in 1867; a French translation of part I appeared in 1878); *On the Causes of Continued Fevers* (Reprinted from the *London Medical Review,* 1863). He had traced the origin of an epidemic of this fever to a milk supply in 1873. His work dealing with cases of gastric-colic fistula appeared in the *Edinburgh Medical Journal* in 1857. Charles Murchison was the son of Alexander Murchison, M.D.; a graduate of Edinburgh, he spent time in Turin, Dublin, Paris, and Calcutta before pursuing his brilliant career at King's College Hospital, the London Fever Hospital, and, after 1871, at St Thomas's Hospital.
56. 'Guy's Hospital. Twelve cases of typhus and typhoid fever treated without stimulants; clinical remarks (under the care of Dr. Wilks),' *Lancet* (Jan. 28, 1865), 90-92, under the general heading of 'A mirror of the practice of medicine and surgery in the hospitals of London.'
57. 'The Alcoholic Treatment of Disease,' *Lancet* (Feb. 11, 1865), 153–54.
58. A. S. Blumgarten, *Textbook of Materia Medica* (New York: Macmillan, 1927, 4th edn.), 132–3.
59. 'Guy's Hospital. Twelve cases of typhus and typhoid fever,' *Lancet* (Jan. 28, 1865), 90–92.
60. See *Encyclopaedia Britannica,* 22 (Chicago: 1943), 650. The references in the article on typhus fever are from the 1920s.
61. Samuel Wilks, letter to *Lancet* (Jan. 8, 1995), 61.
62. Bennett's *The Restorative Treatment of Pneumonia* was in its 3d edn by 1866 (Edinburgh: A. & C. Black). His lectures on clinical

medicine - the title was changed to *Clinical Lectures* in the 5th edn in 1868 - was translated into French: *Leçons cliniques sur les principes et la pratique de la médecine* (2 vols., 1873). Bennett had spent two years in Paris and two more in German medical centers.

63. Samuel Wilks, 'On the Indiscriminate Use of Alcoholic Stimulants in Disease,' *Lancet* (April 27, 1867), 505-07.
64. Gingeot, *op. cit.* (note 36), 25-26.
65. Cod liver oil was a European medical subject, though Maurice Perrin's medical thesis *Sur les effets de l'huile de foie de morue dans la phtisie pulmonaire* (1851) appeared ten years after Bennett's work.
66. *Lancet* (1875), 534. Bennett wrote the article on physiology in the 8th edn of the *Encylopaedia Britannica.* His treatise on *Cod-Liver Oil as a Therapeutic Agent in certain forms of Gout, Rheumatism, and Scrofula* appeared in 1841.
67. J. Hughes Bennett, M.D., F.R.S.E., 'Further observations on the restorative treatment of pneumonia,' *Lancet* (Feb. 3, 1866), 114–116.
68. *Lancet* (Feb. 11, 1865), 153.
69. See Bynum, *op. cit.* (note 18), 10, and Erwin H. Ackerknecht, *A Short History of Medicine* (Baltimore: The John Hopkins University Press, 1967), rev. edn. 1982, 123; the quotation is from Ackerknecht.
70. *Lancet* (Feb. 11, 1865), 153.
71. Samuel Wilks, 'On the indiscriminate Use of Alcoholic Stimulants,' *Lancet* (April 27, 1867), 505.
72. 'The alcoholic treatment of disease,' *Lancet* (Feb. 11, 1865), 153.
73. Gingeot, *op. cit.* (note 36), 8–9.
74. 'Louis-Jules Béhier, 1813-1876,' *La grande encyclopédie*, v, 1162-3. He seems to have been more notorious for beginning the unpopular treatment with cold water in cases of typhoid fever. In 1874 he did a blood transfusion that worked.
75. Gingeot, *op. cit.* (note 36), 31. In his 'Conférences cliniques à la Pitié' (1861-2), Béhier expressed his agreement with the conclusions of Todd's *Clinical Lectures on Certain Acute Diseases* (London: Churchill, 1860).
76. See Françoise Huguet, *Les professeurs de la Faculté de médecine de Paris - Dictionnaire biographique 1794-1939* (Paris: Editions du C.N.R.S., 1991), who quotes Jacques Léonard on Béhier's skill with the needle; and Georges Daremberg, *Les grands médecins du XIXe siècle* (Paris: Masson, 1907), 161–8. Daremberg notes with approval Béhier's fight against the 'habitudes germaniques' that transform the doctor into a naturalist while making him forget that he is a healer.

77. Gingeot, *op. cit.* (note 36), 138–9.
78. 'The alcoholic treatment of disease,' *Lancet* (Feb. 11, 1865), 153.
79. Wilks, 'On the Indiscriminate Use of Alcoholic Stimulants,' *Lancet* (April 27, 1867), 506.
80. *Lancet* (May 18, 1867), 606.
81. *Lancet* (Oct. 19, 1867), 502. Barnes, obstetric physician to London hospitals, has been resurrected by Ann Dally in *Women Under the Knife: A History of Surgery* (London: Hutchinson Radius, 1991), 88–90, for 'one of the weirdest series of lectures ever delivered to a medical audience,' in this case the Royal College of Physicians, on 'The convulsive diseases of women.'
82. This term was coined by William Farr 'to describe diseases ... caused by a process analogous to fermentation.' Bynum, *op. cit.* (note 18), 76. See Dr. Christison, 'The Ætiology of Zymotic Diseases,' a presidential address to the Sanitary Section of the Social Science Congress, published in *Lancet* (1862), 471–6, 501–3. Christison was the first physician to preside over the public health section of the association.
83. Mordey Douglas, letter to *Lancet* (Oct. 26, 1867), 535.
84. *Ibid.*
85. Francis E. Anstie (M.D., F.R.C.P., senior assistant-physician to Westminster hospital), 'On the Theory of Alcoholic Stimulation in Pyrexial Diseases,' *Lancet* (Jan. 25, 1868), 120.
86. Warner, *loc. cit.* (note 20), 253–6.
87. Barnes, letter to *Lancet* (Oct. 19, 1867), 502.
88. Azote is the former name of nitrogen. The French have switched from *nitrogène* to *azote.* It is an essential element of proteins and nucleic acids in living organisms.
89. Mordey Douglas, letter to *Lancet* (Oct. 26, 1867), 535.
90. Quotation is from Stephen F. Mason, *A History of the Sciences* (New York: Collier Books, 1962), 310.
91. The term 'antiphlogistic treatment' hung around long after Lavoisier had made it unnecessary. In Broussais's doctrine, 'Inflammation being the consequence of excessive stimulation, it followed that depletive or antiphlogistic remedies were required' – e.g., bleeding. Bynum, *op. cit.* (note 18), 45. On Bichat's comparison between himself and Lavoisier, see Michel Foucault, *The Birth of the Clinic. An Archaelology of Medical Perception* (1963; New York: Vintage Books, 1975), 131.
92. Mordey Douglas, letter to *Lancet* (Oct 26, 1867), 535.
93. 'The prospects of the profession,' *Lancet* (January 1, 1870), 14–15.
94. *Ibid.*, 14–15.

95. *Ibid.*, 14.
96. *Ibid.*, 15.
97. 'A mirror of hospital practice, British and foreign,' *Lancet* (June 19, 1875), 856–57. The notes for the case were provided by Mr. Garlick, house-physician, University College hospital.
98. *Experiments on the Effects of Alcohol (Ethyl Alcohol) on the Human Body* by E. A. Parkes, M.D., F.R.S., professor of hygiene in the Army Medical School, and Count Cyprian Wollowicz, M.D., assistant-surgeon, army medical staff. (Reprinted from the Proceedings of the Royal Society, 1870.) See *Lancet* (Aug. 13, 1870), 217. According to Sarah E. Williams, *loc. cit.* (note 1), 543–66, the index catalog of the surgeon-general's office, United States army, shows an active publishing industry at work on 'alcohol as a remedy' from the 1860s to the end of the century.
90. 'Recent researches on the action of alcohol,' *Lancet* (Aug. 20, 1870), 265–66.
100. *Lancet* (Aug. 13, 1870), 217. The last point ignores Douglas's odd argument that the capillaries were ruled not by the heart but by the *vis a fronte*. Editorial commentary could not accept the arguments of Parkes and Wollowicz that alcohol did not supply an 'extra force' for 'organic motor life' and that it 'cannot reduce fever-heat.' See *Lancet* (Aug. 20, 1870), 265–66.
101. Joseph Fruton, *A Skeptical Biochemist* (Cambridge, Mass.: Harvard University Press, 1992), 71; *Comptes rendus des séances de la société de biologie*, viii (1856), 30.
102. 'The Uses of Alcohol,' *Lancet* (Dec. 22, 1877), 929.
103. *Lancet* (1864), 417, quoting Wanklyn's brief history, given in a lecture at the Royal Institution. Among the heroes were Wöhler, Pelouze, Kolbe, Wurtz, Perkin, and Duppa.
104. 'Dr. Richardson on abstinence from alcohol in health and disease,' *Lancet* (May 4, 1878), 660.
105. *Ibid.*
106. *Ibid.*
107. A decade later nitroglycerine was being touted as a replacement for alcohol in treating angina pectoris, nausea, spasmodic asthma, opium poisoning, uraemic coma, acute alcoholism, nephritis, death-bed cases, and drowning. See Joseph B. Burroughs, M.D., 'Nitro-glycerine – A Substitute for Alcohol in cases of Emergency,' *Lancet* (June 22 and 29, 1889), 1238–39 and 1297–98.
108. *Ibid.* (May 4, 1878), 661.
109. 'Alcohol in Hospitals,' *Lancet* (Jan. 20, 1877), 102.
110. Letter from Norman Kerr, M.D., on 'The Use of Alcohol in Medical

Practice,' *Lancet* (Jan. 27, 1877), 153. For an early American version of this quarrel over the therapeutic use of alcohol, pitting the economic and moral authority of hospital trustees against the medical authority of the doctor, see Charles E. Rosenberg, *The Care of Strangers - The Rise of America's Hospital System* (New York: Basic Books, 1987), 54–55.

111. OMC has a brief but significant entry for alcohol (ethanol or ethyl alcohol or spirits of wine). 'Ethanol (C_2H_5OH) – many applications in medicine: e.g. as a solvent, antiseptic, and tincture. The pharmacological effects of alcohol itself, chiefly central nervous system depression and peripheral vasodilation, occasionally find legitimate application in therapeutics.'

112. *Lancet* (April 15, 1882), 610–11.

113. *Lancet* (March 3, 1883), 371–72; see the issue of March 24, 1883, 520, for a letter from Dr. T. Morton correcting *Lancet*'s analysis of the report in the matter of lung diseases.

114. George A. Aiken, *The Elements of the Theory and Practise of Physic and Surgery* (London: Dilly, 1783, 2 vols). He also wrote *The Principles of Midwifery or Puerperal Medicine* (Edinburgh, 1784; 3rd edn. 1786). *The Elements* (vol. i, 51, 53) listed wine and ales as nurtrients and antimonal wine as an emetic. According to *The Principles*, relief from the symptoms of amenorrhoea can be obtained from dietetics, wine, peruvian bark, etc. Wine is one of the antihysterics listed for treating chronic hysteria.

115. On doctors and the British temperance movement see Warner, "Physiological theory and therapeutic explanation," 237–9, and Risse, "Brunonian therapeutics," in W. F. Bynum and Roy Porter (eds), *Brunonianism in Britain and Europe* (London: Wellcome Institute for the History of Medicine, 1988), 52, and especially Joanne Woiak, 'A Medical Cromwell to Depose King Alcohol: Medical Scientists, Temperance Reformers, and the Alcohol Problem in Britain,' in Jack S. Blocker Jr. and Cheryl Krasnick Warsh (eds), *The Changing Face of Drink: Substance, Imagery, and Behaviour* (Ottawa: Social History Inc., 1997), 237–70.

4

French and British Wine Therapies

Medicine throws off a fair number of aphorisms, mostly lugubrious. According to an early-nineteenth century sally on comparative medical treatment, the British killed their patients and the French let them die.[1] In contemporary opinion, the famous Paris clinical school, with its twin *idées fixes* of diagnosis and pathology, was not an exception to the rule; indeed, its enthusiasm for experimentation turned some patients into expendable laboratory animals.[2] Therapeutics was the Achilles' heel of medicine, though there were competitors from other medical areas for this distinction. More interested in diseases than in patients, the Paris school came to place an emphasis on 'specific remedies and routine procedures.'[3] (In George Eliot's *Middlemarch*, published in 1872 but set in a period forty years earlier, one of Mr. Lydgate's medical virtues was his training in Paris.) Perhaps the old system had to be destroyed before a new one came into existence; according to Bichat, the old nosology of *materia medica* had to be replaced by a functional knowledge of drugs. The danger, as Ackerknecht makes whiggishly clear, was that new 'rubbish' would replace the old, as in the case of Alibert's *Elements of Therapeutics* (1804). Since by 1826 Alibert's work was in its fifth edition, it is obvious that in this manual he was speaking the 'rational discourse' of the medical community of the day, even if we classify it as nonsense.[4] In the early-nineteenth century medical renaissance one of the results of the new criticism of excessive drug prescription in the British manner was the revival of the more catholic therapeutics of antiquity, with drugs becoming, 'as with Hippocrates and Galen, only one weapon in the therapeutic armamentarium.' Some of the old dogmas and practices remained in vogue. And following Ackerknecht, we may note that novelty brought a renewed interest in the old ideas of preventive medicine, including the use of food as medicine.

The scepticism of the Paris doctors about the scientific foundations of therapeutic knowledge and the curative power of drugs led to a sort of return to 'the belief in the *vis medicatrix naturae*.'[5]

Falling back on the healing power of nature probably indicates that the Paris doctors had enough confidence in their new medicine to indulge in the ancient rhetoric that less well-armed doctors of the eighteenth century felt obliged to reject. The belief in nature also established a safe position in case the disease triumphed over the doctor (and the patient). Nor was the physician likely to become obsolete. In a defence of an old novelty, a doctrine called modern Hippocratic vitalism, A.-L.-J. Bayle defended the idea that in most cases nature cures the patient, who needs only surveillance or support to re-establish his body's equilibrium. The essential and elusive vital force could not be accused of infallibility in its healing processes: sometimes it let the patient die because it did not react to the disease, sometimes it killed the patient by over-reaction, and in other circumstances it reacted too weakly or in a disorganised way. The role of the doctor in treating diseases was thus indispensable, whatever his discourse might have been about the healing power of nature.

In any case, medicine was given a new injection of confidence by chemistry early in the nineteenth century. An 'experimental pharmacology' made a formidable list of drugs available in a pure state, thus making both treatment and experimentation – the two can be easily combined – possible on a scientific basis or at least an impressively quantitative basis.The holy writ of the new therapy was François Magendie's *Formulary for the Preparation and Employment of several new Remedies*, published in 1821 and already in a sixth edition by 1827; it was published in English in 1828. The most significant change in therapeutics came from a new area of scientific work, alkaloid chemistry. The opium poppy, the coca shrub, and the tobacco plant have supplied some of our most popular modern alkaloids, important items of our *materia medica* as well as our *Genussmittel.* When F. W. Sertürner prepared several salts of morphine in 1805 showing that the alkaloid is 'the principle responsible for the physiological effect of opium,' he opened up a flood of drugs whose use transformed the clinic into a place where a patient had as much of a chance of being cured as given an autopsy.[6]

Among the medically important alkaloids discovered between 1820 and 1850 were quinine and cinchonine, atropine, colchicine, codeine, and strychnine. The English translation of Magendie's *Formulary* dealt with over two dozen often powerful and even deadly drugs. Acknerknecht notes that these new remedies were 'added to or replaced the old traditional plant and mineral products.'[7] Wine, especially in its role of excipient in medicinal wines, was a survivor in this therapeutic revolution. Under the heading of 'alkalis obtained from cinchona bark,' Magendie's book listed, e.g., quinine wine: 'twelve grains of sulphate of quinine in one litre of good Madeira – Malaga or almost any wine may be used.' With 164 medicinal wines in the 'Parisian pharmacopoeia,' it seemed that the role of wine in medicine was saved. Indeed, the nineteenth century has been hailed as the great period of medicinal wines. The Lyonnais surgeon Villard, giving more credit than surgeons usually give to helpers, nicely summed up one of the important functions of medicinal wine: 'the scalpel begins the cure, the *vin Mariani* finishes it.'[8]

The basic reference work in the pharmacist's library is the *Codex*, which, as *The Oxford Medical Companion* points out, used to be 'a collection of recipes for the preparation of medicines,' a usage still hinted at in titles like *Pharmaceutical Codex* (British). It used to be the guide of the pharmacist for the preparation of all the official medicaments that he always had to have at the disposal of the doctor. Many of these items – tisanes, potions, pills, for example – required a certain flexibility in preparation in order to accommodate the doctor's therapeutic aim. In the much changed French *Codex*, one of the few continuities was the preparation of medicinal wines or *oenolés*. Let us look at the history of wine in the French *Codex*, which issued from the Revolution, with the first edition appearing in Latin in 1818: *Codex medicamentarius seu Pharmacopae gallica*, transformed into *Codex, pharmacopée française* for the second edition in 1837. New editions, reflecting the latest stage in the marriage of science and the pharmaceutical industry, followed in 1866, 1884, 1908, 1937, and 1965. Before the first national codex there were some codices for the practice of pharmacy in cities such as Paris, Lyon, and Bordeaux. A bitter debate over the value of an emetic wine of antimony as a purgative coloured the early years of the Paris *Codex (1638)*, a creation of the faculty of medicine. Its purgative success in curing Louis XIV of an illness settled the issue in favour of keeping this wine in the *Codex*.[9] The debate was over the chemical substance, not the wine. But most medicinal wines included plant substances, thus escaping from the debate over a growing chemical imperialism in medicine.

The second edition (1837) of the *Codex* justified itself in terms of the need to accommodate the discoveries that had, as the revision commission put it in its scientific *langue de bois*, 'increased the domaine of chemistry and of medicine.' Early codices had described medicaments derived from plants, minerals, and animals and given details on the preparation of chemical products used in pharmacy. This preparation was eventually taken over by industry; by the time of the fifth edition (1908) the function of the pharmacist in this area was reduced to testing the medicaments for purity. These purity tests finally became so complex that only an industrial or a governmental regulatory laboratory could do the job; by 1965 the *Codex* was really a manuel for these laboratories. The descriptions of natural drugs and of the preparations done by pharmacists had disappeared.[10] Six simple and three compound medicinal wines occupied about seven pages of text in the edition of 1837.[11] Wine was lucky to have survived.

The *Codex* of 1866 was the work of a commission of chemists and medical professors, with one botanist from the school of pharmacy thrown in, for 'nature ...continue[d] to furnish new instruments for the art of healing.' The input of chemistry into pharmacy was no longer recognised as the identification of the active therapeutic ingredients in plants but the multiplication of medicaments by means of substitutions for natural substances and the creation of items like chloroform, which had little of their organic origin left. Hoping to establish rules for the doctor to follow in treating patients, modern physiology monitored the precise effect of these medicaments on the body's organs. Five pages or so on medicinal wines seemed to fit into the new pharmaceutical program. A couple of wines were added to the *Codex*, including an iron wine and an emetic wine of Malaga with potassium tartrate and antimony.[12] The medicinal wines of the new *Codex* were more a vehicle for getting various minerals and chemical substances into the body than copies of mom's traditional medicines. Believing in their own future scientific obsolescence, the committee of revision noted that their *Codex* would have the same fate as that of 1837.

In 1884 the *Codex* was reorganised into four parts. The first part included substances drawn from animal and vegetable sources; the second part included products coming from chemical pharmacy; the third part comprised Galenic medicaments; the fourth and new category was veterinary pharmacy, including four medicinal wines. Among the categories of wine listed were ordinary French red and white, about ten per cent alcohol; Lunel (a naturally sweet Muscat wine, one of the *vins doux naturels* from the area between Montpellier and Nîmes) and Grenache (from the sun-loving grape of the same name, used for Gigondas, Tavel, and the naturally sweet wine of Roussillon), about fifteen per cent alcohol. Grenache was adopted as the official wine to replace Malaga, a Spanish fortified wine of about eighteen percent alcohol and fifteen percent residual sugar.[13] Resinous plants or plants whose elements change over time require sweet wines (*vins de liqueur*). Safran, opium, and squill were among the items requiring sweet wines. Wine containing squill was widely used because the bulb of this plant of the lily family was recognised for its cardiotonic, diuretic, and purgative powers. With their high level of alcohol, up to twenty three per cent, medicinal wines were often criticised for causing therapeutic alcoholism. Emile Mauriac, who had seen only one case in his long career, thought that it was rare.[14] Bordeaux's doctors were usually optimistic about any form of wine consumption.

The *Codex* of 1908 collapsed the four categories of 1884 into an alphabetical organisation. Two separate new sections appeared: one for biological products (like those used in serotherapy) and the toxins and vaccines of microbial origin, and another section for veterinary medicaments. Many of the older chemical medicaments, Galenic preparations, and drugs were dropped. Theriac was finally 'relegated to legend.' Wines were now listed in simplified fashion, with their bases given as red and white wines of ten per cent alcohol, muscat wine of thirteen to fifteen per cent, and the more alcoholic *vins de liqueur* such as Malaga and Madera. In spite of the evolution of therapy resulting from 'the incessant progress of science,' the committee of revision retained a small role for the ancient *oenolés.*[15] It was not until the eighth edition of the *Codex* in 1965 that medicinal wines became a sort of marginalia, occupying some space on two pages. Some information was given of a general nature on the wines that were used and their degree of alcohol. In a new development illustrating concern over winemaking, the *Codex* took over twenty pages to deal with oenological products, whose purity had become a matter of public health.

American medicine had led the way in ditching wines from its *materia medica.* Jack Pickleman notes that 'The first U.S. Pharmacopoeia in 1820 listed only nine wine mixtures, including iron, ipecac, opium and tobacco.'[16] In 1905 the *U.S. Dispensatory* listed red wine as a tonic and mentioned seventeen other wines. By 1937 all wines were eliminated. In the 1905 edition of the *United States Pharmacopoeia* the twelve medicinal wines included unmedicated red and white wines and wines of antimony, coca, ergot, ferric citrate, iron, and opium. These wines were jettisoned in 1916, but deceptive labelling hid the fact that certain pharmaceuticals were prepared in wine: 'virtually all of the liquid vitamin formulas' were 'prepared in solutions of white wine.'[17] Other American official lists had succumbed to new therapies and prohibitionist pressure long ago.

Wine remained useful in the practice of medicine because of the important role played in pharmacy by medicinal wines, preparations continuing various dissolved simple substances recognised in pharmacology as medicinal drugs. Why use wine? In *Domestic Medicine*, an eighteenth-century work of immense success well into the nineteenth century, William Buchan (1729-1805) gave a remarkable summing-up of the value of wine 'as a menstruum for extracting the virtues of other medicinal substances.' Wine, 'being a compound of water, inflammable spirit, and acid ... it is enabled to act upon vegetable and animal substances, and also to dissolve some bodies of the metallic kind, so as to impregnate itself with their virtues....'[18] It gives better results than alcohol as an excipient. Two centuries later Lucia added to wine's medical virtues: 'the mild acidity, the buffering action, the desirable range of alcoholic content, and the pleasant flavour provided by the aromatic esters are qualities that combine to make wine pre-eminent among all the vehicles of organic acid nutrients.[19]

Medicinal wines were generally made with white wines, except for the tonic and bitter wines of quinquina and gentian, which were usually made with red wines. The wines had to be pure with a pleasant, fresh taste. No altered or treated wines, like a *vin platré* – wine treated with gypsum (calcium sulphate) to increase acidity and improve colour – were supposed to be used in pharmaceutical preparations. The wine had to be mixable with water in varying proportions without becoming in the least bit cloudy. (The fad for wines of crystal clarity, often achieved by means detrimental to the health of the consumer and the taste of the wine, may have been given a psychological boost by the association that pharmacology made between purity and clarity.) In so far as possible, the nature of the wine had to be related to that of the medicinal substances. Astringent and tonic substances went with tannic red wine. White wines, noted for their diuretic power, were also used to dissolve substances precipitated by the tannins of red wines. Lucia pointed out that the complex chemical composition of wine also explains its widespread use in modern pharmacy, 'which gives it [wine] a whole set of values unavailable in any other menstruum or solvent used for medication.'[20]

Defenders of medicinal wines rejected the idea that a mixture of water and alcohol is the equivalent of wine as a vehicle for medicinal substances. Alcohol is a solvent but it does not contain elements like tannin, organic acids, tartar, glycerine, and sugar, all of which were held to have a special function in the mixture. Tannins, for example, combine with alkaloids, and acids attack metals like iron. It seems that pharmacologists were wrong to ignore the chemical complexity of wine and assume that the alcohol alone is just as efficacious a vehicle for introducing drugs into the body.

All medicinal wines were prepared cold. Defenders of these wines rejected the argument of the advocates of pasteurisation that heat does not alter the composition of wine. The medicinal substances used were dried, except for antiscorbutic plants. Sometimes the ingredients were added to the *marc* (presscake) and the concoction was fermented, pressed, and filtered. Baumé noted that this procedure eliminated the bitterness from squill and absinth wines. Iodised wines were prepared by alternating layers of grapes, with their stems for the extra tannin, and layers of marine plants or kelp. After a fermentation of fifteen to twenty days, the resulting wine contained forty to fifty centigrams of iodine, but amazing as it seems, it did not have a disagreeable taste or irritate the digestive tube. A variety of methods for the preparation of medicinal wines were also specified in the French *Codex*.[21] Though several methods might exist in pharmaceutical literature and lore, the advantages and disadvantages of each procedure were generally pretty well known.

A great disadvantage of medicinal wines was that they deteriorated easily; so only small amounts could be prepared at a time. Medicinal beer was even more alterable and therefore little used. In the early-nineteenth century J.-L. Alibert (Hôpital Saint-Louis) revived a method used by Parmentier to avoid the problems associated with medicinal wines made in the three traditional ways (fermentation, maceration, and steeping). The procedure was to start with an excellent old wine and then add an alcoholic tinture previously infused with the plant element needed for therapeutic purposes. Wines made in this way did not deteriorate and exercised an immediate effect on the patient. The wine was made into the vehicle of the operative element rather than used as a dissolvant.[22]

Knowledge of medicinal wines is now pretty much gone, but perhaps it is easy to exaggerate the historical role of wines in pharmacy. In the medication formulas published in 1697 by P. Garnier, physician of the Hôtel-Dieu de Lyon, wine was an element in only sixteen of the 224 formulas, seven per cent of the preparations. And it would not be long before the apothecaries of the hospital would be using even less wine in their concoctions.[23] The nineteenth century was perhaps a boom period for medicinal wines.

The 'cult of wine' in France has historically given any debate over alcoholism a character different from that in most other countries.[24]

Of course, a number of prominent French doctors have always been critical of drinking, but even some of these critics kept a warm spot in their hearts for wine. A. Richerand, a major Parisian medical figure of the first half of the nineteenth century, professor at the faculty in Paris and chief surgeon of the Hôpital Saint-Louis, was a stern critic of both popular medicine and drinking, but he boasted that the meat and pure wine diet given at the hospital cured hundreds of patients suffering from scurvy and scrofula, two widespread but very different diseases of the time. He rejected a vegetable diet because its considerable volume furnished only a small quantity of curative elements. 'Taken in small quantity, wine stimulates the fibres, stimulates the contractility of the organs, and favours the circulation of the humours; but its abuse is more harmful than its use is profitable.' Even the treatment of fevers posed a problem because the patient's habituation to drink could make him insensitive to this type of stimulant. The more alcoholic the wine, the more harmful it is. Richerand, like many Frenchmen, believed that excessive drinking was more common in England than in France. But he found that in France practitioners of popular medicine often damaged their patients by overprescribing wine. He cited cases of *renoueurs* who treated dislocated shoulders by having the patient drink a big bowl of wine every fifteen minutes and treated broken ribs by having the victim down several pints of a generous wine. Richerand quoted a sour proverb to sum up the dangers of wine: 'qui du vin est ami, de soi-même est ennemi.'[25]

J.-A. Salgues, another early-nineteenth century doctor, also emphasised the dangers of excessive wine consumption while presenting his wine therapy. Salgues was an expert in gerontology, a subject dealing with a small elite in an period when average life expectancy for most people was under forty years. If there is an age when wine offers only advantages, Salgues said, it is old age. True, too much wine produces diarrhoea, drying of the fibres, thinness, dropsy, and feebleness of the intellectual faculties. And irritable old people are punished for their indisposition by their inability to support wine. The choleric are condemned to drink beer, especially if they have kidney stones. For ordinary old folks, however, Plato was right: wine is their milk, producing a gentle excitation in the brain, augmenting and renewing happiness, keeping the mind in constant activity, and in general making the drinker a confident, pleasant person. The authority of Cabanis' *Traité du physique et du moral de l'homme* supported the benefits of lifelong moderate wine drinking. Wine is good for phlegmatics, for people with gas or a hard digestion, and especially in cold and humid weather for the people whose stomachs are overloaded with glairs. Salgues recommended wines we often associate with older people: Malaga, dry Madeira, Muscat, old burgundy. Alicante and good bordeaux would also do, especially 'vin de Graves et de Pontac.' Reds are generally better for old people, except those who are overweight and those afflicted with stones. Salgues retained the old prejudice that champagne is harmful to gouty people. Otherwise, he maintained, wine drinking is one of the few joys of old age, and even a remedy.[26]

In the first quarter of the nineteenth century the medical manuals and treatises gave important roles to alcohol and wine as items in the *materia medica.* C.-J.-A. Schwilgué's *Manuel médical* (1806) identified the tonic qualities of wine and touted it as one of the best means of treating acute diseases, various kinds of fevers, haemorrhages, and neuroses. The therapeutic results of alcohol and wine are seen as rather similar in this manual. Schwilgué was keen on using pure wine that had sufficiently matured; it was administered cut with water. His division of wines was based on sugar, alcohol, acid, and extract. Wines like Madeira and Malaga ('les vins sucrés amers') have a tonic and nourishing effect combined with the power to increase the pulse, warm the body and cause perspiration. Fourcroy had classified old red wines and distilled spirits as fortifying, capable of building up a body run down by illness.[27] Schwilgué held that some wines of Burgundy and the Champagne ('les vins acidulés très-alcooliques) stimulate the appetite, aide digestion, quench thirst, and help transpiration and urinating. Wines of the south, including those of Bordeaux, Graves, and Pontac, and Roussillon ('les vins extrato-alcooliques') combine some of the functions of the other two categories and can have a constipating effect. One of the curious things about items in the *materia medica,* or at least about wine, is that over time the same items changed functions or were assumed to have different effects. A more substantial work, Nysten's edition of the *Traité de matière médicale* noted that *materia medica* itself did not have one definition. Some used the phrase as if it meant medicinal natural history, others meant medicinal chemistry, still others meant therapeutics, and yet another group used it to refer to the science dealing with the action of foreign bodies on living organs. Nysten tried to end this confusion by emphasising the aim of science, meaning the input of different scientific endeavours into 'la science pharmaceutique.'[28] Things did not turn out exactly as Nysten hoped, but perhaps the authority of the text finally produced a general agreement on the therapeutic properties of different wines. More or less what the Hippocratic and Galenic texts had achieved, though with different wines.

Alcohol and wine were still important enough in medicine in the second half of the nineteenth century to earn considerable entries in medical dictionaries and encyclopedias. It was a period that saw the publication of some standard medical reference works. French doctors hatched an impressive brood of works, which seemed more directed at the professional than at the ordinary reader. Alcohol and wine (and even alcoholism) occupied considerable space in these productions, whose publication stretched over the careers of some of the editors.[29] The editors of the *Dictionnaire encyclopédique des sciences médicales* (I, 1864) considered wine important enough to include a section on its chemistry and industrial production; medicinal wines were included under the heading of pharmacology. The *Nouveau dictionnaire de médecine et de chirurgie pratiques* (I, 1864) was respectably technical on the chemical history of alcohol and good on alcoholism but was very limited in coverage of medical information as compared with the long article in the *Dictionnaire encyclopédique* by Béhier. The *Nouveau dictionnaire* gave the standard favourable medical information on the use of wine in medical treatments. Glycerine was given prominence in the *Nouveau dictionnaire* (vol. 16, 1872) and in the *Dictionnaire encyclopédique* (vol. 9, 1883) as a useful medication for treating everything from herpes to haemorrhoids. Garlic, the 'theriac of the poor,' an item used since antiquity and included in the repertory of great men like Sydenham and Cullen, was highly regarded by the editors (H. Baillon and O. Reveil) of the *Dictionnaire encyclopédique,* especially in the external treatment of rheumatic pain, corns, worms and many other ills, but it could not compare with the therapeutic versatility and efficacity of alcohol, wine, and medicinal wines.

The squabble about the merits of wine compared with other alcoholic drinks is an old one in the medical profession. Perhaps the only certain thing that can be said about the debate is that experts in wine drinking areas find wine therapeutically superior, and in spite of upmarket campaigns for single malts and quality beers, wine is easier to identify as the drink of those who believe that they live in higher civilisations. In mid-nineteenth century one of France's leading doctors and most influential medical professors, Apollinaire Bouchardat (1806-86), expert on diabetes, confirmed the bad news about alcoholic drinks and the good news about wine. As professor of public health in the Paris faculty of medicine, Bouchardat taught that 'the aim of hygiene is the conservation and perfection of health

..., which must be based on etiology.' ... 'Knowledge of causes is the most elevated and also the most difficult part of medicine.' Plundering physics, chemistry, and biology, he invented a 'synthetic etiology.' Bouchardat noted that out of 938 admissions in 1859 to the Bicêtre infirmary, 135 were 'victims of alcoholic abuses.' He admitted that the abuse of wine produced the same kind of harm as eau-de-vie or alcohol but, he insisted, to a lesser degree. Even though alcohol 'plays the principal role in the physiological and hygienic action of wine,' Bouchardat insisted that its 'action is modified by other elements' (tannins and acids). He held the conventional view that old wine (five to ten years old) is preferable for therapeutic uses; it had to be served with meals. Sweet and alcoholic wines such as Saint-Raphaël, which had replaced Malaga in Paris hospitals, were to be prescribed, without food, in doses of 120 grams every twenty four hours. Bouchardat, a Burgundian winegrower, believed that good burgundy was the best wine for convalescents. Bouchardat's illustration of the nutritional value of wine was partly based on the idea that the French navy escaped the burden of scurvy because their sailors drank wine instead of the grog issued to British seamen, with the result that the English got scurvy and the French did not. Bouchardat attributed the preventive power of wine to its potassium salts; he did not mention limes or, more to the point, medicinal wines containing plants.[30] Since wine can contain from fifteen to 150 mg of ascorbic acid per litre, Bourchardat might have been right for a different reason.

So it was still possible for an anti-alcohol doctor to retain an important role for wine in his medical therapy on the grounds that it was different in its effects from alcohol and other alcoholic drinks. This would essentially be the position arrived at by French doctors in the early-twentieth century. Doctors were able to cite high-level scientific research in distinguishing the medical effects of wine from those of alcohol. As early as 1868 *Lancet* drew attention to A. Dupin's article (in the *Popular Science Review)* because he was extending the research done by Marcelin Berthelot on the chemistry of wine. The importance of the subject could be illustrated by the fact that 'a single wine may contain twenty-five different kinds of ethers!' Here was 'a circumstance which sufficiently explains the mystery which hangs over the subject of the physiological action of wine as distinguished from alcohol.'[31]

In 1880 the *Lancet* commission on the medical use of wine seemed to anticipate the later French position with a long report on the medical uses of wine.[32] The impetus to the inquiry by the commission came from the government's plan for the reduction of duties on wine imported into England. (The Chancellor of the Exchequer, Gladstone, had an excellent cellar of bordeaux.) The implementation of this plan was supposed to result in a large increase in the importation of wines from different countries and especially of cheap wines from France. This development involved significant consequences for the medical community. The consumption of 'the more strongly alcoholised ports, sherries, and madeiras' would fall. It seems that whereas sherry drinkers were as numerous as ever, the number of port drinkers had not kept up with the increase in population since the 1860s. What could be expected with freely imported wines was a competition between 'beer and spirits as the national beverages' and cheap continental wines, which the Europeans were drinking 'with advantage not only to their character for sobriety but also to their health.'

Lancet was not recommending wine for healthy people. No 'wines whatsoever are necessary for a healthy adult in good physical strength, taking a fair amount of daily exercise, and with no excessive mental strain.' This position was also taken recently by the Canadian medical association. Most light wines taken in moderation with meals were not regarded as harmful, but rather 'as consistent with health as the consumption of drinks such as tea and coffee, which generally take their place. Indeed, strong tea, strong coffee, and, we would add, strong tobaccos have much to answer for in the production of indigestion, nervous palpitation, *et hoc genus omne*, and we should not regret to see them displaced by many varieties of sound wines, free from an excess of sugar, and of feeble alcoholic strength.' The report was limited to the medical use of wines in the treatment of sick people. 'To the invalid the wines are frequently of great value, and in some of the acute fevers the most powerful alcoholic beverages have sometimes to be prescribed, and are more beneficial than any other stimulant. Medical men should know the indications for their use as thoroughly as those for restriction in diet, or for the employment of the various drugs in the Pharmacopoeia.'[33]

One might ask why doctors needed 'an outline of the therapeutic values and indications for the administration of the wines in everyday use,' especially since doctors made up a well-known class of drinkers of quality wine.[34] According to the report, doctors were ignorant of the therapeutic specificity of wines based on their acidity, sugar content, and alcoholic strength. Often prescriptions were based on districts or areas, ignoring the fact that there were light-bodied and full-bodied vintages from the same area. One type of wine might 'be of the greatest advantage to a patient' while another from the same district 'should be imperatively forbidden.' Many medical men forgot there were medically significant wines other than port, sherry, and claret. Minor horror stories abounded, often about ignored dangers of hidden acids and sugar: for example, 'a gouty patient was taking wine with an enormous proportion of fixed acid, and had no idea of the mischief that it was inducing, because the quantity of sugar therein was also large, and completely hid the sour taste....'[35] Given the recognised need for the therapeutic use of wine, the value of a guide for the profession was hard to deny.

The report recognised that in prescribing wine a little science could be a dangerous thing because the chemical analysis so relied on by doctors failed 'entirely ... to show the therapeutic distinctions between wines.' The chemical scheme of classification of wines was only approximate, being of most value in measuring sugar and alcohol and of far lesser value in giving quantities of tannin, which was nevertheless considered a constitutent of wine that was of medical as well as oenological importance. And sometimes knowledge of the structure of a wine was not helpful in advising patients. 'Some choice wines with very little volatile or fixed acid have a great tendency to produce dyspepsia and turn sour in the stomach, and do more harm to a dyspeptic patient than the crudest and most astringent *vin ordinaire*, however rough to the taste this may be....' The report noted that *vin ordinaire* mixed with mineral water could be taken by most invalids instead of the brandy or whisky that doctors frequently recommended. The immaturity of wine, so important in determining its acid properties, was regarded as 'quite beyond the chemist's range.'[36] If the doctor did not know that, he needed, at the very least, the commission's therapeutic guide.

'The patient's daily question, 'What shall I drink?' required more consideration than the stereotyped reply, 'Oh, you can take a little claret'.'[37] Though one could not find a wine of greater clinical value, the problem with clarets was that there was a great variety of them, nearly too much of a good thing, organised into Cartesian complexity by the commercial classification of 1855, with prices ranging from a shilling for a *vin ordinaire* to 'the almost fabulous price' at a public auction of twelve pounds for a dozen Château Latour of the vintage 1858.[38] A doctor who prescribed a red bordeaux could be certain of a consistent product, unlike the whites of Bordeaux and Burgundy. The commission believed that vintage, age of wine, and vineyard determined 'the bouquet and fragrance of the wine' and therefore the price, but had little effect, insofar as could be determined by chemical analysis, on 'the chief constituents' of the wine.[39] This range of variety and price for basically the same wine (clinically) was a great medical advantage, for it meant that the poor could enjoy the same basic medicine as the rich. The patient could 'take either the cheaper or the more expensive varieties [of true not manufactured claret] without running any risk of their having different medicinal effects.' It was obvious to the commission that 'in choosing a red claret, diabetic, gouty, rheumatic, dyspeptic, or anaemic patients have a much more extensive range, with perfect safety, than they possess if the white wines have been ordered for their malady.'[40]

The bouquet of wine was a subject of considerable medical importance, a concept deserving analysis in light of the latest chemical research.[41] A grid presented by Louis Hébert for his fellow physicians divided wines into two families, according to whether the wines were dominated by one of the essential characteristics of wine or mixed wines. The first family was further subdivided into four categories: (1) alcoholic (including dry wines such as dry madeira and dry marsala, sweet wines such as malaga, Banyuls, and Lunel, and the *vins de paille* of Arbois and Ermitage); (2) astringent (including those wines with bouquet such as Ermitage and those without bouquet such as Cahors); (3) acid (including wines with bouquet such as rhines and those without bouquet such Gouais and Argenteuil); and (4) sparkling stuff such as champagne and Saint-Péray. The family of mixed wines fell into two categories: wines with bouquet (the quality wines of Burgundy, the Médoc, and the Midi); and wines without bouquet (the ordinary wines of Burgundy and Bordeaux).

The degree or percentage of alcohol was of vital concern to doctors prescribing wine and alcohol as medicine. Although many of the figures given for Irish and Scotch whiskies and some wines are similar to those today, there is a striking difference in the figures for dry white and red wines, especially for quality bordeaux. About mid-nineteenth century, wine of the Graves (Gironde) and of Beaune (Côte d'Or) were cited at 12.3 and 12.2 per cent respectively, Côte Rôtie at 11.3, red bordeaux (1841) at 11.1, Saumur at 9.9, Margaux (1842) at 9.75, St. Emilion (1842) at 9.21, and Château Margaux (1840) at 8.75. Mâcon white reached 11.0 and chablis 7.33 per cent.[42] Different methods of vinification and chaptalisation have raised levels of alcohol to accommodate the development of different taste models in wine in which the acids are disguised by the alcohol.

Things were simple at the top. In the case of the classified wines the brand of the estate created a confidence in the product difficult to achieve at lower levels, where wines from different areas were blended and even concocted from water, alcohol, and cheap Spanish wine, with a touch of sour claret adding a spurious authenticity. Doctors would rarely be deceived. 'In true claret the taste is astringent and subacid, never really sour, and even in the roughest samples the peculiar vinous bouquet is well-marked.'[43] The commission described a model of fine wine in which quality was determined by vintage as well as age; if the wine had sufficient tannin and over eleven per cent alcohol, it had to be kept for at least ten years to develop fully its best qualities. The classified wines were distinguished by 'superior flavour, soundness, and bouquet.' After 'the exceptionally fine year of 1864,' the best vintage was that of 1875, followed by 1870, 1868, and 1865. The commission showed its superb command of the arcana of the commerce and civilisation of wine, including judgment of its aesthetic qualities. A patient would be fortunate to find a doctor who knew as much about health and disease.

The gastronomic knowledge of the doctor was of medical use because a wine recommended for medical purposes had be a good drinking wine, endowed with the traditional virtues. In 1883 *Lancet* recommended a champagne (*cuvée exceptionnelle*) sold under the label of Hedges and Butler as 'a fair representative of the champagne which is best for medical use. It is dry, with excellent bouquet and flavour, and is well matured by age. Such wine is of the finest of stimulants, without being what is often called 'heady'.'[44] The doctor's socio-oenological knowledge also helped the patient who could not afford the medical benefits of the champagne that he needed. In an analysis of a sparkling Saumur in 1905 the taster for *Lancet* called attention to the excellence of sparkling wines produced in Saumur, which were 'in no way dietetically inferior to the wines produced in the Champagne district. The highly trained palate will detect a difference in the aesthetic qualities and that is all, but the majority of people [would find the Saumur] just as pleasing as is a high-class and a high-priced champagne.'[45]

The commission recognised the clinical value of red clarets as 'exceedingly great,' optimistically noting that every therapeutist was 'fully aware of the marked benefit ... derived from their use in most cases in which tonics are indicated.' Taken with meals, clarets were 'true tonics ... with neither a stimulating nor a sedative effect.' Red bordeaux had a reputation for being 'much less stimulating than the

Sauternes' and both the red and white burgundies. The commission thought it probable that the tonic effect of clarets was due to 'the peculiar combination of tannin with a certain but low percentage of alcohol.'[46] (It is not likely that the doctors of the commission would be happy with the increase of several degrees in alcohol content of the new model claret of the second half of the twentieth century.[47])

For treating anaemia, ordinary debility from overwork, feeble digestion, and similar organic weaknesses, the commission declared the reds of Bordeaux to be 'almost as good a prescription as most of the tonic drugs in the Pharmacopoeia' as well as always being 'an advantageous adjunct to this class of remedies.' A maximum of half a bottle was allowed with the meal, thus limiting the patient's intake of alcohol. Claret was considered especially useful in stimulating the appetite and aiding the digestion of patients who could eat little and so lost strength, especially in hot weather.

Some groups of patients were wrongly excluded from the company of wine-drinkers. Diabetic patients were an obvious category one would expect to be prohibited from drinking wine because of the danger from unfermented or residual sugar. But the diabetic patient could 'safely take an occasional glass of red claret' because of its low grape-sugar content. The commission seemed pleased that this meant that the diabetic patient would therefore not have to 'be prohibited from the more expensive wines of this class, whereas Sauternes and white burgundies of high class would inevitably aggravate his malady.'[48] Gouty and rheumatic patients were usually condemned to consume alcohol only in the form of whisky, gin, and brandy, thus being deprived of the joy and benefits of claret. The commission declared this to be 'certainly a mistake.' The comparatively low amounts of fixed acid and alcohol in claret made it possible to permit patients with atonic gout to benefit greatly from a glass or two daily. Its low level of residual sugar also made claret a good wine for 'persons with a tendency to obesity. The astringency derived from the tannin separated 'the thin red clarets from the thin white ones' and rendered the reds 'available for so many more forms of disease.' The astringency made it a wine 'of great advantage in treating cases of atonic and so-called bilious dyspepsia, anaemia, and patients with any tendency to relaxed or chronically congested mucous membranes.'[49] Perhaps only red burgundies could come close to the red bordeaux in clinical value.

The commission began its analysis of red burgundy by noting that the numerous red wines of the Côte d'Or, 'great favourites with connoisseurs,' were not so well known in England as the clarets. The

Burgundian soil, 'remarkable for the large quantity of iron with which the carbonate of lime is pervaded,' supposedly develops the perfect characteristics of the pinot noir grape. The model of burgundy known in England was far from perfect. Burgundies, though 'deeper in colour, more full-bodied and generous,' possessed 'a more typically vinous, if somewhat less delicate flavour and bouquet than other red wines of similar quality and price,' but they did not keep their best qualities beyond ten or twelve years, after which many of them become 'somewhat thin.' Santenay and Corton held up longer. These opinions were probably typical of contemporary commercial opinion of burgundy in nineteenth century England.[50]

Instead of considering wines from the six main wine-producing regions of Burgundy (our conventional division), the commission divided the wines for practical medical purposes into three groups.[51] The groups were, first, the relatively cheap ordinary wine, such as inferior growths of Mercurey and Beaune, or 'very new specimens of some of the higher classed wines'; second, the better Beaunes, and the wines of Nuits, Volnay, and Pommard; third, the superior burgundies, meaning the biggest names in Burgundy, such as Romanée, La Tâche, Richebourg, Musigny, better known Chambertin, and Clos de Vougeot. Corton and the better known Volnays were somewhere between the second and third groups. The wines of the Mâconnais and the Beaujolais – 'popularly, though erroneously, classed with the true burgundies' – were considered separately, which made some sense oenologically and more sense medically.[52]

The wines of the Beaujolais, made from the Gamay grape, were found to be very astringent, with 'a marked proportion of tannin,' reasonable levels of grape-sugar and fixed acid, and a level of alcohol a little below that of the clarets analysed by the commission. Georges Duboeuf's drinker-friendly beaujolais had not yet been invented. So beaujolais was the wine to prescribe when one of 'marked astringency' was indicated. The cost-effective opinion of the commission was that there was no reason why beaujolais could not be drunk in all cases in which clarets were recommended.[53]

High-priced burgundies, the wines forming the basis for the medical use of red burgundy, had very little to distinguish one from the other *medicinally*. The cost of these wines almost precluded 'their being prescribed medicinally, but since they could 'exceptionally be of importance,' the commission analysed two: a Chambertin and a Romanée, both of the vintage of 1870. Both were low in tannin, almost completely without sugar, and high in alcohol. Such were 'the chemical characteristics of these grand wines.' In view of the wine's having a degree of alcohol well over thirteen per cent, the commission warned that the potency of the effects of these wines 'must make physicians somewhat cautious in recommending them, although in many types of disease no class of wine will produce so great benefit.' It remained to decide in what cases to make use of this very marked therapeutic value of red burgundy.[54]

With practically no residual sugar, the top red burgundies were considered 'especially well fitted' for rich diabetics. They were equally 'well fitted for convalescents from fevers and other acute affections.' They were also 'superior to all other wines in cases of anaemia, general debility, feeble development, and mal-nutrition not depending on gastric or intestinal irritation.' They could be drunk in the last case, though sparkling wine was recommended if the irritability was 'a marked symptom.' With an amount of fixed acid much the same as in clarets and with a lower percentage of grape-sugar, red burgundy could be 'even more valuable in many case of rheumatism and neuralgia.'[55] Keeping in mind the fact that these burgundies contained more alcohol than the clarets, doctors could still find many uses for them in treating their better-off patients.

Red burgundy was regarded as stimulating at first but with a 'markedly sedative' after-effect, which made it better than most other classes of wines for patients 'weak in physical powers, but excitable and highly nervous in temperament.' An added bonus was that in some cases this sedative influence permitted the patient sometimes to dispense with the ordinary soporifics (chloral, opium, and bromides). And who could deny that a glass or two of good burgundy is 'an excellent adjuvant in most cases in which iron and cod-liver oil form the routine treatment.'[56]

Red burgundy was not for everyone. Gouty patients were better off with other wines. A curious myth held that gout was not found in Burgundy. Bilious and plethoric people were advised to avoid the wine, for even a small amount could give 'patients headache and a sense of fullness and discomfort.' Burgundy was also 'said to favour the development of obesity' but the commission, while doubting that medicinal quantities would made people fat, noted that the fat in Burgundy probably came from the 'excessive eating with which burgundy-drinking is generally accompanied.'[57] (Conventional wisdom had never regarded burgundy as good as claret for the digestion.) Red burgundy had many medicinal virtues but its high alcohol made it a wine to prescribe with care in spite of its great therapeutic value.

Except for chablis, most of which was not 'true chablis,' white burgundies were little known in England, 'even less known than white clarets.' The commission idly speculated on this curious preference of the English for what James Joyce called beefsteak wines over less astringent and thinner white wines. The prevalent lack of interest in expensive white burgundy by the drinking monied class was perhaps to be accounted for by the fact that the more expensive and full-bodied ones were 'certainly sweeter than the English palate [was] accustomed to.' A more medical explanation was that 'dyspeptics, with a tendency to acid fermentation,' could drink red wines freely and with benefit, which was not possible with French white wines. It seemed that the older, well-matured whites were generally too sweet and the thinner ones were 'very apt to cause, or at any rate aggravate, those forms of indigestion which give rise to acidity, heartburn, etc.'[58] White burgundy had limited therapeutic use.

Even authentic chablis was not of much use. In the specimen analysed by the commission, there was more fixed acid than in the cheaper white bordeaux, but there was also less alcohol and less total solids, with nearly no unfermented sugar. The last point established at least the special medical importance of chablis. A diabetic could drink diluted chablis as a thirst-quencher 'or undiluted as a dinner-wine, with even more impunity than most white clarets.' Chablis was not recommended for dyspeptics or gouty patients. Because both chablis and white bordeaux were thought to have 'a slightly aperient rather than a constipating effect' the doctor had to be careful not to trigger an unfortunate incident in prescribing these wines 'for delicate invalids with any tendency to diarrhoea.' In fact, the cheaper white bordeaux wines were considered medically preferable to ordinary chablis, in spite of the latter's being 'much fuller in flavour, mellower, and more exciting.'[59]

The commission declared that the best white burgundies were 'vastly superior in most cases in which stimulants should be ordered' to 'the crude fortified ports and sherries so freely prescribed.' For a wine with 'a primarily stimulating and afterwards slightly sedative effect, an old Montrachet was as good as the best sauternes, including Yquem. An analysis of the Montrachet of 1870 vintage found that it had too much residual sugar to permit consumption by a diabetic. Its chief value seemed to be as a restorative, and the commission seemed eager to recommend it as preferable to the fortified wines so much in vogue. 'The advantage of such a restorative as a good Burgundy wine, in which the alcohol is less than fifteen per cent by volume, must be ... obvious to every practitioner who has to deal with tardy convalescence after fevers, operations, etc.' The availability of the 'remarkably delicate and sound' Montrachet of 1876 vintage at thirty shillings per dozen also showed that white burgundies were cheaper than any reasonably mature fortified wine. The surprise was that 'these valuable wines' were 'so seldom prescribed.'[60]

In discussing white bordeaux, the commission made an obvious division into two classes of wines: dry whites, described as thin wines with a slightly acidulous taste; and the high-class sauternes, 'full of delicate fragrance and flavour,' much sweeter and more alcoholic than the other class. The physician was warned not to forget in advising patients that their medical uses were 'so very opposite.'

The sauternes, like the great white burgundies, were believed to stimulate and then have a sedative effect on the drinker. So they were 'valuable to nervous, excitable patients,' for whom they did good when the use of stronger stuff, including port and sherry, was unwise. Because of a high sugar content they were absolutely forbidden to diabetics and people with a tendency to obesity; they were also to be avoided by gouty and bilious people. They supposedly aggravated dyspepsia. 'In cases of lung disease in which the patient ... [was] exhausted by coughing and ... [wanted] to sleep,' but for whom opiates were dangerous and chloral was inadvisable, sauternes could be beneficial, even though 'many other wines would be positively harmful.' But 'except as a calmative, and occasionally as a restorative in convalescence from acute disease,' the commission found little use for sauternes in medicine.[61]

The commission was enthusiastic about dry white Bordeaux wines. These 'pleasantly tonic' wines were prescribed to excite the fitful and delicate appetite. They were especially useful in the treatment of 'bilious' indigestion as well as helpful in the digestion of fatty foods. Diluted with mineral water and iced, white claret gave relief to 'a patient parched with the thirst of fever' more than did 'most of the remedies usually recommended for this purpose.' These wines, having a low level of residual sugar, could be taken by diabetics for an occasional change in a strict diet. And they were also a good weapon in the fight against fat, whether corpulence already acquired or threatening to arrive. White wines were not for the anaemic or 'people of lax fibre,' who should cleave to the astringent reds. They tended to be aperient for people prone to diarrhoea. Above all, the clarets were not for people having 'any tendency to acid types of dyspepsia' because these wines would likely turn acid in stomachs having feeble digestive powers. 'In the dyspepsia of gouty invalids they require to be used with much caution, but they can be consumed with less fear of increasing the amount of uric acid in the blood than most of the wines in general use.'[62] But in the end these wines added another useful, cheap drug to the doctor's therapeutic arsenal.

The role for wine in medical therapy fitted in nicely with the idea that wine was a better drug for the lower classes than drinks containing high doses of industrial alcohol. Part of the medical profession believed that the health of the poor would improve if they could be seduced into switching from these drinks, especially gin, to wine, even artificial wine. In 1868 *Lancet* praised the proposal to open shops of the Victoria Wine Co. in poor areas of London. An analysis of the company's sherry and port led to medical approval of them even though the wines examined were not made wholly from grapes. This preference for the wine-store over the gin-palace was historically founded: 'our ancestors were able to drink with impunity so much port and claret not so much because of their constitutions as the excellence of the liquor imbibed.' Louis Pasteur would have been pleased had he known that English doctors essentially agreed with his idea that the English working class should be persuaded to drink pure and pasteurised wine, thus adding a good food to their diet.[63]

The quality as well as cost of wine consumed by poor and destitute patients was a issue of some importance. In 1862 medical attendants at the East London Union, dispensed over 130 gallons of wine and spirits to 134 patients at a cost of slightly over £140. In commenting on this 'consumption of wine by pauper patients,' *Lancet* approved of the evidence of 'a wise economy on the part of the guardians.'[64] The poor quality of the wine given to the sick poor sometimes made news. In 1864 the medical officer of the Risborough district of the Wycombe Union complained that the only wine supplied was tent (*vino tinto*), a Spanish red wine of low alcoholic content. A decision was then taken to replace this plonk with good port.[65] Good medicine required good wine.

A quite different medical opinion, emphasising the insalubrity of wine, was coming into existence during this same period. *Lancet* was reporting in 1860 that it was so difficult to find pure wine in Paris that many families were drinking beer. The consequence of importing cheap wine into England was expected to be that Parisians would 'largely adopt the use of English beer.'[66] The idea that much of

French natural wine was an adulterated product, with an enormous amount of what was sold as natural wine really being artificial wine, created a sensation in 1860, when Gladstone was arguing for a reduction in wine duties on the grounds that high taxes tempted the wine trade to adulterate their products. Only the rich could afford pure and wholesome wines. Low prices through a reduction of taxes were seen as a way to turn some luxuries of the rich into necessaries of life for the poor.

Much excitement was generated by Gladstone's description of the bad wine served to sick sailors:

> I happened to be on board the ship Scourge when one of the sailors, who had met with a severe accident, was recovering from a surgical operation. I asked the surgeon whether it was not necessary to give him some good wine. He told me that it was, but that he had to supply it from their [officers'] own mess. He asked me to taste some of the wine from the ship's stores, and I did with difficulty manage to drink part of a glass.

Though the wine served to sailors was duty-free, Gladstone used the incident not a lesson in social distinction but as an illustration of the difficulty of obtaining wholesome wine. *Lancet* commented that the difficulty faced by the ship's surgeon was felt more strongly by infirmary surgeons, by parochial medical officers, and especially by practitioners among the working class. 'To order wine for a working man is very often to give him a vile and semi-poisonous compound, the therapeutic effects of which differ very sadly from the generous juice of the grape.' Hospitals had very large wine bills when they bought good stuff. An unintended consequence of Gladstone's unpleasant dégustation was that the Admiralty began an investigation of the quality of wine supplied to the navy for medical purposes, 'unfit for invalids, although exempt from duty.' Since drugs were supplied from the Apothecaries' Hall, it was assumed that this guaranteed that they 'were not of an equally adulterated and deleterious description.'[67]

In the early-1870s doctors Thudichum and Dupré were busy alarming wine drinkers about the chemicals in wine and warning sherry drinkers about dangerously large quantities of potassium sulphate in sherry. After Thudichum delivered a lecture on wines to the Society of Arts, *Lancet* declared that 'everyone, whether in the medical profession or out of it, should study the facts which he brings forward concerning the 'manipulation' of different kinds of wines....'[68] In this period the French were also debating the danger of high levels of the same chemical found in wines of the Midi because of the prevalent practice of plastering southern wines.

When Thudichum and August Dupré published their *Treatise on ... Wine* in 1872, it received attention in *The Times* under the rubric 'the chemistry of wine.'[69] In his classic book *Sherry* Jullian Jeffs deplores the fact of general acceptance of the shoddy science used to alarm the public about the amount of sulphuric acid (present as potassium sulphate) produced in wines, especially sherry, by plastering, which supposedly had 'the object of removing from wine its natural acidity, and making it smooth to the taste.' In reality the aim was to achieve a balanced wine by increasing acidity in wine made from grapes that had become sugar-laden in the sun; picking grapes when less ripe would have obviated the need to use *yeso* (plaster) in making sherry, and this procedure is now followed by some firms. Jeffs notes that Thudichum carried out experiments with 'musts produced in London from imported Lisbon grapes' and used 'plaster in vastly greater quantities than ever used in the vineyards.'[70] Thudichum and Dupré had followed the general strategy of comparing the chemical composition of natural wine with the commercial wine generally available to the consumer. What struck the medical reporter for *Lancet* about the review was that it denounced 'the messes now fabricated in France and Germany under the name of wine.' Nor did the reviewer spare the chemists, who, 'perhaps by reason of a professional love for artificial products,' defended the scientific manipulation of wine and advocated more of it. Both writers for *The Times* and *Lancet* recommended Greek and Hungarian wines as pure wines, that is wines having the chemical characteristics of pure wine.

From the 1880s on, the consumer was perhaps more threatened by artificial wine than by manipulated natural wine. And the continuing spread of phylloxera in France and then other wine-growing countries only increased the amount of artificial wine on the market. Early in 1889, English authorities, acting on suspicion, seized 1500 casks of wine. All casks contained artificial wine concocted of water, an inferior quality alcohol, a little glycerine, Chilean colouring matter, marine salt, and a large quantity of plaster.[71] Dupré had gone 'so far as to say that the depressing influence of ... [potassium sulphate] might more often than not counteract all the stimulant action of the alcohol upon the heart, and might thus actually knock a debilitated patient down rather than pick him up.'[72] Prescribing wine was getting to be more trouble than it might be worth.

The presence of potassium sulphate in sherry was still important enough as a medical issue for *Lancet* to send an investigator to Jerez to see what was going on in the sherry business. His report completely vindicated real sherry, 'vinum Xericum, the vino de Jerez,' which was found not to contain 'a single ingredient foreign to its composition.' None of the changes found in the plastered wine were regarded as a threat to the health of the drinker. Even taken in large doses, much more than in a bottle of sherry, potassium sulphate was known to have only a laxative effect. The analysis following gives the results of the commissioner's investigation. Column (1) is for a treated must and column (2) for an untreated must.[73]

The analysis of (1) 'Mosto' previously treated with Sulphate of Lime and (2) of 'Mosto' not so treated

	(1) %	(2) %
Solid Matters	**2.16**	**1.88**
Sugar	**0.37**	**0.23**
Potassium bitartrate	**0.093**	**0.28**
Tartaric acid	**0.338**	**0.21**
Acetic acid	**0.09**	**0.05**
Mineral matter	**0.37**	**0.23**
Potassium sulphate	**0.34**	**0.085**
Potassium phosphate	**–**	**0.041**
Alcohol by weight	**11.62**	**10.85**
Alcohol by volume	**14.37**	**13.43**
Proof spirit	**25.18**	**23.54**
Alcohol by volatile ether	**0.0214**	**0.0071**
Alcohol in volatile ether	**0.0382**	**0.0172**
Total alcohol in ethers	**0.0596**	**0.0243**

One of the dangers in the medical use of alcohol was that patients would become addicted to alcohol. In the nineteenth century this was a particularly strong argument for doctors who felt that they had a clear duty to deal with a new social pathology, namely, the excessive consumption in western society of cheap, highly alcoholic beverages produced by the modern fermentation and distillation industries. Since public health measures and preventive medicine were reducing the mortality from many diseases and practically eliminating some altogether, the need for alcohol therapy was difficult to justify. The chemical and pharmaceutical industry produced alternative medicines which doctors were eager to test on patients. And above all, there was the problem of internal inconsistencies in the paradigm of alcohol therapy, which were more difficult to ignore as the nineteenth century wore on. Even some early defenders of the therapy had worked on 'the problem of treating pyrexial diseases simply by hygiene and proper food.'[74] An effective case could finally be made for limiting the therapeutic use of alcohol or for eliminating it altogether.

Closure of the medical debate over alcohol and wine therapy was attempted at approximately the same time in both Great Britain and France. In 1907 *The Hospital* published a therapeutic guide based on the solid science of the day. The part dealing with wines was eventually translated into French.[75] The guide tried to escape from the impasse produced by the condemnation of the therapy by anti-alcoholic doctors clashing with the positive recommendation by doctors supporting the moderate use of alcohol. The authority of its verdict was based on material facts, issuing from impartial scientific work done according to the rigorous methods of research laboratories. Like history, science had its noble dream. In this case the science was a series of meticulous and conclusive pharmacological experiments on the complex issue of the therapeutic effect of wine on diseases.

It was easier to come to negative conclusions than to positive ones. Given the scientific state of physiology and pharmacy, it was impossible to predict on the basis of the chemical data that one specific wine would help and another wine would harm a patient. It was only possible to indicate the category of wine that might be suitable for a certain kind of illness. There was a prevalent belief that the abuse of wine produces less serious diseases (gout, plethora, apoplexy) than alcohol (cirrhosis, neuritis, diseases of the central nervous system). This was an illusion based on the fact that the first group of diseases was treatable whereas the second group was practically incurable. The abuse of either wine or alcohol could produce the second group of diseases.

Positive results seemed merely a confirmation of old arguments, regardless of how comforting it was to have these beliefs confirmed by scientific experiments. In three categories of artificially produced digestion (diastatic, peptic, and pancreatic), experiments showed that the effects of alcohol making up to three per cent of the foodstuffs in a diet acted rather favourably on the digestive chemical phenomena. So eight to ten ounces of wine or a little less than half a bottle with a meal in no way hindered the digestion. The wine had to be consumed in small amounts at a time, preferably with an equal amount of alkaline mineral water that was neither too effervescent nor too cold. The dilution of wine by water could just as well take place in the stomach as in the glass, thus avoiding the gastronomic crime of changing the colour of the wine by mixing it directly in the glass with water.

The Hospital declared French light wines the most likely to be natural. The 'bordeaux' of Australia and California did not fall into the recommended category but were compared to port, sherry, and madeira, impeding digestion because their high acid and sugar contents hindered the digestion of proteins, though more in the case of pancreatic than peptic digestion. The quantity of their extract elements and tannic compounds provoked a further unfavourable influence on digestion. The tannin in tea, especially Indian, could also have a harmful effect on the digestion, even in its pancreatic stage. The 'tannin and its derivatives form insoluble compounds with the food proteins and, in addition, precipitate the inorganic ferments that make food soluble and ready to digest.' This was alarming news.

Champagne also did poorly in the experiments, 'leaving much to desire from the medical point of view.' One reason was that drinking champagne violated *ex hypotesi* a fundamental law of gastronomy against mixing alcoholic drinks, for champagne had a complex liqueur added in order to produce the sweetness preferred by the targeted consumer. A less ascetic age than ours did not seem much interested in *brut zéro*. Whatever one says about this ingenious argument, it shows the remarkable degree to which the medical mind was guided by its own social rituals. 'With meals the gastronomic art has to be considered as well as dietetic science.'

More susceptible of scientific proof was the charge that champagne hinders pancreatic digestion. On the positive side, one can praise its stimulation of peptic digestion. Indeed, *The Hospital* praised a good brand of champagne as very useful in treating cases of atonic dyspepsia because wine is an energetic stimulant of gastric digestion as long as it is drunk slowly to permit a thorough mixing with the contents of the stomach. Champagne was not a recommended drink for people who had trouble digesting starches or were afflicted with deficient pancreatic functions. A dose of alkaline water could neutralise the paralysing effect of champagne on the pancreatic digestion, but *The Hospital* warned that champagne has a bad effect on the digestion because it causes disturbances in the duodenum. Beer and ginger ale were also accused of stopping digestion in the duodenum, though without any effect on digestion in the stomach. An age that took eating seriously was necessarily obsessed with its digestive processes; a later age would have a similar obsession because it did not take eating seriously.

While the medical debate went on, administrators of hospices and hospitals had to decide on whether to give patients and employees wine with their meals. The decisions about wine in hospitals took place within the context of discussions about diet and nutritional content of food items as well as about the therapeutical implications of meals. Diets necessarily changed over long periods of time, though wine was always present in the hospital. If hospitals are, as Jacques Tenon said, the measure of a people's civilisation, then one would expect to find wine – a key element of French civilisation – conspicuous in the hospital diet.[76] In one sense the medical debates find little echo in the daily life of the hospital, though the outcome of these debates determined long-term policy in hospitals. Let us look briefly at wine drinking in the hospitals of Paris since the early-nineteenth century.

Governmental agencies in the Restoration needed to remind themselves that France had not returned to the system of weights and measures of the ancien régime. In 1825, as a preliminary to issuing new rules on the provision of food in the institutions under its control, the general administrative council of Paris hospices and hospitals reminded its personnel that in 1806 the ministry of the interior had issued a decree imposing the metric system on France. After receiving from its commission a report on food in these institutions, the council issued detailed regulations on the feeding of employees and patients.[77] The rules formalised a structure of eating and drinking in state institutions that was based on the social hierarchy of employees and the age and sex of residents and patients. In the hospices one ate the *régime gras* during the first five days of the week and the *régime maigre* (meatless) the other two days as well as during Ember days. Meals looked good, at least on paper: milk, cheese, and fruit for breakfast; soup and meat for lunch; and meat, vegetables or rice, and fruit for supper. Male employees and service personnel got one litre of wine per day; their female counterparts got half that amount as well as less bread. People at the bottom of the personnel hierarchy (workers, men who did hard labour, cooks) received three quarters of a litre, with the cook's being rewarded with an extra twenty five centilitres (cl). In the Maison de retraite at Montrouge the male boarders got half a litre and the females got forty cl of wine daily. The inmates of the Hospice de Bicêtre were limited to twelve cl of wine daily, but living longer increased the allowance, which went up to a generous thirty eight cl daily for people who could hang on beyond eighty five years. In the Hospice des incurables men got forty and women thirty cl daily. Children in the Hospice des orphelins et orphelines were limited to one decilitre every Sunday. The diets in hospitals and in the sick-wards of hospices were based on the same regulations, except that the visiting medical man (a health officer rather than a doctor) could prescribe the amounts of wine for patients. A sick person might have to follow a prescribed diet with wine absolutely forbidden. The sick generally had wine prescribed according to a quarter, a half, or three quarters of of a portion of fifty cl; the full portion for a sick child was twenty cl. Judging from the amount of attention it received, wine was an important item in the *régime alimentaire* of state institutions in the Restoration.

A new regime is obliged to produce new regulations. In 1841 the ministry of the interior in the July Monarchy (1830-48) modified the rules governing eating and drinking for the people in hospitals and hospices, including those on an unrestricted diet or a modified one based on the nature of the illness. Wine continued as an important element in the diets of the employees, patients, and shut-ins. Pregnant women and wet-nurses were identified as deserving twenty five cl of wine daily. Children between two and six years of age were limited to 10cl daily. Male employees in first and second class categories received a full litre daily; those in third class dropped to 60cl for men and 40cl for women; women in the second class also got 40cl. There was no first class employment category for women. The pleasant custom of increasing wine allowance with age continued and even rose to half a litre for certain categories of patients who passed the age of eighty.[78] In the *règlement* of 1841 one can detect a fine tuning of rules as well as a mild emphasis on economy. The ultimate authority of the doctor in deciding on the diet the patient had to follow was clearly restated.

During the last third of the nineteenth century the alimentary regime of the hospital sick and of inmates of hospices and retirement homes as well as the meals served to personnel working in these institutions was determined by a Second Empire regulation issued on 20 December 1867.[79] The basic diets were classified as (1) unrestricted, (2) simple *or* only bouillons, (3) potages, and (4) solid food; each of these diets could also be sub-divided according to the therapeutic requirements of the patient. The new regime was promulgated after several years of 'experimentation' by an administrative commission of divisional directors and financial heads of medical institutions. As a result of the introduction of a scheme based on 'four degrees of alimentation,' there was no need for supplementary prescriptions once a person had been medically assigned to the proper feeding level. The sick were divided into categories of children, adults, and old people, with males and females separated. Other categories could be based on 'physiological needs' –

e.g., pregnancy and wet-nursing. The quantity and quality of the meals of the employees were based on position in the bureaucratic hierarchy. Hospital personnel with an official rank went to one dining hall and those without rank went to another. Wine was part of the Second Empire's alimentary regime, but it had been designated, in a ministerial circular of 15 December 1859, as optional for two types of diets in hospices. Wine rations in hospices and hospitals were moderate (from a French viewpoint); only children had a generous allowance, including even 25cl for those under thirteen. The other allowances varied from 25cl for a convalescing male patient to 10cl for women giving birth. Old folks in hospices got a 20cl (males) or 15cl (females). Wine production was low and prices not cheap in the 1850s because of powdery mildew in the vineyards.

The Second Empire model regulation for hospices and hospitals was established by an administrative commission in agreement with the medical personnel of the establishment. Any modification required a medical recommendation transmitted through the commission to the prefect for his approval. It is tempting to see here a French model of medicine in which the certainty of medical science justifies the authority of the physician over the patient's regimen in an institution whose rules are largely established by an enlightened bureaucracy. In 1906 Gustave Mesureur, head of the Assistance publique de Paris noted that the regulation of 1867, which was based solidly enough in science to last thirty five years, marked real progress for the period. This friendly judgment really meant that by the early-twentieth century the program established towards the end of the Second Empire needed to be replaced. It no longer satisfied the needs of the medical services and, above all, no longer reflected the progress that had been made in medical science.[80]

In July 1901 an Assistance publique commission headed by Chauffard of the Hôpital Cochin presented a project to the Société médicale des hôpitaux on the improvement of hospital diets, which needed gastro-aesthetic as well as scientifically-based improvements.[81] Too much boiled beef and bouillon were served to patients, probably because of the literature on the fortifying property of beef, the convenience of preparation of these items, and the opportunity of using cheap cuts of beef. Wine was not a drink of any special importance to this commission. To the contrary, it suggested that to milk, wine, and beer, there could be added a healthful, inexpensive drink that was becoming increasingly popular, namely light cider, which in the hospital could be cut with water as required. Above all, carafes of filtered drinking water should be made available for the sick, who would thus escape being 'submitted to the obligatory regimen of pure wine, or even wine cut with a tisane. The commission wanted to medicalise hospital eating by replacing the old 'degrees of alimentation' with 'regimens of a medical order' based not on the old system's quantities of raw food but on the nutritional data of science.

The available data on alcoholism had a considerable influence on the report made by Chauffard's commission.[82] First, there was a proposed reduction of the daily wine allowance to thirty cl for males and twenty five cl for females, though beer and cider would increase alcohol consumption slightly. Secondly, an awareness of the existence of alcoholic children led to the limitation of wine consumption to a daily fifteen cl for the flexible category of 'grands enfants.'[83] It seems that hospital doctors and medical professors (the two categories often overlapped) were more conscious of the need to reduce alcohol consumption than was the medical profession at large. No doubt the hospital doctor saw more alcoholics than the general practitioner.

Implementation of the new diet, officially described as 'a rational application of the rules of modern alimentation,' adopted by the hospital central administration in 1902, began as an experiment at the Hôpital Cochin in November 1903. A major aim of the trial was to establish the cost of extending the diet to the Paris hospital system. The diet itself did not need to be tested, for its therapeutic superiority to the old diet had already been established. Patient opinion, regarded as important by administrators and doctors, was favourable to the diversity of menus and the higher quality of food in the new diet. Although other hospitals soon clamoured for the new diet, its increased cost (400,000 more francs) precluded any wholesale switch in diets. Many small changes added up to a surprising increase in expenses. Even a simple matter of providing a choice of beer along with the ubiquitous wine increased the cost of feeding patients. And there was the extra dessert for some sugar lovers. Though money was saved when it was found to be medically unwise to give old people a full meal at night, that saving was offset by an increase in the wine ration for them. Extension of the new diet had to be a gradual process extending into 1904.

Hospital personnel had been experimenting with and changing their own diet since 1897. The two separate dining halls, dating from the consolidation of 1867, were given the same menu, except that the first class employees got less but better quality meat and extras such as more milk, sugar, and vegetables, and a second dessert. Both dining halls could choose their drinks: milk, beer, and red or white wine. The personnel, especially those in the first class refectory, found the new regimen a great improvement over the old one.

The provisioning of the hospitals of Paris from its central establishments in Les Halles was not entirely satisfactory. The meat supplied by the *Boucherie centrale* would have been of higher quality if the administration could have afforded it. In the early-1900s the quality of eggs and cheese was improved. Moving centralised hospital provisioning out of the 'gut of Paris' would have made it easier to improve the quality of most supplies.[84] Even the central bakery's supposedly nutritional bread had a sour taste, not popular in non-sourdough country. Yet no product was introduced into the provisioning system without passing expert inspection at the *Magasin central*. Only one part of the supply system seemed perfect, the central wine cellar. *La cave centrale* supplied good wine cheaply to all the medical establishments of Paris. In 1906 the average price of red wine was 0.236 francs a litre. Quality control of the wine supply was ensured by a team of professional wine tasters. Out of all the photographs in the archives of the Assistance publique it would be hard to find a picture of a happier group of professionals than that of these tasters. Most people condemned to a hospital stay would probably agree that the *dégustateurs* performed a serious therapeutic duty.

The evolution of hospital diets depended to a large extent on advances in nutritional science and on the cost of implementing dietary changes. By the early-1920s time was ripe for another modification of hospital regimes. But it was not immediately clear exactly what the new regime would be. René Gaultier confessed that nutritional issues were complex, especially when it came to correlating experimental results with the daily reality of feeding patients.[85] The old scientific certainty exuded by Chauffard and his colleagues had been replaced by a certain caution. Of course the carefully repeated experiments of the Société scientifique d'hygiène alimentaire supported by the opinions of the Société des médecins inspecteurs des écoles furnished some solid guidance for the introduction of modifications making diets 'more in agreement with modern ideas.' Thus superalimentation and hyperalbuminism needed to be 'calculated in terms of energy or calories, vitamins, minerals, and amino acids (a recent actor on the nutritional scene). According to Louis-Joseph Landouzy, Marcel Labbé, and Armand Gautier, little was known about daily human food requirements. Gautier noted that great progress had been made in feeding animals scientifically, whereas scientific knowledge of feeding humans was in such a primitive state that even the principles were contested.[86] Gautier was a firm supporter of the Pasteurian view of wine as a safe, healthful drink, though the project for the new alimentary regimen of the 1920s put no emphasis on this idea. The recommended wine consumption for patients dropped to 15cl for sick males and 10cl for sick females. The convalescent male's allowance rose to 25cl but that of the convalescent female did not change. Children over fifteen years of age could get 10cl of wine daily. Old men in hospices had to get by on 20cl; old women were limited to fifteen cl, the same as the allowance for epileptics. Wine had lost its therapeutic halo.

A debate within the Conseil supérieur de l'Assistance publique in January 1924 revealed that political compromise rather than expert opinion was often the basis for decisions on regimens.[87] In a report to the Conseil supérieur de l'hygiène de France, Marcel Labbé recommended some changes in hospital and hospice alimentary diets, including a wine allowance of 25cl. In the Assistance publique council some people wanted only 15cl. The compromise agreed on in the hospital administration was 20cl. In certain regions beer or cider could be substituted for wine. An interesting argument, based on the concepts of flexibility and authority, was made in the council for returning to the low level of 15cl: the basic allowance of wine should never be generous, thus allowing the doctor to increase the amount for special diets. Léon Mirman was not convinced of the solidity of the recent science undergirding the doctrine of daily requirements. Very few doctors knew anything about daily nutritional requirements. Only a succession of changing opinions existed: 'l'ignorance totale.' In 1899 the Conseil supérieur de l'Assistance publique believed it was competent to establish a precise alimentary regimen. Mirman suggested in 1924 that if the council declared itself incompetent to do so, it would make great scientific progress.

The only answer to scientifically based doubt is scientifically based authority. The general secretary of the council escaped from Mirman's trap by declaring that it was because of the council's incompetence that it relied on the advice of the Conseil supérieur de l'hygiène publique de France for implementing changes in hospital and hospice diets. To head off another sceptical attack, the secretary invoked the example of the situation of the hospitals in Grenoble, where patients were happy with their diets, though the report on Grenoble admitted that from the viewpoint of nutritional science, this did not show that they were well fed. The happy, ill-informed patient: what every hospital is tempted to wish for. Medical attempts to limit wine consumption, however feeble they were generally, seemed to be paying off. Between 1912 and 1922 the daily consumption of wine in the Grenoblois hospitals dropped from just over 25cl to 18cl. But this modest if significant drop corresponded to declining consumption nationally, which makes it difficult to know whether to praise (or blame) doctors for the drop in hospital wine consumption. A quarter of a century later, wine would be of little significance in an authoritative guide to hospital diets.[88] It was the end of a cycle. The issue of wine drinking by patients would not become a matter of debate on the basis of medical science until about a quarter of a century later, when the elusive French paradox would stimulate interest in a subject that most doctors thought of no scientific importance.

Notes

1. Erwin H. Ackerknecht, *Medicine at the Paris Hospital* (Baltimore: The Johns Hopkins University Press, 1967), 129. The remarks I make about therapeutics at the beginning of this chapter draw on Ackerknecht's analysis, 129–38.
2. Joan Sherwood, 'Syphilization: human experimentation in the search for a syphilis vaccine in the nineteenth century,' *Journal of the History of Medicine and Allied Sciences*, 54 (1999), 371–2; see Ann La Berge and Mordechai Feingold (eds), *French Medical Culture in the Nineteenth Century* (Amsterdam: Rodopi, 1994).
3. Ackerknecht, *op. cit.* (note 1), 129.
4. Michel Foucault, *Naissance de la clinique* (Paris: Presses Universitaires de France, 1963), deals much more successfully than Acknerknecht with this problem in the mutation of medical thought when, e.g., he analyzes the differences between the discourses of Pierre Pomme and A.-L.-J. Bayle. See Ramunas Kondrates, 'The Brunonian Influence on the Medical Thought and Practice of Joseph Frank,' in W. F. Bynum and Roy Porter, editors, *Brunonianism in Britain and Europe* (London: Wellcome Institute for the History of Medicine, 1988), 77, on the 'significant change ... taking place in the perception, description, definition, and ordering of medical knowledge.'
5. Ackerknecht, *op. cit.* (note 1), 133–4.
6. See entry for alkaloids in Clifford A. Hampel and Gessner G. Hawley, editors, *The Encyclopedia of Chemistry* (3d edn, New York: Van Nostrand, 1973).
7. Ackerknecht, *op. cit.* (note 1), 137. See Pierre Boussel et Henri Bonnemain, *Histoire de la pharmacie ou 7000 ans pour soigner*

l'homme (Paris: Editions de la Porte Verte, 1978), 206, for a useful list of men and their discoveries in the 'pharmaceutical arsenal.'

8. See Michel Montignac avec la collaboration du Dr Hervé Robert, *Boire du vin pour rester en bonne santé* (Paris: Flammarion, 1997), 92–4.
9. The *Pharmacopoea Burdigalensis seu descriptio medicamentorum ...* of 1643 was reprinted in 1979. It lists some 300 simple medicaments, mostly from plants, and thirty nine mineral products. On the Parisian debate see Allen G. Debus, *The French Paracelsians. The Chemical Challenge to Medical and scientific Tradition in Early Modern France* (Cambridge: Cambridge University Press, 1991), ch. 3, especially 95–99.
10. Boussel et Bonnemain, *op. cit.* (note 7), 244.
11. *Codex, pharmacopée française* (Paris: Béchet, 1837), 290–97. The simple medicinal wines were each based on a substance such as absinth, gentian, quiquina, and squill; the compound wines included two opium wines and an anti-scorbutic wine. A section on medicinal vinegars follows that on wines.
12. 'Vins médicinaux,' in *Codex* 1866, 394–9. The work also contains information on *alcoolatures* and *alcoolats.*
13. The *Codex* of 1884 also reduced by two thirds the digitalis in the famous compound digitalis wine (diuretic) of Trousseau, turning it into the 'vin de digitale composé de l'Hôtel-Dieu.' The 'vin diurétique de la Charité' contained no digitalis.
14. Emile Mauriac, *Le vin au point de vue médical. Sa composition chimique, ses propriétés thérapeutiques, ses indications et ses contre-indications dans le traitement des maladies* (Paris: Doin, 1903), 22.
15. The *Codex medicamentarius gallicus* of 1908 was revised by a committee including representatives of the Paris faculty of medicine, the school of pharmacy (by then part of the University of Paris), the veterinary school of Alfort, and the hospitals of Paris. The power and prestige of the University of Paris was symbolized by the president of the committee, the director of higher education, Louis Liard.
16. See Jack Pickleman, M. D., 'A glass a day keeps the doctor ...,' *The American Surgeon,* 56 (1990), 397.
17. Salvatore P. Lucia, M. D., *A History of Wine as therapy* (Philadelphia: Lippincott, 1963), 148–53.
18. William Buchan, *Domestic Medicine. A Treatise on the Prevention and Cure of Diseases, by regimen and simple medicines* (London: J. Smith, 1803; London, n.d., a new Stereotype edition), 540.
19. Lucia, *op. cit.* (note 17), 148–153.
20. *Ibid.*, 198–199.

21. *Codex medicamentarius gallicus - pharmacopée française* (1866; 1884; 1908; 1911; 1926 - supplement; 1937; 1949). See also E. Leclair, *Ce qui intéresse les médecins* (1908), and A. Andouard, *Les nouveautés du Codex de 1908* (Paris: Baillière, 1910).
22. J.-L. Alibert, *Nouveaux élémens de thérapeutique et de matière médicale...* (Paris: Béchet jeune, 1826, 3 vols.), iii, 136–7.
23. Georges Durand, *Vin, vigne et vignerons en lyonnais et beaujolais* (Lyon: Presses Universitaires de Lyon, 1979), 26–7.
24. Patricia E. Prestwich, *Drink and the Politics of Social Reform: Antialcoholism in France since 1870* (Palo Alto, CA: The Society for the Promotion of Science and Scholarship, 1988), 48.
25. A. Richerand, *Des erreurs populaires relatives à la médecine* (Paris: Caille et Ravier, 1812), 115–8, 271–3. In his *Histoire des progrès recens de la chirurgie* (Paris: Béchet, 1825), Richerand, who devised the chest operation named after him, was listed as professeur d'opérations de chirurgie à la Faculté de Médecine de Paris as well as chirurgien en chef de l'Hôpital Saint-Louis.
26. J.-A. Salgues (Médecin et professeur d'anatomie et de physiologie à l'Institution académique des nations européennes, etc.), *Hygiène des vieillards ou conseils aux personnes qui ont passé l'âge de cinquante ans* (Paris: Méquignon-Marvis, 1817), 115–26.
27. Fourcroy, *L'art de connoître et d'employer les médicamens dans les maladies qui attaquent le corps humain* (Paris: Simon et Nyon, 1785), ii, 47–8.
28. *Traité de matière médicale* (2 vols, Paris: Brosson, 1818), 3d edn, revised, corrected, and expanded with notes and formulas of the new *Codex pharmaceutique* by P.-H Nysten. The first edition of 1805 carried a forty-page preface by Schwilgué. Section on alcohol and wines, i, 363–8.
29. See, e.g., Adolphe-Benestor Lunel, *Dictionnaire universel de médecine* (3 vols., Paris: Chez l'auteur, 1861-3); *Nouveau dictionnaire de médecine et de chirurgie pratiques,* edited by Bernutz, Richet, A. Tardieu, Troussseau, etc. – (Paris: Baillière, vol. i appeared in 1864 and vol. 39 in 1886); and *Dictionnaire encyclopédique des sciences médicales,* vol. i, A - ADE, (Paris: P. Asselin), edited by Raige-Delorme et A. Dechambre with L. Lereboullet taking over in 1886, when the monster work was in its fifth series.
30. A. Bouchardat, *Traité d'hygiène publique et privée basée sur l'étiologie* (Paris: Alcan 1887), 3rd ed. Bouchardat's *De la glycosurie ou diabète sucré, son traitement hygiénique* (Paris: Baillière, 1875) was for a period the best work on the diabetic diet.
31. *Lancet* (August 15, 1868), 645.

32. 'The *Lancet* Commission of the Medical Use of Wines,' *ibid.* (June 26, 1880), 1001–03; *ibid.* (July 3, 1880), 17; *ibid.* (July 24, 1880), 145–7; *ibid.* (Oct. 23, 1880), 660–1.
33. *Ibid.* (June 26, 1996), 1002.
34. The quotation is from *ibid.* (June 26, 1880), 1001.
35. *Ibid.* (June 26, 1880), 1001.
36. *Ibid.* (June 26, 1880), 1001–2. See also *ibid.* (July 3, 1880), 17, on comparing two white burgundies, similar in terms of chemical analysis though one was far superior to the other and consequently serving different clinical purposes. Often the clinical use of the wine was based on elements established by analysis.
37. *Ibid.* (July 24, 1880), 145.
38. On the classification of red bordeaux into *premiers*, *deuxièmes*, and *troisièmes crus* or growths, see Edmund Penning-Rowsell, *The Wines of Bordeaux* (4th edn, London: Penguin Books, 1979), p. 228, and David Peppercorn, *Bordeaux*, (London: Faber and Faber, 1982), chapter 3, 'Classifications old and new.'
39. The *Lancet*'s commission judged these to be total solids, grape-sugar, fixed acid, volatile acid, tannin, and absolute alcohol by weight and by volume. An analysis of the second growth Saint-Estèphe wine Cos d'Estournel gave the following results:
    In 100 vols.

Total solids	1.93
Grape-sugar.	.09
Fixed acid	.35
Volatile acid	.22
Tannin	.24
Absolute alcohol	
by weight	9.29
by volume	11.52

40. The commission used the terms white claret and red claret for the dry white and red wines of Bordeaux. *Lancet* (July 24, 1880), 146–7. The commisssion stated that 'The seven analyses which we have given as typical of wines of different degree, from the high-priced classified samples to the cheapest *vin ordinaire*, show a difference of only 1.3 per cent. by volume of absolute alcohol (from 10.21 volumes to 11.52), of .1 per cent. in tannin, of .05 per cent. of grape-sugar, and .7 per cent. of fixed acid, whilst the sum of total solids only varies from 1.64 to 2.14 parts in 100 volumes.'
41. Louis Hébert, 'Boissons,' *Nouveau Dictionnaire de Médecine et de chirurgie pratiques* (Paris: Bailliére, 1864; 1886), v, 330–1; for a

history of research on bouquet, see Harry W. Paul, *Science, Vine and Wine in Modern France* (Cambridge: Cambridge University Press, 1996), 306–10.

42. These figures are from Alphonse Chevallier and Er. Baudrimont, *Dictionnaire des altérations et falsifications des substances alimentaires* (4th edn, 1875); they were used by Michel Lévy in his *Traité d'hygiène publique et privée* (Paris: Baillière, 1879), 2 vol., 6th edn, i, 838.
43. *Lancet* (July 24, 1880), 146.
44. *Ibid.* (March 3, 1883), 370.
45. 'Analysis of Crémant du roi (Saumur Veuve Amiot),' *Ibid.* (1905), 32-3. The analysis gives the alcohol by weight and by volume, the extractives, mineral matter, volatile acidity reckoned as acetic acid, fixed acidity reckoned as tartaric acid, sugar, and ethers reckoned as ethyl acetate. *Ibid.* (1905), 367, gives an analysis of Offley's 'Duke' Very Old Port.
46. *Ibid.* (July 24, 1880), 146.
47. See Paul, *op. cit.* (note 41), 144, 148–51.
48. *Lancet* (July 24, 1880), 146.
49. *Ibid.* (July 24, 1880), 146.
50. See Paul, *op. cit.* (note 41), chapter 8.
51. For a brief description of the six regions (from north to south: Chablis and the Auxerrois, the Côte de Nuits, the Côte de Beaune, the Côte Chalonnaise, the Mâconnais, and the Beaujolais), see Anthony Hanson, *Burgundy* (London: Faber and Faber, 1982), 17–23.
52. *Lancet* (Oct. 23, 1880), 661.
53. *Ibid.*
54. *Ibid.*
55. *Ibid.*
56. *Ibid.*
57. *Ibid.*
58. *Ibid.* (July 3, 1880), 17.
59. *Ibid.*
60. *Ibid.* The percentage of absolute alcohol in the 1870 Montrachet was 12.08 by weight and 14.93 by volume.
61. *Ibid.* (June 26, 1880), 1002.
62. *Ibid.*
63. 'The Wine-Store versus the Gin-Palace,' *Ibid.* (August 15, 1868), 227.
64. *Ibid.* (1862), 398.
65. *Ibid.* (1864), 562.

66. *Ibid.* (1860), 592.
67. 'Medical annotations,' *ibid.* (1860), 177.
68. See *infra*, chapter 5, on pathogenic disorders caused by plastered wine, and *Lancet* (Feb. 12, 1870), 241.
69. J. L. W. Thudichum and August Dupré, *A Treatise on the Origin, Nature and Varieties of Wine, being a Complete Manual of Viticulture and Oenology* (London: Macmillan, 1872). See also Thudichum, *On Wines, their Production, Treatment and Use* (London: W. Trounce, 1873) and *A Treatise on Wines* (London: G. Bell, 1894). Wine was not the only liquid on which Thudichum was an expert: see *A Treatise on the Pathology of the Urine* (London: Churchill, 1877).
70. Julian Jeffs, *Sherry* (London: Faber and Faber, 1961; 4th edn, 1992), 92.
71. *Lancet* (April 27, 1872), 600.
72. *Lancet* (Feb. 12, 1870), 241
73. Jeffs, *op.cit.* (note 70), 171–3, 270–1; Jeffs also includes the analysis made for the lees.
74. Anstie, 'On the Theory of Alcoholic Stimulation in Pyrexial Diseases,' *Lancet* (Jan. 25, 1868).
75. 'Composition chimique et valeur diététique des vins,' *Revue de la société scientifique d'hygiène alimentaire*, vii (1909), 361-90; translated from *The Hospital* ...(15 June 1907).
76. Jacques Tenon, *Mémoires sur les hôpitaux de Paris* (Paris: Royez, 1788), 1.
77. *Régime alimentaire des hôpitaux et hospices civils de Paris* (1825), copy in the Archives de l'Assistance publique - Hôpitaux de Paris.
78. *Règlement sur le régime alimentaire des hôpitaux et hospices civils de Paris, approvée par le Ministre de l'Intérieur, le 30 novembre 1841,* copy in the Archives de l'Assistance publique - Hôpitaux de Paris.
79. Gustave Mesureur, 'Le régime alimentaire des hôpitaux et hospices,' *La revue philanthropique*, xx (1906), 120–29.
80. *Ibid.*, 120.
81. 'Le régime alimentaire dans les hôpitaux de Paris,' *La revue philanthropique,* xi (1902), 630–32.
82. 'Projet de règlementation nouvelle du régime alimentaire dans les hôpitaux ...' (12 July, 1901), copy in the Archives de l'Assistance publique - Hôpitaux de Paris.
83. See Dr Antony Rodiet, 'Les enfants alcooliques,' *La revue philanthropique*, xi (1902), 654–73.
84. See Emile Zola, *Le ventre de Paris* (Paris: Fasguelle, 1873).
85. René Gaultier, 'La détermination du régime alimentaire pour les établissements d'assistance publique', *La revue philanthropique*, 42

(1921), 24–30.

86. *Ibid.*, 27–30.
87. Conseil supérieur de l'Assistance publique: report by M. Brizon, session of 31 January 1924. Two annexes contain the reports by Labbé for the hygiene council and Dr. Hermite on Grenoblois hospitals. Document in the Archives de l'Assistance publique - Hôpitaux de Paris .
88. *Guide de diététique hospitalière* (Paris: Carnet de l'économe, 1946), by Dr J. Trémolières (head of the nutrition section at the Institut national d'hygiène) and Thérèse Dupont (dietitian).

PART III

IATROGENIC TALES

5. The Debate over the Pathogenic Nature of Plastered Wine

6. Debates over Wine Alcohol, Prussian blue, and Sulphur Dioxide

5

The Debate Over the Pathogenic Nature of Plastered Wine

Wine is a living liquid susceptible to many diseases. Since antiquity producers and sellers have added various substances to wine to keep it in a healthy state. But a healthy wine does not necessarily make a healthy consumer. Some of the wine additives have been suspected of harming consumers and others have been identified as downright dangerous to consume in any quantity. Two of the most controversial additives have been sulphur dioxide and Prussian blue or potassium ferrocyanide. But the great medico-scientific debate relating to wine consumption in the nineteenth century was over plastering the wine, which really refers to sprinkling plaster on the grape crush. We have seen how, in the 1870s, Thudichum stirred up English sherry drinkers by drawing attention to the chemical practices of the master mixers of Jerez. This briefly famous medical chemist claimed that dusting the crush with plaster and fumigating the casks with sulphur produced a dangerous amount of sulphuric acid in the wine. Thudichum's muddled research and his errors were soon exposed, but he was on to a hot topic in the drink business and had made a bumbling entry into a drama that had been playing in France for twenty years.[1]

In the late-nineteenth century the legal manipulation of plastering wine generated a serious debate, which ended in a discussion of the functioning of the liver, an organ of great importance and even greater sensitivity in a wine drinking society. Plaster of Paris or calcined gypsum is a white powder consisting essentially of calcium sulphate. Pro-plastering propaganda claimed that since antiquity Mediterranean wine makers had been sprinkling plaster on the grapes before pressing them. It seems, however, that plastering is really a recently invented tradition, a convenient historical fiction for innovators who did not wish to alarm consumers about a new additive to wine. And it may be irrelevant to quote Falstaff on lime in the sack.[2] It is still legal to add calcium sulphate to wine.[3] The accepted reasons for its use at mid-nineteenth century were that it produced a total fermentation in a shorter time than without the use of plaster, increased the acidity of the wine (important for the low acid wines of southern climes), brightened up the colour, clarified the wine quickly, preserved the wine, and made its transport easier. Some of these justifications were aesthetic, but some concerned the protection of the health of the wine, thereby making the addition of plaster a useful sanitary measure in food production. Although there has been some debate recently over sulphured wine, the debate over the salubrity of plastered wine gradually disappeared along with the practice. Yet it was a great affair in its day, involving major economic interests (wine producers in the Midi), various levels of government, the consultative committee of public hygiene, the Academy of medicine, and a pack of scientists, especially the viticultural luminaries of Montpellier.

The investigation of the practice of plastering wine was part of a general concern for public health that had animated governments, professional classes, and especially the medical profession since at least the Restoration, and, in some ways, since the old regime.[4] The impetus to debate, the consultative institutions, the regulative bureaucratic mechanisms, and the government's will to act on the basis of a professionally defined concept of public health might all have had their roots established before Second Empire, but the beginnings of experimental investigation to provide a scientific basis for the implementation of governmental regulations for the protection of public health began after 1848 and ran on into the Second Empire. It is not unreasonable to claim that since the 1850s it has been recognised that using too much plaster produces a controversial if not dangerous level of potassium sulphate in the wine.[5]

The argument that plastering and sulphuring wine are empirical procedures carried out since antiquity implies that they are safe. When these practices were called into question, the winemakers called upon experts to show that their opponents were wrong, even if they could not show that winemakers were right, or at least to show that their plastered wine was not poisoning the public. As early as the mid-1850s the chamber of commerce of Montpellier was worried enough about plastering to constitute a scientific committee to answer the important and accusatory questions of the day about plastering the harvest. A professor of general chemistry and toxicology of the faculty of medicine (J. E. Bérard), and professors of chemistry of the faculty of sciences (G. Chancel), and of the school of pharmacy (B. Chauvy) examined the issues. Perhaps the most serious worry of the winegrowers of the Hérault was that the army would decide that the plastered wine the department supplied to the soldiers posed a health risk. In November 1853 the ministry of war asked the Commission supérieure et consultative des substances militaires to see if plastered wines were a health threat and to formulate its proposals quickly. Michel Lévy, one of the big names in military medicine, and A.-B. Poggiale were given the job of quickly carrying out experiments in the laboratory of the military Hôpital du Val-de-Grâce (Paris). Though the commission did not come up with anything new on the subject, Lévy wrote a report recommending that the army avoid buying plastered wines, at least until the Comité consultatif d'hygiène publique could carry out a related investigation being requested by the ministry of the interior. Lévy repeated the sinister observation made by the prefect of the Pyrénées-Orientales that plastering was widespread in his department though the winegrowers themselves drank unplastered wine.[6] The one general question tormenting the chamber of commerce was whether adding the plaster could give 'deleterious qualities' to the wine, thus 'constituting a fraud punishable by law.'

In a short masterpiece of scientific reasoning, the chemists gave the chamber the answer it hoped for: plastering, as generally practiced in the Midi, could not make wine harmful to the health of the consumer.[7] The basis for this answer was a series of experiments of pre-Pasteurian simplicity that concentrated exclusively on wine's inorganic substances. Since adding calcined gypsum or plaster to wine did not alter its organic composition — a big but reasonable assumption for the science of the period — all that the experiment required was to compare the inorganic substances of a natural wine with those of a plastered wine.

Although confident in their science and certain of the innocuity of plastered wine, the experimenting professors recognised that a serious criticism could be levelled at their work. They had worked with fully fermented wine whereas in the real world winemakers sprinkled plaster on the grapes before the wine was made. This difference between laboratory science and the world of production was the basis of a common criticism of science when it was used to justify new laws and regulations. Bérard and his colleagues had a simple and effective reply to this criticism. 'The principles of science authorise us to think that from the viewpoint considered in this operation, the results would be the same in both cases.'[8] In cases where the courts had asked them for analyses of plastered wines of producers, the researchers found the wines the same in composition as those that had contact with plaster for only a few days, as in their experiment. In fact, in two cases the action of the plaster was not so complete as in the experiments. To be exempt from all criticism, the team planned to carry out experiments directly on the next harvests. Viticulture was turning into a profitable area of research for scientists. And the supposedly ancient practice of plastering the harvest would be a topic of intense medical and scientific debate as the nineteenth century moved into its final quarter.

Plastering wine was an issue that divided politicians, bureaucrats, doctors, and scientists nearly as soon as it became a quasi-public issue. Discussion of the practice took place in the national society of agriculture in 1857, when its bad effects were talked about, and in 1860, when reference was made to the opinion of Victor Rendu, author of the classic *Ampélographie française* (1854 and 1857), that plastering is an unnecessary practice. Rendu pointed out that one skilled winegrower-oenologist produced good wines without adding plaster or salt, which was also a conventional and still legal preservative.[9] After 1856 the Comité consultatif d'hygiène took the matter under consideration. Its recommendation to the government led the ministry of justice to issue a circular (25 July 1858) saying that in the current state of scientific knowledge and given the data available on plastering, neither chemical analysis, nor induction, nor direct experience could justify considering traditional plastering, in comparison with other procedures, as causing 'appreciable health trouble.' This opinion was reassuring, especially for producers and their politicians. But the reassurance was not contagious. The old suspicions and doubts festered into new quarrels over the salubrity of the process and further expert investigations of its effects. And it was not long before the research of Bérard and his colleagues was challenged by other scientists.

It is probably of some significance that plastering was a relatively new process in the Midi, spreading in the Hérault only after 1849 under the banner of a 'new method of vinification.'[10] So the debate over its safety was contemporaneous with its rather rapid diffusion, which is best explained by its success in making wine a better commercial product. A better consumer product is often another matter, and is of less concern to producers for the mass consumption market. It seems that the hygiene committee itself was not fully convinced of the safety of the procedure because it proposed that the government carry out an investigation in viticultural departments through hygiene and health committees or councils with the help and supervision of agricultural societies. Perhaps this set-up was not a case of asking the fox to look after the chickens, but of introducing a balanced system of investigating a controversial subject. Adumbrating the whole discussion was the fact that, as Hippolyte Marty pointed out, 'competent men were disturbed' because it was known that plastering does modify the chemical composition of wine.[11] This fact would be at the core of a long debate in public health.

In a circular (1858) to the *procureur-général* giving the opinion of the hygiene committee, the minister of justice said that it was useful to take account of the committee's scientific solution to the problem. But no matter how much research had been done, no clear answer had yet emerged on whether plastered wine was a threat to the consumer's health. Finding a lack of agreement between experts, politicians and governments were free to endorse the views of the people with political clout in winegrowing regions. Scientific reports could also be selectively exploited for partisan purposes. Indeed, it might be easily argued that some scientific reports were written to support clearly defined constituencies.

No one was more critical of plastered wine than Michel Lévy.[12] His arguments against the wine and its scientific supporters summed up the case for the opposition. Plastered wine was bad wine that would be undrinkable by the time it reached consumers if it were not treated. Winegrowers were reported not to plaster the wine they drank themselves, though supposedly an anguished agrégé of the faculty of medicine and pharmacy in Montpellier had to stop drinking the plastered wine given to him by his father-in-law, a winegrower in the Aude.[13] In plastered wine the beneficial salt potassium tartrate was replaced by potassium sulphate, 'an irritating and purgative salt, which was not even used therapeutically.' Lévy identified potassium tartrate as one of the most characteristic elements of the natural composition of wine. In order not to deceive the consumer, plastered wines should not be sold under the label of natural wine. If solid medical evidence on the bad effects of the second salt were lacking in France, it was not the case for Africa, where French military doctors had noticed its irritating and diarrhoea-producing effects. 'No informed doctor will admit that it makes no difference if a drink containing two to six grams of potassium sulphate is introduced into [people's] daily diet.'

Experiments were carried out on alcoholised solutions and on wine already made, but it was not certain that they had any validity for wine made from grapes to which the plaster was added before they were crushed (the standard procedure for making *vins plâtrés*).

Again, a question arose on the relation between science and reality. According to Chancel, known for his work on vinification as well as the chemical constitution of wine, the results would be different because grapes contain eight to nine grams and wine two to 2.5 grams of potassium bitartrate - most of what is 'lost' remains in the *marc* or presscake. Nearly all of the potassium bitartrate in the *marc* is introduced into the wine as bitartrate or acid potassium sulphate. Therefore the acidity of the wine is raised, its colour enhanced, its stability ensured, and its resistance to bacteria increased. In a memoir published in 1866, Chancel found this process very different from adding plaster to wine, a liquid already saturated with potassium bitartrate: 'this salt is transformed into neutral calcium tartrate, which is precipitated, free tartaric acid remaining in dissolution, with all the potassium as neutral sulphate.'[14] No change was found in the acidity of the wine. Chancel's research excited interest among hygienists in confirming the presence of sulphuric acid (in the state of acid potassium sulphate) in traditionally plastered wines. Marty was quick to point out that this was 'the capital point of the question' because it established the potential danger of heavily plastered wines. The tartar of the presscake could release three to four times more potassium and sulphuric acid into these wines than what was contained in natural wine. The hygiene committee could hardly ignore this disturbing news.[15]

About ten years after Chancel's results were published, the Conseil de santé des armées convinced the ministry of war to modify its decision of 1859, which had permitted up to 4 grams of potassium sulphate per litre in army wine. Since on-going research changes the basis of scientific and medical advice on issues, it is not necessarily a bad thing that bureaucracies proceed cautiously and slowly in their actions. Medicine seems particularly vulnerable to the danger of repenting at leisure if it proceeds with haste. After 1876 army wine could contain only two grams of potassium sulphate per litre. The army's decision may have intensified, if it did not precipitate, a flurry of medico-legal activity concerning plastered wine. Some courts in trying suits over the excess of potassium sulphate in wine accepted the two-gram limit of 1876 while others referred to the four-gram limit of 1858. Once the danger of large amounts of potassium sulphate became known, afflicted consumers started bringing lawsuits against merchants who sold them the plastered wines. Courts in Grenoble, Vienne, Melun, and Paris condemned excessive plastering. Other courts, like the tribunal of Montargis (Loiret), falling back on the ministerial circular of 1858

(21 July), accepted the harmlessness of plastered wines.

Typical of the cases coming before the courts was that of Madame L, landowner in Orbec (Calvados). Her doctor asked a pharmacist to analyse a wine that he suspected of causing early symptoms of poisoning in his patient. Madame L had heart trouble. After drinking this wine, supplied by a departmental wine merchant, her palpitations increased. She also became dyspepsic with a considerable loss of weight. Stopping the wine stopped the sickness. The pharmacist found the wine to be normal in appearance and taste, although after swallowing a sample, he felt a constriction of the throat and a sensation of very intense heat in the epigastrium. In testing the wine for fuchsine, added alcohol, alun, and plaster, he found that it contained the enormous amount of 6.226 grams of potassium sulphate per litre. This salt could reasonably be assumed to be the cause of Madame L's palpitations and dyspepsia, especially if she drank a litre a day, which was not then regarded as an excessive amount for a serious moderate drinker.[16]

Medical opinion shifted increasingly against plastering after the 1860s. In 1879 the hygiene committee took up again the issue of plastered wines: innocuous or harmful? Taking into account the research done since 1862, the committee decided that it was time to change its opinion. The committee unanimously adopted a report accepting the idea that the daily use of wine with 'a certain quantity of potassium sulphate has a bad effect on the digestive system.' The report, written by Legouest, an army surgeon, took into account people's complaints about plastered wines and the fact that this salt (acid potassium sulphate), unlike neutral potassium sulphate, was rejected in therapeutics as one of the worst purgatives of the *materia medica.*[17] The committee recommended that the amount of potassium sulphate, whatever its origin, be limited to two grams per litre of wine. Legouest admitted that the recommendation was a matter of 'scientific supposition' based on what was medically accepted about the action of the salt on the body. Medical observation of the phenomenon was difficult, for the 'indispositions caused by the use of plastered wines were usually minor enough to be treated by the drinkers themselves.'

In medical experiments it is difficult to establish clear-cut connections between diet and disease. So the hygiene committee was probably wise in its prudent recommendation that people limit their intake of potassium sulphate. Over a century later we follow the same principle. Although no clear experimental link has been established 'between fat intake and the risk of breast cancer' or even heart disease, it seems reasonable for medical researchers to advise us to avoid pigging out on fatty foods.[18] In the case of advising the government to limit the amount of potassium sulphate in wine, the hygiene committee took into account the peremptory nature of its arguments and the requirements of the wine industry. The health of the consumer was not likely to suffer unduly from the political necessity of the committee to avoid an absolute proscription of *plâtrage*.

Pro-plasterers were dealt a heavy blow in the 1880s by the chemist Magnier de la Source, who, like many other scientists, was willing to accept *plâtrage* because of its commercial advantages provided that it resulted in no more than two grams of potassium sulphate per litre of wine. In establishing the chemical composition of 200 wines of current consumption in Paris, he found forty per cent to be heavily plastered and seventeen per cent dangerously plastered, up to nearly three and nearly six grams per litre respectively.[19] In spite of his acceptance of the process, Magnier de la Source was emphatic on the dangers of prolonged consumption of heavily plastered wines, especially those rich in alcohol and tartaric acid, which produce free sulphuric acid in a dangerous drink also loaded with potassium sulphate. Hardly anyone was idealistic enough to call for the banning of plastering. Most participants in the debate hoped for regulation of the process and a law enforcing the limit of two grams per litre.[20] Most scientists and doctors can live with the idea that the ingestion of small amounts of commercially convenient additives does not threaten public health, that is, most consumers.

The general plastering inquiry of 1884, carried out by the ministry of commerce operating through the prefects, produced 652 documents for the hygiene committee to study. The ministry wanted to know whether the opinions of various commercial and business organisations (including wine dealers), and health councils could provide the basis for the committee to modify its previous recommendation. The ministry was probably disappointed, for the committee, upholding its three previous reports, stuck to its opinion that there should be a legal limit of two grams of potassium sulphate per litre of wine. Out of the 652 organisations consulted, 550 gave their opinion, with seventy per cent favouring the limit of two grams per litre. Another forty seven bodies were against any kind of plastering. Only commercial organisations were against the limit, but not overwhelmingly, while agricultural and especially hygiene councils were strongly against *plâtrage*.

The report of the hygiene committee was written by Richard, professor at the Val-de-Grâce hospital.[21] He gave a great deal of supplementary information on the well-known medical lore concerning the effects of plastered wines on the organism. Both popular and medical opinion attributed a series of digestive disasters to the consumption of plastered wine ('accidents de superpurgation, coliques, diarrhées répétées, indispositions, maux d'estomac assez sérieux, un pyrosis, dyspepsie, affections chroniques viscérales'). 'The digestive tube is kept in a permanent state of irritation.' Like Bussy earlier, Dr. Duval of the hygiene council of Arles experimented on himself and his family. He drank daily a litre of plastered wine containing 2.5 grams of potassium sulphate. The expected symptoms appeared. Duval observed the same symptoms in other consumers of plastered wine. The producer and seller of the wine, Dr. Bouzinac, used to make a special vat of unplastered wine for his personal consumption.[22]

By the late-1880s Germany and the Swiss canton of Zurich were sufficiently convinced of the dangers of plastered wine to impose legal limits on its sale. More serious, at least as an example for France, was the Italian defection from the plastering camp in 1887, when Italy imposed a limit of two grams of potassium sulphate per litre of wine. Although in France the measure had been long advocated and even decreed, the political reasons for a delay in its implementation put French wine producers in the same category as their fellow producers in Portugal and Spain, countries that also had no legal limits on plastering. When in 1887 the Spanish ambassador to France protested that a limit of two grams per litre would discriminate against French importation of Spanish wines, especially sherry, the government turned once more for advice to the hygiene committee.

The committee's report, written by Dr. Gabriel Pouchet, pointed out that it was less the famous sherry wines that would be affected than the cheap, highly coloured, alcoholic reds used in France for *coupage* or mixing with *piquettes* and raisin wine. If they were kept out, all the better. Besides, the good wines of Spain, those that could compete easily against the wines of the Midi, had no need of excessive plastering. Pouchet's report gave the committee another opportunity to reiterate its recommendation of a two-gram limit on potassium sulphate, now supported by 229 provincial hygiene councils and 129 agricultural organisations. The minister of commerce then declared another delay (of a year's duration) while waiting for action to be taken on yet another inquiry on *plâtrage.*

This was to be an inquiry with considerable scientific clout, based on research by top people in the faculties at Montpellier and, as requested by the minister of agriculture, orchestrated by its Ecole nationale d'agriculture (E.N.A.M.).[23]

The research undertaken by the commission of the Montpellier school tried to answer three questions. The first two need not detain us long. Bouffard analysed plastered and non-plastered wines of the region to see how much potassium sulphate existed in each category of wine. He was surprised to find that wines producers gave him as unplastered wines could contain substantial amounts of the suspected salt. In analysing this work, Marty found that the source of Bouffard's odd results was in believing the winemakers.[24] Between 1865 and 1878 Marty and a colleague (Coulier) had analysed ninety two wine samples guaranteed to be pure. They found that sixty five of the samples were unplastered. One has to believe the analysis, not the declaration of a winemaker intent on fooling the researcher in order to show the similarity if not the complete identity of the two categories of wine.

Is plastering really useful in winemaking? This was the second question taken up by the commission and answered positively by the viticulturalist Gustave Foëx in the second part of the report. Since the historical use of plaster was part of the scientific case in favour of the additive, Foëx made customary if careless use of the authority of Pliny, who was often misquoted to justify commercially convenient winemaking practices. A more careful reading of Pliny showed that he was far from approving the practices of his time for correcting faults in wine or denaturing it.[25]

Foëx's position as head of the national school of agriculture in Montpellier, source of agronomic enlightenment in the Midi, probably influenced his views. Most of the winemakers in the Aude, the Pyrénées-Orientales, and the Hérault, and some in Provence, as well as most of those in Spain, Southern Italy, Greece, and Algeria were convinced plasterers. Their political, commercial, and professional representatives made sure that national institutions were keenly aware of their views. But even at the departmental level in France, medical and public health opinion and even political opinion were not necessarily prisoners of the self-proclaimed economic interest of the winemakers. This became clear in a vote of six to four against *plâtrage* in the health conscious Conseil général of the Gard in 1884, but in 1887 the council returned to political orthodoxy on the issue when the departmental society of agriculture and Foëx asked for its (new) opinion and was not disappointed to find that it then accepted plastering. The high priests of scientific objectivity asked for political support and by coming up with the right results showed that they deserved it.

Foëx's arguments were heavily supported by scientific references, some to research that was peripheral to his pro-plastering position.[26] Audoynaud's experiments on the favourable role of plaster in fermentation gave Foëx some support for the view that plastering was 'a useful and sometimes indispensable operation' in the Midi. Marty and other enemies of unlimited plastering were able to use the same experimental results in favour of the position that there should be a limit of two grams of potassium sulphate per litre of wine. The argument that plastering was indispensable could at best be applied only to wine produced, especially in years of bad weather, in low, humid vineyards, which is where most Midi wine was produced after phylloxera destroyed the vines on the hillsides. The new wine was a product for mass consumption, produced by big companies and shipped to the cities by the railroads, essentially the same economic forces that supported the attempt to eradicate phylloxera by the use of pesticides. And even in the case of this wine Audoynaud showed that there was no need for plastering more than would result in exceeding the limit of two grams per litre.

Anti-plasterers could also point to the fact that non-plastered wine was produced for those people who did not want to drink the standard stuff. One of the best known producers in the Hérault, Gaston Bazille, gave up plastering, without any drop in the quality of his wine, after a client offered him a higher price for unplastered wine. It was commonly accepted that the fine wines of Bordeaux and Burgundy could not be plastered without modifying their taste. This argument was irrelevant to the mass market situation in Paris, where cut or mixed wines were the rule and most people's taste was undiscriminating. In Bordeaux and Burgundy, according to Marty, people were still used to drinking natural wine. In the second half of the nineteenth century many people got used to drinking plastered wine, which in 1887 was declared by the Cour d'appel de Montpellier not to be natural wine. Since Chaptal's rejection of the possibility of a natural model for wine, few scientists had accepted the idea that a fermented and manipulated product like wine could be called a natural product, even though that term might be ambiguous. And perhaps Foëx and his scientific band were also convinced that the law would sooner or later conform to the science of the pro-plasterers.

The third part of Foëx's report dealt more directly with plastered wine as an issue in public health: was drinking such wine really dangerous, as claimed by the members of the hygiene committee and many others? An effective use of the word 'really' seemed to imply that opponents of the process were not dealing with reality, the territory of science. Foëx declared that only a series of medical experiments based on modern scientific methods could answer the question. In his memoir on these 'clinical experiments,' Dr. Bourdel, the physician at E.N.A.M., noted that all conclusions were previously based on 'reasonable guesses,' with comparisons being made, in experiments on animals, between the more or less toxic action of potassium salts or similar salts. Sometimes sick people who were given the salts as remedies were also observed. 'Never before,' boasted Bourdel, 'has one had the occasion to experiment directly on the physiological and toxic action of determined doses' on people drinking plastered wine for a prolonged period.[27] One admirable aspect of this gastrointestinal experiment was that the agricultural school carried it out on its own personnel, including the director. Perhaps a matter of convenience. The school was also an ideal place for the experiment because the personnel it fed were served non-plastered wine. The irony of this situation was not missed by commentators like Marty.

Subjects of the month-long experiment were divided into two groups of ten, with each person drinking a litre of wine daily. Foëx included himself in the group (A) drinking the wine containing four grams of potassium sulphate per litre. When the group began suffering from fatigue, the problem was solved by changing from a wine with thirteen per cent alcohol to one with eight per cent. No significant symptoms were observed in this group that were not observed in the group (B) drinking non-plastered wine. Even two subjects with heart trouble in group A did not have their conditions aggravated. Analyses of the urines of the subjects in group A, done by Audoynaud, showed no significant deviations from the profile of normal urine.[28] From this skimpy data, it could be inferred that no functional trouble was produced because the potassium sulphate was eliminated daily by the kidneys. Foëx concluded that the daily ingestion of 4 grams of potassium sulphate in plastered wine presented no danger for a month and probably for an indeterminate period.

Marty and his commission, unconvinced by the science of Montpellier's national school of agriculture, easily identified numerous weak parts of the report by Foëx as well as the separate memoirs by Bourdel and Audoynaud. Marty also politely called attention to several pieces of shoddy reasoning before moving in for the kill.[29] Since there was overlapping and some repetition in Marty's critique of the different documents, it is more convenient and economical for us to consider the criticisms topically rather than according to each document as Marty does with Bourdel's and Audoynaud's memoirs. The documents were all based on the same research project, of which Marty also made damaging general criticisms.

The two major problems with the experiment were the small number of subjects and the short time of the experiment. How reliable were results based on ten males drinking plastered wine for a month? No one remarked that the study included only men, although women were often listed among the numerous wine drinkers diagnosed as suffering from ailments whose cause was traced to drinking such wine. If more people had been studied over a longer period, it is probable that the results would have generated more confidence. Whether the results could have been any more certain is by no means clear. After all, a recent study of more than 120,000 men and women taking 'large doses' (about 100 international units daily) of vitamin E over more than two years still needs clinical trials to confirm a strongly suggested preventive value in reducing the risk of heart disease.[30] Foëx himself was aware of the shortness of the time allowed for the experiment. Dr. Bourdel was interested in the effect of plastered wines on muscular force even though he admitted that the experimental period was too short for any conclusion; he concluded, however, that the suspected wines did not cause a reduction of muscle power. Marty noted the impossibility of recognising 'in these conditions the morbid phenomena that can slowly attack general nutrition, kidney functioning, and the circulation.'[31]

It became clear that what seemed scientifically solid to the pro-plastering group seemed sloppy science to the anti-plasterers. The experiment may have been done at the wrong time of the year, at the end of winter, when changing temperatures bring big changes in eating habits with accompanying body reactions, which could be confused with the effects of plastered wine on certain phenomena - e.g., body temperature and the elimination of urea. Louis Ravaz, who was in the group drinking non-plastered wine, suffered from a light fever one day because he ate too much salad.[32] This criticism led into a more serious one, a dual criticism in fact. The diet of the subjects was not the same. Nor had the condition of health of the subjects been established in detail at the beginning. And a subject's normal urine was determined by only one analysis. Marty wanted to know if the subjects were usually drinkers of plastered wine, for that would make a difference in their reaction. Marty was not happy that nearly all the subjects were in good health. What would be the effect of plastered wines on people with kidney and liver diseases? (At least one of the two subjects with heart trouble in group A (drinkers of plastered wine) emerged unscathed from the adventure.) Would these sick people eliminate nearly all the potassium sulphate in their urine, like the ten healthy drinkers in group A according to Audoynaud's analysis? For Marty the research of the professor of chemistry was as useless as that of the professor of medicine (Bourdel).

It is not unreasonable to argue that Foëx's experiment turned up some evidence in favour of the toxicity of plastered wine. A lymphatic person in group A found it difficult to get used to the wine. Bourdel blamed excessive alcohol, but after the wine was reduced from thirteen to eight per cent, the difficulty persisted. Marty turned the tables on Foëx and his colleagues here by arguing that one out of ten is something to note. It also turned out that, contrary to Bourdel's claim that no one had significant digestive problems, two other members of group A experienced epigastric pains and colic for a short time. Bourdel thought that he was justified in claiming that none of the subjects on plastered wine had 'appreciable digestive troubles.' It was easy to take another view of the results. When Bourdel moved beyond the Foëx commission's research he noted that a dose of 7.5 grams of potassium sulphate per litre of wine would produce stomach cramps, intestinal colic, and diarrhoea in subjects not used to drinking such wines. If the subject was foolish enough to continue ingesting such a high dose, his body got used to it, Marty was quick to point out that this showed how bad these wines were for the people of northern France, unused to the *vins plâtrés* of the Midi. And was it a good idea to have a daily dose of a substance whose effects were so dangerous at a high dose? It was hard to establish safe limits because the amount of potassium sulphate ingested would vary with the amount of wine drunk.[33]

The hygiene committee accepted the recommendation of Marty's report, which allowed it to uphold its previous position of a limit of two grams of potassium sulphate per litre of wine. It was a compromise between the demands of production and commerce and of hardline defenders of public health. From the 'exclusive viewpoint of hygiene,' no medical group could 'in principle, approve the plastering of wines,' but Marty took into account 'the necessities of production and commerce.'[34] Accepting the commercial argument that moderate *plâtrage* improved the wine, Marty saw the lower limit as an advantage for the consumer. Here was a clear statement of what has become a familiar commercial argument, that additives protect the consumer as well help the seller. The commission thought it better that consumers drink plastered *petits vins* (ordinary wine) than artifical wine made with raisins and sugar, *piquettes*, or simply watered wine. It was estimated in the early-1880s that these 'artificial' wines made up about a third of the approximately sixty million hectoliters of wine consumed annually in France.[35] The Académie de médecine, agreeing with Marty's reasonable compromise, gave its prestigious support to the limit of two grams of potassium sulphate per litre of wine and recommended that the ministry of justice enforce this limit, already stipulated in a governmental circular of 27 July 1880.

The polite protests and reasoned rejections generated in the Midi and even in Bordeaux by Marty's report and its approval by the Académie de médecine show that the doctors and their institution were taken seriously. One of the more curious actions was taken by the Société de pharmacie in Bordeaux. It accepted the experimental work done at the agricultural school in Montpellier and sent a report to the Académie de médecine recommending a limit of four grams of potassium sulphate per litre. Marty was astonished that such a proposition could come from an area famous for its healthy winemaking traditions. This seems to have been a temporary loss of viticultural sanity in Bordeaux, whose oenophilic propaganda had little to do with that of Montpellier. The Bordelais also suggested that heating and filtering might provide a future alternative to plastering as ways to keep the germ count low in wine of the Midi.[36]

The heavy artillery against Marty's report was lined up by the Société centrale d'agriculture de l'Hérault. The two major items were memoirs by Joseph de Girard, a chemist who was professor at the faculty of medicine in Montpellier, and Justin Cot, a member of the Académie de médecine who did a report for the agricultural society of the Hérault. Marty found that most of the arguments were not new and had already been adequately answered ; what was new could be easily refuted by more science. Cot's report, adorned with some creative quoting and full of hasty deductions, was demolished at some length by Marty because it represented the voice of the powerful agricultural society of the Hérault and perhaps also because of Cot's national status as a spokesman for wine in the chamber of deputies. Marty's task was made a little easier by the fact that many producers in the Hérault and the Aude were closer to his position than to Cot's demand for a limit of four grams per litre. After the appearance of Marty's complementary reply to the critics of his report, the Académie de médecine unanimously approved on July 10, 1888, the limit of two grams per litre.[37]

Marty's report was politically definitive, though squabbling and manoeuvring continued for a couple of years. Then on July 11, 1891 the Griffe law imposed a two-gram limit on wines and their liqueurs. Politics invites paradoxes. Griffe, a senator for the Hérault after 1879, was a defender of natural wines against the industrial or artificial wine made from raisins. Adding to wine a substance suspect in the mind of many doctors and scientists was hardly consistent with the gospel of natural wine; no one remembered that Chaptal had pointed out that natural wine itself is a sort of convenient fiction. The limit on potassium sulphate in wine was part of a package providing what might optimistically be called safeguards for consumption. Ten years of determined resistance by the winegrowers of the Midi ended with the adoption of the law of one of their greatest defenders. Wine could be pushed as a *boisson hygiénique* once again, until a debate arose over the effect of even two grams per litre on the the health of the consumer. As in the debate over sulphur in wine, many critics wanted a 'poison' eliminated from wine, not limited in quantity. And of course the debate over the effects of wine alcoholism had already emerged by the end of the nineteenth century. The two debates converged on the etiology of cirrhosis of the liver.

Notes

1. Julian Jeffs, *Sherry* (London: Faber and Faber 1961; 4th edn, 1992), 91–3.
2. It is always possible to find some historical precedents for plastering, however; see, e.g., Jeffs, *op. cit.* (note 1), 170–1, for a reference by Pliny to plastering as an African practice, a discussion in the Castilian Cortes in 1570, etc. Jeffs also points out that it is probable that Shakespeare was not referring to the practice of plastering the crush but to a practice of English vintners and taverners, who 'reduced the acidity of badly made wines ... by adding lime.'
3. Bernard Blanchet, *Code du vin et textes viti-vinicoles français et communautaires* (Montpellier: Ed. de la Journée viticole, 1970), 16. Le décret 55-672 du 20 mai 1955, art. 1er, ajoute: 'En ce qui concerne les moûts: l'emploi du plâtre dans une limite telle que le produit ne renferme pas plus de 2 grammes du sulphate de potasse

ou de soude par litre.'

4. Jacques Léonard, *La médecine entre les pouvoirs et les savoirs* (Paris: Aubier Montaigne, 1981), ch. ix, 'De l'hygiène à l'anthropologie.'
5. L. W. Marrison, *Wine and Spirits* (3d edn, London: Penguin, 1973), 82.
6. M. H. Marty, *Le plâtrage des vins* (Paris: Masson, 1888), 8–9.
7. *Sur le plâtrage des vins*, rapport fait à la chambre de commerce de Montpellier par MM. Bérard, Chancel et Cauvy (Montpellier: C. Coulet, 1856).
8. Bérard *et al, op. cit.* (note 7).
9. *Séance publique annuelle de la Société impériale et centrale d'agriculture de France* (5 août 1860), 36–37.
10. Marty, *op. cit.* (note 6), 7.
11. *Ibid.*, 11. On pages 13–14 Marty analyses a report by Poggiale in the *Journal de pharmacie et de chimie*, 3d series, xxxvi (1859), 164–70, condemning plastering.
12. Michel Lévy, Inspecteur du service de santé de l'armée, was directeur de l'Ecole d'application de médecine et de pharmacie militaires (Val-de-Grâce). His disapproval of plastered wines was repeated in his *Traité d'hygiène publique et privée* (Paris: Baillière, 1879), 6th edn, 2 vols., i, 843.
13. Marty, *op. cit.* (note 6), 73.
14. G. Chancel, *Etude de la composition des vins et des procédés de vinification* (Mémoires de l'Académie des sciences et lettres de Montpellier, 1866).
15. Marty, *op. cit.* (note 6), 20–22.
16. The amount consumed by Madame L was not given by the pharmacist, G. Lugan, in his note, 'Accidents occasionnés par l'usage d'un vin plâtré,' *L'année médicale. Journal de la société de médecine de Caen et du Calvados*, 2e année (1877), 105–107.
17. 'On est loin d'être ... bien renseigné sur l'action que peut exercer, à l'intérieur le sulphate avec excès d'acide sulfurique, sel caustique et d'une saveur acide intolérable lorsqu'il est en dissolution concentrée.' Legouest, *Rapport sur les vins plâtrés* ..., cited in Marty, *op. cit.* (note 6), 24.
18. A recent study found 'no statistically significant relationship between any of the constituents of fat or levels of antioxidants and ... women's chances of having breast cancer or benign breast disease.' *The New York Times* (May 19, 1993), A1, 9. Yet it is probably prudent to include moderate doses of vitamin E in one's diet in order to reduce the risk of heart disease. See 'Vitamin E greatly reduces risk of heart disease, studies suggest,' *The New York Times*

(May 20, 1993). Both articles are by Jane E. Brody. For the scientific basis of the articles, see Meir J. Stampfer and others, 'Vitamin E consumption and the risk of coronary disease in women,' *The New England Journal of Medicine*, 328 (May 20, 1993), 1444–9, and, equally important, the correspondence in *ibid.* (Nov. 4, 1993), 1424–6.

19. Magnier de la Source, 'Le plâtrage des vins, ses avantages, ses dangers,' *Répertoire de pharmacie and Journal de chimie médicale, de pharmacie et de toxicologie*, new series, ix (1881), 357; Marty, *op. cit.* (note 6), 30–33.
20. Magnier de la Source, 'De l'influence du plâtrage sur la composition et les caractères chimiques du vin,' *Journal des connaissances médicales* (January 10 and 11, 1884), 11 and 21.
21. Richard, 'Rapport sur le plâtrage des vins' (15 June 1885), *Recueil des travaux du Comité*, xv (1885), 363; Marty, *op. cit.* (note 6), 33–39.
22. Marty, *op. cit.* (note 6), 37.
23. The commission of E.N.A.M. chosen by the head of the school, Foëx, who was president of the commission, included A. Audoynaud (chemistry), Bouffard (oenology, technology), François Convert (rural economy), André Crova (physics), Pierre Viala (viticulture), Adolphe Bourdel (medicine). From the viewpoint of the history of science, the biggies were Foëx and Viala, though the others were known in their day. See G. Foëx, 'Rapport sur le plâtrage des vins,' *Bulletin du ministère de l'agriculture*, vi (1887), 483–522.
24. Marty, *op. cit.* (note 6), 47–49.
25. Marty cites the Latin text and Littré's translation of Pliny's *Natural History.* An analysis done by Marcelin Berthelot of a wine from the Roman period, discovered near Arles, found no evidence of plastering: 'Ni chlorures, ni sulfates sensibles.' Berthelot, 'Analyse d'un vin antique,' *Journal de pharmacie et de chimie*, 4th series, xxvi (1887), cited in Marty, *op. cit.* (note 6), 56–57; for the citation of Pliny, see 51–52.
26. Dumas' famous memoir on alcoholic fermentation (*Annales de physique et chimie*, 1874), for example. See Marty, *op. cit.* (note 6), 54.
27. Dr. A. Bourdel, *Du plâtrage des vins. Expériences cliniques sur l'homme soumis à l'usage du vin plâtré* (Paris: Coulet, 1888), 4th edn. Bourdel had published forty other items in several areas of medicine by this date.
28. 'Le poids de l'urée et celui des phosphates alcalins et terreux n'ont pas sensiblement varié ...,' quoted in Marty, *op. cit.* (note 6), 64.

29. Two examples: first, misuse of the research by Antoine Rabuteau, who showed that fifteen to twenty grams of potassium sulphate is a toxic dose but speculated that lesser amounts are unhealthy; second, the argument that Bouchardat's solution, used to treat uric gravel, contained eleven grams of potassium salts per litre, the maximum amount ingested daily. Marty observed that, first, the potassium is not in the state of acid sulphate; second, a daily food (plastered wine) cannot be compared to a medicine given for a short period. *Ibid.*, 64–65.
30. Jane E. Brody, 'Vitamin E greatly reduces risk of heart disease, studies suggest,' *The New York Times* (May 20, 1993), A1, 9.
31. Marty, *op. cit.* (note 6), 65. Bourdel's clinical observations were on (1) body weight, (2) temperature, (3) muscular strength, (4) circulatory function, (5) respiration, (6)digestion, and (7) urinary secretion. Bourdel, *op. cit.* (note 27), 17 ff. Marty found all the observations unsatisfactory, with major questions unanswered, whether because of failure to record variations in weight or to explain variations in temperature, etc.
32. 'Un léger état fébrile dû à un abus de salade'. Marty, *op. cit.* (note 6), 66, note 1.
33. *Ibid.*, 68, 70–73. Marty used cases reported by a doctor at the Ecole de médecine de Nantes and by P. Hugounenq, departmental councillor in the Hérault.
34. Ambroise Andouard (corresponding member of the Académie des sciences), 'Le plâtrage des vins,' *Annales d'hygiène et de médecine légale*, 3rd series (1888), cited in Marty, *op. cit.* (note 6), 76.
35. A. Gautier, *La sophistication des vins* (1884), cited in Marty, op. cit. (note 6), 77, note 1. Between 1860 and 1870 annual wine production was 60 to 65 million hl, dropping to 48 million hl in the next decade, and then to 30 to 35 million hl in the early-1880s. Exports dropped by two million hl and imports went up by seven million hl; so if one adds five million hl to a production figure of 35 million hl, the natural wine available in the 1880s was about 40 million hl; this means that about 20 million hl of the annual consumption of about 60 million hl was made up of artificial wines.
36. Marty, *op. cit.* (note 6), 84, note 1.
37. 'Rapport complémentaire,' appendix to Marty, *op. cit.* (note 6), 89–99. Joseph de Girard, 'De la partie chimique du rapport présenté par M. Marty ... (1888, reprinted from the *Bulletin de la Société centrale d'agriculture de l'Hérault.* Dr. Justin Cot, *Observations relatives au rapport de M. Marty* ... (1888, also reprinted from the *Bulletin ... Hérault*). A. Bouffard replied to Marty: 'Remarque sur la

proportion de sulphate de potasse naturel dans les vins non platrés — Réponse au rapport de M. Marty ...,' *Annales de l'Ecole nationale d'agriculture de Montpellier*, iv (1888-9), 174–184 (presented to the Académie de médecine on 5 June 1888).

6

Debates over Wine Alcohol, Prussian Blue, and Sulphur Dioxide

1. Wine alcohol and cirrhosis of the liver

The wine drinker needs a good liver and a steady supply of B vitamins, especially thiamine. Among the liver's many functions are the making of 'clotting factors and other vital proteins that go into blood serum' and the metabolising of alcohol and other drugs.[1] The liver has several potentially deadly enemies, including hepatitis, cancer, and cirrhosis. In western countries cirrhosis or interstitial chronic inflammation of the liver 'most commonly results from chronic heavy intakes of alcohol' rather than from a virus.[2] Though a description of the disease and its alcoholic etiology were given by Matthew Baillie in his work *Morbid Anatomy* ... (1793), the term cirrhosis was introduced in the early-nineteenth century by R. T. H. Laënnec; alcoholic cirrhosis of the liver is named after him – *cirrhose de Laënnec.*[3] By the mid-nineteenth century there was an intense medical interest in cirrhosis. Some of the leading researchers and clinicians of the day did experiments, made observations, and cut out diseased livers to display to their colleagues in learned societies.[4]

Lynn Payer pointed out that the *crise de foie* used to be the French national pathology. Not that the phrase means much any more, except digestive trouble.[5] As a direct factor in contemporary French mortality, cirrhosis of the liver produced by alcoholism puts on only a mediocre performance: in 1974 it stood fifth on the list of chief causes of mortality, causing 3.79 per cent of deaths.[6] Smoking was recently killing about 60,000 people per year, accounting for ten per cent of France's mortality. Alcoholism is blamed for 40,000 deaths a year and costs the state about eighty billion francs annually. Two million people are hooked on the drug alcohol. Nor does the French paradox prevent heart disease from being the primary cause of death in France.

Historians of medicine generally give short shrift to cirrhosis as they take the high whiggish road to topics such as Claude Bernard's discovery of 'the glycogen-forming function of the liver.'[7] But practising nineteenth-century doctors were much more concerned with cirrhosis than with the conversion of excess glucose into glycogen as a food reserve. By the early-twentieth century the debate over types and classifications of cirrhosis had come to a confusing climax. As early as 1897 Desoil had despaired of agreement: 'Each author creates his own cirrhosis: it's anarchy.'[8] Hepatology developed late as a medical science. Nearly a hundred years later, researchers are still seeing through a glass darkly on some aspects of the disease.[9]

In his *Clinical Lectures on Diseases of the Liver* (1868), Charles Murchison noted that cirrhosis, or the so-called gin-drinker's liver 'can almost invariably be traced to the abuse of strong spirits, and especially the habit of drinking them neat, and accordingly it is most common in those countries and towns where such a habit prevails.' By contrast, chronic atrophy was elusive in etiology because it presented 'several diseases, which in their etiology and anatomical characters, are essentially distinct, but which often present symptoms so similar that it may be impossible during life to distinguish them.'[10] Bichat's old Parisian clinical program of opening up a few corpses still had its uses.

In a later work on malfunctioning of the liver (1874), Murchison did not offer much comfort to pro-alcohol doctors. He attributed primary functional derangements of the liver principally to 'errors in diet' and 'various alcoholic drinks,' including wines. In bourgeois Britain it could be claimed that many people were eating more food than needed to maintain the nutrition of the body. 'There can be no doubt that the present system of living, and especially the consumption of even what are regarded as average quantities of rich food and stimulating drinks, contribute largely to derange the liver.' Murchison identified alcoholic drinks as being 'most apt to derange the liver.' They did so in two ways. First, by causing 'persistent congestion of the liver'; even in healthy persons small amounts were capable of producing 'a temporary hepatic congestion.' When alcohol is 'taken in excess, or too frequently, the congestion of the liver becomes permanent and the functions of the organ are deranged.' Long congestion could produce 'structural disease.' And doctors should remember that 'certain persons ... may ... have a constitutional intolerance of alcohol.'[11]

Unlike many French doctors, Murchison did not find that wines had any advantages over pure alcohol; quite to the contrary, they could be more dangerous.[12] Wines and other alcoholic drinks could 'often cause derangement of the liver, which a corresponding quantity of pure alcohol would not produce.' No blame could be placed on 'any one ingredient of the offending liquid – neither by the free acid, the ether, the salts, gum, sugar, nor extractive matter.' There was an identifiable culprit, however: sugar. Murchison here arrived at every scientist's goal, the establishment of a general rule. 'The injurious effect of alcoholic beverages upon the liver increases in a direct ratio with the amount of sugar plus alcohol which they contain.' It was the mixture of sugar and alcohol that did the damage, for larger amounts of sugar or alcohol with food did not produce the same 'injurious results.' Bad news for lovers of famous bourgeois fetishes: Trockenbeerenauslese, Sauternes, Barsac, Banyuls, Port, and all their relatives with high residual sugar. Murchison's experience showed that the alcoholic drinks 'most apt to disagree with the liver are malt liquors of all sorts, but especially porter and the stronger forms of mild ale, port wine, madeira, tokay, malaga, sweet champagne, dark sherries, liqueurs, and brandies, whilst those which are least likely to derange the functions of the organs are claret, hock, moselle, dry sherry, and gin or whiskey largely diluted.' So in the end the doctor was left with the wherewithal to practice alcohol therapy and the drinker had a goodly choice of drinks to produce euphoria safely if they were consumed in moderation.[13] (Murchison would be pleased to learn of the fact revealed by recent research that Californian alcoholics, unlike their counterparts in Paris and New York, have large deposits of iron in their livers. There is a large amount of fructose in the wine consumed by the Californian boozers, and the sugar is a chelating agent making iron more readily available to the liver.)

By the late-nineteenth century the medical community generally agreed on the etiology of cirrhosis in drinkers: it is caused by alcohol. Members of the Académie de médecine were therefore surprised in 1897 to hear one of their most distinguished colleagues deny this dogma. The heretic was Etienne Lancereaux, an expert on alcoholism and a specialist in pathological anatomy. In the opinion of his former students at least, he was a star of the Paris faculty of medicine.[14] How did he arrive at his position of denial? Lancereaux, a keen observer (or constructor) of facts and a formidable clinician, was surprised to find that drinkers suffering from cirrhosis of the liver presented few signs of alcoholic intoxication. His search for an explanation of this anomaly led him to the idea that the cause was the potassium sulphate ingested as a result of excessive wine consumption rather than the abuse of spirits. Somewhat dubious of this general proposition, he added 'at least in France.' Lancereaux's clinical evidence, based on his personal observation of 210 cases of cirrhosis over thirty five years, led him to attribute the disease to various alcoholic excesses, with wine being the sole culprit in sixty eight cases and strongly present with liqueurs, rum, and absinth in 126 others.

Combined excesses of wine and beer accounted for twelve cases and cider for only four. He identified wine as the efficient cause of cirrhosis in Paris, for excessive wine drinking was present in all cases, and wine was often the sole source of the alcohol consumed. Lancereaux's patients drank from two to six litres - usually three litres - of cheap red (the mythic *gros rouge*) at eighty centimes a litre, in a twenty four hour period. To put a proprietary stamp on his discovery Lancereaux wanted to describe his category of cirrhosis as *cirrhose oenolique* or *vinique*. Perhaps he dreamed of eventually being honoured by the invention of a new diagnostic category in hepatology – *cirrhose de Lancereaux*.

Like most medical arguments outside the elite towers of experiment, Lancereaux's case was based on an appealing and reasonable mixture of clinical observation and anecdotal evidence as well as a simple experiment producing what turned out to be ambiguous results. There was the geographical or regional argument. In wine country, where alcoholism was held to be unknown or at least rare, men drank three to four litres of wine daily without signs of intoxication but did end up with cirrhosis, as on the shores of Lac Léman with its seductive *vin d'Ivorne*, the Anjou, and the Vendée (Pays Nantais). Lancereaux found cirrhosis to be relatively rare in Normandy – land of calvados, applejack with fifty per cent alcohol – and Brittany, two areas where there were more drinkers of *eau-de-vie* than of wine. This surprising revelation was backed up with data supplied by his former students. Dr. Baley, practising in Châteaudlin (Finistère), where lots of *eau-de-vie* was guzzled, had not seen a case of cirrhosis in four years. Critics of Lancereaux's thesis would not be long in finding other medical practitioners whose experience would be quite different from that of Dr Baley.

But Lancereaux, a faculty man, also had an experiment up his sleeve to help his argument. It was generally believed that the alcohol in different spirits is the common element causing pathological disorders when people abuse hard liquor. Two distinct diseases could result from that abuse. First, Lancereaux established by clinical observation and discussion with his patients that fatty degeneration or steatosis of the liver is characteristic of the drinker of alcohols. Secondly, he established experimentally that cirrhosis of the liver is special to drinkers of excessive amounts of wine containing potassium sulphate or of sulphated drinks. Normal wine drinking was not implicated here. From 1893 on Lancereaux and his intern in pharmacy (Coturieux) did a set of experiments to see if potassium sulphate causes cirrhosis. Several animals (guinea pigs, rabbits, and dogs) were fed two to seven grams of this salt every twenty four hours.[15] The dogs hated it and died in a state of depression after a period ranging from six to eighteen months. Autopsies showed tumefaction of the liver and the spleen, with the liver changes being identical with those observed in humans as 'cirrhosis of the wine drinker.' He was happy to find that a lifetime's observations were corrobated by experiment: the potassium salt produced the same effect on the livers of animals as he had found in the livers of wine drinkers.

In reviewing the relevant literature (including Ludger Lallemand, Maurice Perrin and Duroy, Dujardin-Beaumetz and Audigé, Strassmann), Lancereaux became even happier because of the contradictory results reported on the effect of alcohol on the liver. Disagreement between colleagues left the way open for his hypothesis on potassium sulphate as the agent in the etiology of cirrhosis. He did not wish this new etiology to result in suspicion being cast on all potassium salts, for the evidence was conclusive only against the sulphates. In emphasising the limitation of their conclusions, scientists hope to achieve a greater certainty and limit spurious squabbling.

French medical research has always been fortunate in having available a large Parisian reservoir of disease. Lancereaux drew attention to the prevalence of cirrhosis among the wine drinkers of Paris, where, he argued, the wine was usually plastered. With four to six grams of sulphate per litre, the wine in Paris could be identified 'as especially responsible' for cirrhosis. The time needed to develop wine cirrhosis could vary greatly according to the quality and quantity of the drink consumed and the profession of the drinker. A labourer in Paris could abuse his liver for ten to fifteen years before being laid low.[16] The younger the drinker, the quicker the disease developed. Lancereaux had successfully treated two five-year old girls for advanced tumefaction of the liver. And on one occasion he cured a retail wine merchant's six-year old son, whose mother had been giving him lots of wine to strengthen him but ended up giving him cirrhosis with ascites instead. Beer with sulphites (compounds containing the radical groups SO_3 or HSO_3, salts of sulphurous acid) and sulphates could also be dangerous if, like the waiters in brasseries, one drank eight to ten litres per day. In Lancereaux's opinion, an effective cure for alcoholic cirrhosis had to be based on avoidance of an excess of wine, particularly plastered wines, which were the most dangerous. So the amounts of plaster and sulphur added to beverages had to be reduced if not prohibited. And certainly another method of preservation had to be found. It seemed that Lancereaux had made a convincing case against potassium sulphate and even cast suspicion on wine itself.

But Lancereaux's case was soon submitted to the merciless scrutiny of his colleagues, who quickly recovered from the shocks of novelty of argument and denial of solid old dogma. The discovery that potassium sulphate in wine causes cirrhosis was soon found to be defective in method and evidence and use of statistics. It was in some ways a typical scientific quarrel.

The criticism of method came chiefly from J.-V. Laborde and Emile Vallin. Vallin, a member of the section of hygiene in the Académie de médecine and editor of the *Revue d'hygiène et de police sanitaire*, pointed out the fatal flaw in Lancereaux's argument based on the Paris statistics. It could easily be argued against Lancereaux that the 126 subjects who drank different sorts of alcoholic drinks got their cirrhosis from alcohol and that the remaining sixty eight, who drank only wine, perhaps drank so much of it that they too got their cirrhosis from alcohol. One of the basic problems with the statistical argument correlating potassium sulphate and cirrhosis in drinkers was that the population base was too small. Nor did the addition of Châteaulin make much difference because the total population of this town was less than 4000. In Vallin's opinion this was another case of statistical work being done *a posteriori*. The clear need was to get the research of hospital doctors in cities with a male working class population of several hundred thousand. In the great thirst-creating industries like glass and steel, some workers drank even more than ten litres of wine a day, which was the equivalent of drinking about two litres of *eau-de-vie*. In this case potassium sulphate would seem superfluous as a cause of cirrhosis. But the matter remained uninvestigated. (Like most of his colleagues, Vallin did not consider female alcoholism to be statistically significant enough for inclusion in this experiment.) Perhaps the most glaring statistical omission was the Midi, a gigantic reserve of men who had long been heavy consumers of plastered wine.[17] Vallin's familiarity with the use of statistics in medical and health issues may have further encouraged members of the academy of medicine to regard his criticism as a serious blow to Lancereaux's argument.

Given the cultural status and economic importance of wine in France and the tax revenues it generated, it is perhaps surprising that a debate about the dangers of wine drinking was held at all in an official institution. Indeed, there was a widespread medical opinion denying any danger. (Both Lancereaux and Vallin approved of moderate wine consumption.) So there is probably not much point in wondering if doctors pulled their punches in discussing vinism. And, after all, medicine, like wine, was part of French civilisation, not a set of external, objective criteria by which behaviour could be judged. Vallin defined moderation as a litre of wine a day. This was a typical reasonable medical opinion of moderation, but the medical wine model was based on a far less alcoholic wine than the typical wine of today. Vallin and many of his colleagues also believed that wine was less dangerous than other popular drinks, even when they contained the same amount of alcohol. A comparison with absinth ('la fée verte'), which usually contained seventy degrees of alcohol, gave the advantage entirely to wine. Ten glasses or 300 grams of absinth, the equivalent of 210cm^3 of alcohol at 100 degrees, contained the same amount of alcohol as two litres of wine, but the absinth was believed to produce 'a more dangerous drunkenness.' Vallin compared absinth drinkers to consumers of opium and hashish.[18]

The academy of medicine split into two groups on the issue of the etiology of cirrhosis, one group accepting the evidence that potassium sulphate was to blame and the other group clinging to the classic view that the culprit was alcohol, especially bad alcohol, that is non-wine alcohol.[19] Some members thought that much confusion would be cleared up by an inquiry to find out if cirrhosis were spread equally over France or limited to certain provinces. Such an inquiry would also have to establish the category of drinkers especially affected by the disease.

The statistical problem with Lancereaux's human samples was not the only vulnerable area of his case. His method of animal experimentation was also open to criticism. This criticism was more serious, for a study could always be extended, redone, or refudged to accommodate statistical sniping by critical colleagues. But if the experiment itself were basically flawed, little could be done to save the conclusions of the study. The scientific virility of the experimenter himself was under attack in this sort of criticism. Vallin scored a few points against Lancereaux on both general and detailed levels of criticism. To say that animal experiments were not conclusive and that more details were needed did not mortally wound Lancereaux's argument. Danger lurked in the detail: however ingenious the hypothesis that potassium bisulphate caused the death of his animals and cirrhosis of the liver in humans, the extrapolation to humans of the amounts fed to the animals gave the equivalent of sixty to 350 grams for adult males. Not even Lancereaux's exaggeratedly high estimates for the amount of potassium sulphate in wine could produce such a feast of potassium bisulphate for humans. Yet within the limits of scientific argument Lancereaux's new theory on alcoholic cirrhosis of the liver survived Vallin's critique of its experimental basis better than it stood up to the exposure of its statistical weakness.

Laborde's attack on Lancereaux's experiment was quite a different matter, based essentially on the reproducibility of experiments as a basis of solid science. For Laborde, as for other big-name professors like Jaccoud, Dieulafoy, and Conil, cirrhosis of the liver was the end of a general pathological process brought on by alcohol. Laborde began his attack with a few rhetorical flourishes to show his expertise, general knowledge, and modernity: experimentation has its rules, which cannot be ignored without endangering the validity of the experiment, and Lancereaux's work showed what can go wrong when the experimenter ignores the rules. In his discussion of diagnostic techniques, Laborde included 'examination by the new method of X-rays' but did not explain how this new technique might have saved Lancereaux's experiment. No doubt the total absence of such novelty in the experiment was enough to arouse the suspicions of men running on the experimental frontiers of science.

Laborde's most damaging blow came with the presentation of his own experiment on animals which did not produce the same results as Lancereaux's experiment. Several years before the debate in the academy of medicine, Laborde had carried out an experiment on two dogs of about the same weight. After drinking up to half a litre of wine each per day for two weeks, the dogs lost their appetite and showed signs of 'wine inebriety,' defined as titubation and a lack of motor coordination, rather than alcoholic drunkenness, defined as complete 'ivresse' with the dogs in a stupor and unable to stand up because of paresis of the hind quarters. This is a traditional French cultural distinction that emphasises the joy given by wine compared to the morose stupor produced by other (often foreign) alcoholic beverages. Laborde's dogs ingested an amount of potassium sulphate that would be the equivalent of six grams for a man of sixty kg. When he spoke to the academy, Laborde was stuffing a dog of eleven kg with fifteen grams daily, the equivalent of ninety grams for the sixty-kg man. After eighteen days the dog still seemed to be in excellent health. The experimental method is not reluctant to fall back on an *a fortiori* argument.

Laborde did not hesitate to conclude that the guilty agent in cirrhosis of the liver was alcohol, not potassium sulphate. He did not think that the debate was closed, for 'from the viewpoint of deduction and application truly convincing experiments have to be done with a commercial plastered wine and a normal non-plastered wine.' Lancereaux, a firm adherent to the school whose doctrine was 'open up a few corpses,' remained convinced that he was right. In the autopsies he had done on over 1000 drinkers he had never found either arteriosclerosis or interstitial nephritis. Alcohol was therefore not dangerous for heart or kidneys. Both Laborde and Lancereaux were convinced of the solid observational and experimental bases of their conflicting opinions on the role of potassium sulphate in the etiology of alcoholic cirrhosis.[20]

Both groups debating this etiology thought it important to look at the evidence in various regions of France and in other parts of the drinking world. Usually rigorous scientific minds seemed gullible enough to believe the most amazing assertions supporting their case. Serious people could accept the fantastic idea that there was no cirrhosis in Burgundy. Apple-growing Normandy had the reputation of being one of the leading centres of alcoholism in France, but Normans guzzled apple jack and industrial alcohols rather than wine. Such examples were cited repeatedly against the attribution of cirrhosis to potassium sulphate in wine.

The Vendée provided ammunition for both camps. In support of his position Lancereaux was able to cite letters from doctors, including Baratier, author of the memoir *L'alcoolisme au village* (1897). A letter from Dr Berthet of Le Croisic was more valuable than most letters because the doctor said that Lancereaux's position corresponded to what he had observed in hospital patients and in autopsies. Since the white wine of the gros plant and muscadet vines was the regional drink of the *pays nantais*, it could not be the cause of cirrhosis, or else the disease would be widespread. Lancereaux subscribed to the widely accepted view that cirrhosis was rare in wine country, even if alcoholism was strikingly present, if natural wine were drunk. (Defining natural wine was a moot point; our version of it is an invention of the late-twentieth century.)

Laborde doubted that the argument centring on white wine showed that alcohol was not the etiological culprit in cirrhosis. True, Dr Terrien of Essarts, a small town in the Vendée, reported that the *paysan du bocage* believed that five to six litres of wine a day seemed a reasonable amount to drink. (This wine had only seven to eight degrees of alcohol.) Cirrhosis was rare in these white wine drinkers. Terrien found that in the Vendée, as in Normandy, cabaret drinkers of industrial alcohol were the ones with damaged livers.

Laborde's position on the etiology of cirrhosis of the liver was strengthened towards the end of 1897 by a report in the *Gazette médicale de Nantes* on a survey done by Dr P. Aubrey in the departments of lower Brittany reporting that the numerous alcoholics in rural Morbihan generally drank hard cider and *eau-de-vie.* Aubrey, perhaps surprised to find only rare cases of cirrhosis, speculated that the disease required the presence of a specific social class, the retailers of cheap drinks (*débitants de boissons*), who provided drinkers with a constant ingestion of different, generally impure hard liquor or strong stuff. Dr Aubry also believed that a necessary condition of cirrhosis was the absolute absence of exercise. Potassium sulphate was unimportant because there was so little of it in the *cidre du pays.* Between the ages of thirty and fifty years, most alcoholics succumbed to various infections, especially pneumonia, accompanied by numerous nervous afflictions. Alcohol – 'bad' alcohol – caused cirrhosis in cider and calvados country.[21]

Laborde's position was also supported by a study of cirrhosis in the Yonne.[22] The three regions of this department made it a good case study. The area in the Champagne drank mediocre acidic wines. The Orléanais stuck to cider and *poiré* (perry or fermented pear juice). Plastering was unknown in both districts, but a tiny percentage of the middle classes drank the plastered wines of the Languedoc, the Hérault, and the Gard. In the canton of Toucy (near Auxerre), drinkers of these wines had no cirrhosis. Peasants who drank cider and moderate amounts of *eau-de-vie de marc* showed no signs of the disease. The only victims were artisans, small business owners, and sellers of alcoholic beverages who drank large quantities of the local acidic white wines and also abused aperitifs and bad quality liqueurs. Drinking large quantities of wine and *eau-de-vie* rarely led to cirrhosis. Yet another optimistic medical report on the grape. An element of subtlety was introduced by the notion of quality: the better the wine, the less chance of the drinker's getting cirrhosis. But the conclusion favoured Laborde's position, not Lancereaux's, on alcohol as a cause of cirrhosis.

A vaguely epidemiological argument was implicit in this study of the Yonne. Intending to cover as much of the entire drinking population as possible, the author of the memoir presented to the academy had sent out a questionnaire to departmental doctors, forty two of whom replied, with fourteen of them taking part in a subsequent discussion in the medical society of the Yonne. Rendu, who presented Roché's memoir to the academy, noted that provincial medical colleagues were better able than Parisian doctors to do the sort of work involved in establishing an etiology of cirrhosis. Provincial doctors, knowing their clients better and being aware of their hygienic habits, could give precise details in their observations. That type of practice was unusual in the big city. (Dr Louis Destouches of Montmartre might have disagreed.) Of course this study of the Yonne said little about the direct influence of sulphates because only a tiny percentage of the population drank plastered wine. Alfred Riche rightly complained that the question at the origin of the quarrel remained unanswered.[23]

The French liver does not have a monopoly on cirrhosis. Members of the academy on the lookout for foreign research to support their positions had no difficulty in finding sick alcoholic livers all over western civilisation. Throughout much of the nineteenth century the great authority on alcoholism was the Swedish professor Magnus Huss, whose classic study of chronic alcoholism was invoked by Lancereaux to support his own argument. But Lancereaux made a hash of Huss' findings, including the conclusions on the danger of *eau-de-vie* and other alcoholic drinks except wine and beer. Vallin exposed Lancereaux's ignorance of Huss's work by quoting the German translation of *Chronic Alcoholism* and then tried to damage Lancereaux's case more by citing Frerichs on the notorious English gin drinker's liver.[24] Lancereaux's position was further weakened by evidence from the United States. Dr Eugene Dupuy, a member of the Société de Biologie, who had practiced in the United States, identified the high alcoholic content of whisky as the agent producing cirrhosis in the American liver. This thesis was illustrated by the existence of cirrhosis in Maine, a state addicted to whisky, not wine. Vallin also quoted a letter from Dr A. Britto of the faculty of medicine in Bahia, Brazil, where the cirrhotic drunks were rum drinkers. An impressive case had been built up to defend the classic thesis that excessive alcohol consumption causes cirrhosis of the liver.

But the case appeared to be only empirical, even when distinguished authorities were cited. Perhaps this procedure encouraged the medical opposition to use the same tactics in counterattacking; since it had the same training and shared the same logic and scientific principles, it could hardly have chosen any other course. Lancereaux could easily counter the rum-in-Brazil example with a rum-in-Haiti one. Dr Audain, who practiced in Haiti, where there was 'an excessive consumption' of tafia and rum, declared that cirrhosis was rare there. Perhaps drinkers did not live long enough to get cirrhosis. Still, it was remarkable that in twelve years he had seen only five cases of cirrhosis, two of which were of syphilitic origin. Two of the afflicted were wine drinkers.

Lancereaux's major blow to the opposition came from Italy. Giacinto Viola of the medical clinic in Padua was about to publish, in the *Archives générales de médecine*, a major study on the province of Venezia. Viola argued that Laennec's atrophic cirrhosis, practically unknown in Venezia in the past, had become common since southern Italian wines had displaced local wines. Jumping to the conclusion that here was a significant correlation, Viola argued that the higher level of alcohol in the southern wines was less important in the etiology of the new disease than their high extract and their potassium sulphate content from plastering.[25] (Contrary to some pro-wine propaganda, 'the Italian prevalence of alcohol-related diseases is among the highest in the world.' Differing in distribution from area to area, the cirrhosis rate is about forty per 100,000 inhabitants annually in northern areas and about twenty per 100,000 in southern areas. Though there is no clear explanation available, the disease seems related to the bad habits of fathers, especially drinking and smoking more than ten cigarettes daily. Students in Calabria begin drinking earlier than in Veneto but they drink with a higher frequency.[26])

Instead of confronting the logical and factual basis of Viola's argument – difficult to do before it appeared – Laborde shifted the argument to the equally treacherous grounds of epistemology and changing models of wine. Appearing to be caught off guard by Lancereaux's clever use of Viola's study, Laborde pointed out that it is easy to cite contradictory results from wine country that are supplied by the most competent observers. Dr Lejeune of Meursault, who had been in practice in Burgundy for twenty eight years, wrote a letter stating that cirrhosis was common in wine drinkers. Then he defused this bombshell by adding that very few people drank natural wine anymore. All wine had its level of alcohol increased a couple of degrees by chaptalisation. Most households (nine out of ten, according to Lejeune) consumed 'spoiled wines,' wines that in most cases had 'second wines' added to them. These second wines got much of their alcohol from chaptalisation. The serious wine drinker took lots of *petits verres* of all sorts of wine and wine liqueurs in addition to matching the heavy amount consumed by the normal drinker. Lejeune did not need to give any evidence that the alcohol of chaptalised wine was more dangerous than that of 'natural' wine. Nearly everyone not connected with the sugar and commercial alcohol producing industries was willing to accept this idea, although there was little or no evidence to support it. The myth of the 'national drink' carried with it the corollary of the distinctiveness and healthier nature of alcohol derived only from grape sugar without added cane sugar. Whatever the scientific standing of Lejeune's observations, he had put alcohol back in the spotlight as the cause of cirrhosis, while exonerating 'natural' wine.

Acceptance of wine as a food and therapeutic agent did not necessarily preclude an awareness of possible dangers of wine consumption in addition to the extreme danger of *vinisme*. In 1929 the *Bulletin de l'organisation internationale du vin* (BIV) carried a pro-wine article by Maurice Loeper, professor at the medical faculty in Paris, and J. Alquier, general secretary of the Société scientifique d'hygiène alimentaire. After dealing with the chemical composition of wine, including the implications of the presence of certain substances for the human organism, they took up the touchy subject of the toxicity of wine. Not a common topic in the BIV, except for indignant refutation. It turned out that wine alcohol was the least toxic of alcohols. Experiments had shown that wine alcohol did not cause the same lesions as sugarbeet alcohol did in the liver and intestines of a drinking pig. Dogs slept a few hours after drinking wine but went into a coma of twenty four hours with grain alcohol and three days from sugarbeet alcohol. True, it should not be forgotten that four cc. of wine alcohol could kill a rabbit, but the wine was injected into a vein, which could not be compared to the effect of wine that passed into the digestive tract. Of course a human male who drank three to four litres of wine daily would eventually get gastric and liver lesions. One had to stick to five gr. per kilo of weight to be on the safe side, or at least this was the latest good news from medical research. (Lucy Randoin would shortly recommend less than twenty five per cent of the generous allowance recommended by the BIV.)

Promoters of wine consumption usually try to argue that wine is not in the same consumption category as hard liquor. Is there a difference between the effects of fermented and distilled beverages on the body? There is research that shows that when comparable aqueous solutions are administered, wine is absorbed more slowly into the blood stream and maintains a lower peak in blood alcohol than whisky or gin. This seems to be the result of wine's buffering agents. By increasing the alkaline reserve, these natural buffering agents prevent the acidosis that alcohol alone produces. (Natural buffer systems like haemoglobin and carbonic acid in the blood are partly responsible for keeping an acid-base balance, that is the pH, within a physiologically accepted range.) It has even been shown experimentally that wine cures cirrhosis, an incurable disease it can cause. As early as 1929 Maurice Loeper showed the value of sweet wines and white table wine in treating liver disorders. In 1938 Jean Miquel's thesis showed to the satisfaction of the medical faculty of Toulouse that alcoholic liver cirrhosis resulting from excessive wine consumption occurred in areas where wine was made from hybrid grapes, especially the variety Noah, and was nonexistent in areas planted with *Vitis vinifera.* The factors used to explain this curiosity were the sometimes typical doses of methyl alcohol and the high level of manganese in wine from hybrid vines. Wines made from Noah grapes could had up to five times the level of manganese in wine made from *Vitis vinfera* grapes, which were not completely exonerated, however. Good wine coming from normal French varieties of vines was never the *exclusive* cause of cirrhosis, though there were excesses of goodness.[27]

In the 1950s and 1960s work by Emidio Serianni in Italy and John Carbone in California pursued the paradox. Loeper's work showed that wine facilitates the assimilation of nitrogen and stimulates deamination of the liver. This was a specific confirmation of a general thesis widely accepted in French medicine to the effect that wine does not cause cirrhosis; or how else could one explain the low rates of the disease in wine country? Doctor after doctor in practice in wine producing areas affirmed that he had never seen a case. Anecdotal evidence seems as unreliable as statistics. Serianni's work showed that red wine with meals speeded up detoxification action by the liver in the excretion of hippuric acid. Carbone experimented with the diet of five chronic alcoholics with severe cirrhosis: his startling medical procedure was to give them each a litre of red wine daily. Liver biopsy showed 'a marked clearing of the fatty and cellular infiltrations characteristic of this disease.' The patients' health improved strikingly.[28] Healing is a mysterious process.

Even a whisky maker could find experiments casting doubt on the dogma that alcohol and cirrhosis are related. True, statistical evidence points to more liver damage from cirrhosis among alcoholics than in the general population. But one line of research has shown that in rats that 'this type of liver damage is not the direct result of alcohol ingestion since the same changes were produced on the same basal diet when sugar was given instead of alcohol.' The liver changes may have resulted from insufficient 'lipotropic factors in the diet' or vitamin deficiencies characteristic of alcoholics due to their poor diet.[29] Speaking from his *Chaire de thérapeutique* in the medical faculty of Paris in 1933, Loeper pleased the defenders of wine by proclaiming that wine is not a luxury foodstuff. Sometimes a medication, it is a useful stimulant to both somnolent brain and enervated body. [30] No doubt. And James Joyce agreed, to excess. 'Come dinner time, he would drink white wine, bottle after bottle, until he was oblivious to the cigarette burning his fingers.'[31] Joyce died at the age of fifty eight of a perforated ulcer and generalised peritonitis, but according to the postmortem report his spleen, liver, heart, kidneys, and genito-urinary tract were all normal. Joyce didn't care for red wine, which he insulted as beefsteak, and loved white wine, 'electricity,' especially the Swiss wine Fendant de Sion, whose aesthetic properties included a colour like the 'orina ... di un'arciduchessa.'[32]

2. Potassium ferrocyanide and the dangers of clarity

Consumers like or have been convinced by wine makers that they like absolutely clear white wine and non-murky red wine. Clarity pleases the consumer and is convenient for the maker. 'Haze and sediments can form several ways in wine,' chiefly by five types of precipitation through the presence of potassium and calcium salts, protein, protein-complex, pigment, and metals (iron and copper).[33] Traditional fining agents such as egg albumin, gelatin, isinglass, which are unreactive compounds, have been used for centuries to give an acceptable clarity and stability to wine. After wine was brought into the chemical empire other products became available to solve old problems more cheaply and effectively: a polymeric resin, silica gel or kieselosol, bentonite, and potassium ferrocyanide, the last item being 'used to precipitate iron and copper from wine.' It is illegal to use potassium ferrocyanide in the United States because of the danger that an excessive amount could produce cyanide poisoning. American wine makers can use 'a much safer proprietary formulation called Cufex, which includes compounds that reduce the risk of leaving a toxic residue.'[34] In most other countries, including France, potassium ferrocyanide can be legally used in making rosé and white wines.[35]

The right to use this chemical, which today hardly anyone knows about, was the subject of a medical debate in France in the late-1930s.[36] Wine interests in Bordeaux and their allies carried out a vigorous campaign to get the use of potassium ferrocyanide legalised in the making of white wines. The basic argument was geographical: the Champagne and Burgundy had less trouble with vinification because they were able to harvest grapes later, in cooler weather, than

Bordeaux. In September 1934 the Fédération du Commerce des Vins, Spiritueux et Liqueurs supported a change in the law. Various wine-making and commercial organisations petitioned the ministry of public health in favour of getting governmental approval of 'collage bleu' (Prussian blue), which had supposedly become a widespread method of clarification of whites in other countries, thus putting the French at a commercial disadvantage. The national argument was put to good use. German firms were accused of buying and clarifying white bordeaux by this method and then selling them at a great markup. In fact, only ordinary wine was treated in Germany. The excited discussion in the Académie de médecine seemed to assume that all white Bordeaux, including the great Graves and Sauternes, would be treated.

No threat to public health could be shown. Even a massive dose of fifty grams of the stuff would have only a purging effect, always a good argument in a Dr Kellogg-less country where constipation was a frequent complaint. If there were any small amount of ferrocyanhydric (or ferrocyanic) acid left in the wine, it could be tasted and this alone would, in a gastronomically acute group like the French, prevent any abuses. At the Congrès des Médecins Amis du Vin held during the summer of 1935 in Lausanne an experiment was carried out on volunteer tasters. These guinea-pig physicians drank both treated and non-treated wines for several days without being able to tell them apart. Nor did 'detailed observation' of the drinkers of wine treated with potassium ferrocyanide reveal the slightest physiological problem. On the basis of these strong arguments, the pro-treatment forces perhaps hoped for a favourable opinion from the Académie de médecine when the government asked for its opinion.

The academy appointed a commission of six of its members to study the issue and report back with a recommendation. This was not the first time that the academy had given its opinion on the use of potassium ferrocyanide. It had always been against its use, and this time the commission was of the same opinion. There were three basic reasons, with many implications, some medical, some gastronomic-cultural, for refusing to approve the treatment. First, treated wine would be no longer pure but adulterated.' Secondly, the wine could retain a residue of ferrocyanhydric acid, which required expert detection. Even a small army of chemists would be able to test only part of the wine produced for export; family production would not be tested at all. Thirdly, the acid is poisonous. The academy maintained a healthy suspicion of experiments. A toxicological study published in Bordeaux had failed to find any ferrocyanhydric acid in heavily treated wine. A congress of the Oenotechniciens de Bordeaux in 1927 recommended the use of blue fining, and oenologists soon went from opposition to support of the procedure.[37] The main reason for the academy's refusal to approve the treatment was the lost of purity; the second (which included the third) problem could, at least in theory, be handled in the same way it was handled in Germany. France was famous for its 'crus naturels,' and doctors regarded this a good reason not to add another chemical to them. There was also the fear that the failure to observe short term effects did not mean that there would be no long term effects on serious wine drinkers. The idea of inflicting this chemical on a large population of French citizens seemed revolting to the medical conscience, tempting though it might have been to welcome a new group of patients as a gift from the chemists.[38]

Looking at the issue from 'a more elevated viewpoint' than the results of technical studies – medicine was, after all, an art as well as a science – the commission decided to uphold its ancient principle of refusing to approve the addition of any new chemical product to foodstuffs. Indeed, it found so excessive the list of chemicals already authorised that it declared it time to revise and reduce the list. In a rather old fashioned opinion, the commission declared that 'the wines of France are not and must not be industrial products.' It could be and was observed that many industrial products were of higher quality than many of the wines of France. Still, the opinion was valid for the best wines of France, the ones that the top doctors are likely to drink.

In order not to show themselves completely hostile to scientifically-based changes in food and drink production, the Académie de médecine left open the possibility of another discussion by the commission with new members added. The protests from the Gironde were sufficient to ensure that the commission discuss the issue again, this time with outside experts added. The commission did not change its mind; nor did the Académie change its recommendation against clarifying white bordeaux with potassium ferrocyanide. In Edouard Barthe's opinion, which carried political as well as medical weight, there were adequate existing methods to filter wines. And he insisted that not all oenologists protested against the refusal of the ministry of agriculture to authorise blue fining.[39] No argument, whether chemical, oenological-gastronomic, or commercial, could convince the doctors that the process was needed. Neither the Champagne nor Burgundy wanted authorisation to use potassium ferrocyanide. It seemed that Americans would have to forego drinking those *grands* Sauternes which, according to J.-L. Faure, they were returning unopened because they looked more like purulent urine than the *orina* of Joyce's archduchess. Meanwhile, the great whites of Bordeaux had been saved from chemical pollution, just as the quality of French bread had been narrowly saved earlier when the government turned down a request for permission to add chemical substances to the baguette. No one seemed to remember at this point that French bread had been corrupted long ago and that some doctors had sounded an alarm in vain.[40]

3. Sulphur dioxide - a threat to the drinker's health?

The wisdom of the traditional practice of preserving wine by using sulphur dioxide (SO_2) was not much questioned before the end of the nineteenth century. The debate over potassium sulphate has disappeared and no one knows much about Prussian blue, but the debate over SO_2 is still with us because of the widespread use of the product and the near universality of sulphuring wine, at least until recently, when 'organic' unsulphured wines started to come on the market. Sulphur, a yellow, non-metallic element, common in nature, is one of the 'basic raw materials of the chemical industry.' Living organisms cannot do without sulphur, vital in the growth of plant and animal tissues. 'It is a constituent of foods and of practically all animal fluids, secretions, and excretions.'[41] SO_2 is an acid anhydride, a non-metallic oxide that can combine with water to form sulphurous acid (HSO_3) – or so chemistry and oenological texts used to say; received chemical wisdom now is that only an aqueous solution of SO_2 is formed, or at least no molecules of sulphurous acid have ever been detected. Since 'sulphurous acid *per se* does not exist,' the phrase just means an 'aqueous solution of sulphur dioxide.'[42] (We continue to use the phrase as a convenient narrative fiction.) Controversy over SO_2 has come chiefly over its use as a preservative in food production with consequent questions about the results of its ingestion into the human organism.

Sulphur and wine: a traditional marriage whose utility is undeniable though its necessity has become debatable. A nasty debate over its use enlivened the end of the nineteenth-century, when sulphur dioxide and sulphites (salts or esters of sulphuric acid) were coming to be widely used to preserve foodstuffs. Several accidents occurred as a result of excessive doses in food, and there were a few fatalities. The Conseil d'hygiène de France, after discussing the issue on several occasions, became alarmed enough over the high doses found in meat, milk, and beer to prohibit the addition of sulphur dioxide to meat and milk. Beer drinkers were presumed immune or else to deserve their punishment. But a later decision did limit the amount that could be used in fermented liquids. For beer and wine the maximum was 200mg. of free and combined sulphur dioxide per litre. An ostensibly moderate compromise.

The wine business was noisily indignant. Some producers of *grands vins* protested because their complex product was the result of several manipulations each requiring the addition of sulphur dioxide. Agricultural associations squealed in protest against a regulation that threatened to stop the ancient ritual of burning the sulphured wick, vital for purifying wine casks and helping conserve the wine. Wine science rushed in to agree with the users of sulphur dioxide. Roos, head of the oenological station of Montpellier, speaking to the Société centrale d'agriculture de l'Hérault, a strongly pro-sulphur group, took the position that the restriction was unworkable. A two-year old wine that had been racked twice a year in a sulphured cask contained more than the legal limit of 200mg. per litre. Sulphur was finally giving a headache to the producer as well as to the consumer.

Some chemists became alarmed that they might be branded as poisoners of the public. In 1894 the Swiss society of analytical chemists united in declaring that in sulphured wine and cider the free sulphur dioxide should not exceed 20mg. per litre, though the total amount of free and combined forms could go as high as 200mg. (total of acids transformed and measured as sulphuric acid (HSO_4). The later decisions of the Conseil d'hygiène de France were based on the same assumptions. What caused alarm in the French wine business was the method imposed by the Conseil to determine the total amount.[43] Roos ruthlessly criticised the method imposed by the mandarins of the Conseil because it could result in the paradox of the rejection of a wine as being strongly sulphured although none had been added.

This mystery was cleared up by a little more science than the usual minimum required for bureaucratic decisions. Louis Hugounenq, professor in the faculty of medicine of Lyon, after doing analyses of a great number of wine samples along with their ashes, concluded that wine, like a great number of natural products, contains sulphur in three forms.[44] Hugounenq found in several natural wines enough organic sulphur to give, when oxidated, a quantity of from 190 to 243mg. of potassium sulphate per litre of wine: this corresponded to 88mg. of sulphur dioxide. Roos showed that a wine of the grape variety Alicante-Bouchez, which he had prepared himself without sulphuring, showed a dose of 125mg. (measured as sulphuric acid) per litre when submitted to oxidation by means of bromated water. Paturel got up to 75mg of potassium sulphate per litre for the wines of the Mâconnais. Variety of grape and soil counted for a great deal. So the violent method of titrating sulphuric acid by oxidation was not reliable because it ignored the amount of natural sulphur in the total amount used as a basis of rendering a legal decision. The bureaucracy seemed to be doing sloppy science, even if it was the science of scientists. It was assumed that what is natural is safe; the same was assumed for the unnatural, up to a certain point. The solution to the problem was embarrassingly simple: use of Bunsen's elegant method (oxidation of sulphurous acid by iodine, etc.) as applied to the analysis of wine by Ripper. There was one procedure for whites and another for reds and sweet wines, the last two requiring direct distillation, with a modification proposed by Paturel.[45]

Oenologists (and chemists) agreed that from 100 to 150mg. of sulphur dioxide per litre of wine was required for the total destruction of organisms harmful to wine. Because the Swiss limited the free form to 20mg. per litre and the French wanted a limit of 100mg. per litre for the total amount of sulphur dioxide in a wine, the method of determination of amounts meant the difference between legally and illegally dosed wines. Method created reality.

Let us sum up the wisdom of science about 1900 on the complex issue of sulphuring wine? Total sulphur dioxide content has little meaning for determining the sanitary state of a wine. The health of a wine depends upon the amount of free sulphur dioxide available. Scientists tied directly or indirectly to the wine industry (mostly scientists in university faculties and related organisations) emphasised that a slight excess of sulphur dioxide could produce only minor troubles for the health of the consumer, who, in theory, had a choice of more and less sulphured wines, though no information was on the label. An excessive amount of free sulphur dioxide was hardly likely to be ingested, for even a dose lower than the legal limit gave the wine an atrocious taste of sulphur as long as the free agent was not transformed. The combination of sulphur dioxide with the elements of the wine caused a nearly total disappearance of its harmful properties. Again science had provided producers with a justification of a chemical practice if it were done with precision according to the rules devised by scientists for the manufacture of a safe and healthy wine. Within the parameters imposed by modern consumption and its regulation by means of laws based on reasonable compromise, it is not easy to offer a workable alternative.

It is difficult to make any of the charges against sulphur dioxide stick, especially when it is used in moderate, legal quantities, and even less in many cases today because of an increasingly aseptic technology of wine production. Fourcade and Peynaud (1952) recommended putting potassium metabisulphite (a salt of SO_2 containing fifty seven per cent SO_2) in a canvas sack into the wine as the best method of using sulphur.[46] True, doctors have been known to worry about its effects, but given competing threats to health, including the danger of alcohol in cases of excessive wine consumption, SO_2 seems a trivial concern except for the few people exceedingly sensitive to it.

The old standard reference of the table wine industry, *Table wine* (1951) by Amerine and Joslyn, gives an extensive analysis of the use of sulphur dioxide in winemaking, including a few lines on the chemical's toxicity. The authors note than in spite of the 'voluminous literature on the possible toxic effects of drinking wine containing sulphur dioxide,' and the 'long controversy as to the toxicity of sulphites,' only minor problems have ever been attributed to the 'ingestion of sulphite.' The two problems they mention are 'a significant decrease in excretion of thiamine [vitamin B_1] and an increase in urinary excretion of calcium'. And referring to the inevitable experiment on rats, *Table Wine* notes that the abused animals 'with a deficiency of all B vitamins were more susceptible to sulphur dioxide toxicity than those not deficient or deficient only in thiamine.' Not much for the ordinary consumers to worry about, unless they become addicted to wines 'approaching the 450mg. per litre limit.' An unlikely event, even for a lover of Sauternes.[47]

In 1977 Pierre Simonis, as part of the thesis for his doctorate in medicine did a review of the medical case against sulphur dioxide.[48] Accepting the old dogma that wine is a food, he included wine in the daily food supply of the average Frenchman. Simonis stated that most of the SO_2 ingested by a large part of the French population came from wine. Although we now know that this was probably not true, this reasonable mistaken belief was generally accepted by the medical community until the 1980s. Simonis was unable to find any solid evidence of the danger of SO_2 that would justify a medical warning. 'The chronic toxicity of sulphites seems weak for most animal species' was his comforting conclusion.

And yet there was enough evidence for researchers to cast suspicion on sulphur dioxide as a factor in the malfunctioning and perhaps even the damaging of some organs. Much seemed to depend on the nutritional state of the body ingesting the chemical. A well-nourished body would not be affected by an amount of SO_2 that could be toxic to a body suffering from malnutrition. Sulphur has a higher toxicity for persons whose diet is poor in vitamin B_1. Simonis cited the research done by Lhuissier in 1966 showing that sulphites destroy thiamine in sulphur-treated products – of little importance for wine because wine contains little thiamine – and, more important nutritionally, also destroys the thiamine that comes from food during digestion. SO_2 seems to have disruptive and damaging effects in the digestive process and system. Sulphites have been found to inhibit the activity of digestive enzymes. Experimentation on animals provides most of the information, thus leaving the results open to the classic criticism that the effects of sulphites on humans might be different and have not been scientifically demonstrated. (The same warning applied to a positive effect. It seemed that SO_2 was shown to offer protection against dental cavities by modifying micro-organisms in the mouth, particularly those on the surface of teeth. This has been shown scientifically only for rats.) Simonis could only say that SO_2 had been shown to irritate the digestive system. This gastrointestinal malfunctioning probably came from the liberation of sulphurous acid in the stomach. A last specific accusation against SO_2 was its potentially dangerous effect on the excretion of calcium in urine and feces because of its intervention in the process of calcic metabolism. Simonis had concocted a strong case showing the potential dangers of sulphur to wine drinkers.

This negative assessment of sulphur dioxide, although hedged with the cautious remarks on the limitations of the research backing it up, would hardly have been an appropriate judgment in a thesis on *L'hygiène du vin d'Alsace*, defended at the Château de Kientzheim.[49] So Simonis' summing-up on the subject emphasised that in spite of the recent increase in knowledge of the nutritional and physio-pathological effects of ingesting SO_2, no definitive conclusions could be established concerning its effect on the human organism. Simonis seemed to accept the prudent French policy of limiting the quantity of SO_2 to a total of 250mg per litre of wine, a limit wine producers could easily live with. Simonis agreed with Brugirard's view that 'Wine, the national French drink, is certainly the most analysed, the most tasted, classified, and regulated of all food products.'

In the 1980s some researchers as well as some wine producers concluded that wine was taking a bum rap in the case of the charge that sulphured wines were endangering the health of consumers.

'The potential health problems' arising from the use of SO_2 came, it was argued, 'largely from misuse of the product in other food processing applications.'[50] A report on how much SO_2 Europeans ingest claimed that it came from many sources, including wine. Studies of the intake of SO_2 in Italy showed that the main quantities were 'to be found in fresh and frozen shrimp, chopped meat, dried potatoes, and wine ... mainly white wine.' The French situation was shown to be 'very similar ... to Italy, both in relation to the levels of SO_2 found in wine and to habits of consumption.'[51]

This optimistic view eagerly spread by the wine industry and its learned friends was admirably summed up in a magisterial 'special report' by the well known oenologist Cornelius S. Ough in 1987.

> Many studies have been undertaken to determine if sulphur dioxide is harmful to humans. For the most part, they show it to be harmless to normal people at the legal levels in wine – 350mg total sulphur dioxide (free and bound) per L[iter]. Most table wines contain less than 100mg. per L. At this level, the only persons who appear to be affected are asthmatics and – from preliminary experiments – those who are steroid-deficient. The very few people who, in addition to having these problems, are deficient in the normal sulphite oxidase enzyme that converts sulphur dioxide to sulphate for elimination are sensitive not only to free sulphur dioxide but to its bound form as well. The bound forms may hydrolyse in such persons' small intestines, where the pH is higher, which may put a more severe load on their sulphite elimination system.[52]

It is convenient that the amounts of sulphur dioxide needed for the protection of wine correspond to the amounts that normal persons can easily tolerate. If normal persons did not have a medical existence, they would have to be invented to justify industry's needs.

Notes

1. Denis Grady, 'Scientists growing livers to order in hope of successful transplants,' *The New York Times* (10 Sept. 1996), B6.
2. *The New Encyclopaedia Britannica,* vol. 17 (Chicago: Encyclopaedia Britannica, 1989), 302, and the *Concise Science Dictionary* (Oxford: Oxford University Press, 1987), 404–405.
3. *'Cirrhose,' Nouveau dictionnaire de médecine et de chirurgie pratiques,* vol. xv (Paris: Baillière, 1864-86), 115–29. The *Nouveau dictionnaire* recognised three categories of cirrhosis: inflammatory, cardiac, and specific. For the curious history of Laennec's relation to cirrhosis, see Jacalyn Duffin, *To See with a Better Eye. A Life of R. T.*

H. Laennec (Princeton, N. J.: Princeton University Press, 1998), 70–3.

4. See Alf. Becquerel, 'Recherches anatomiques et pathologiques sur la cirrhose du foie,' *Archives générales de médecine*, 3rd series, vii and viii (1840); Cl. Bernard et Laboubème, 'Sur deux cas d'altération du foie (état graisseux et cirrhotique du foie),' *Comptes rendus des séances de la Societé de biologie*, vol. iii (Oct. 1851); J. Cruveilhier, 'Cirrhose du foie – nature de la cirrhose,' *Bulletins de la Société anatomique de Paris*, 3rd series, vii (1852); Ed. Monneret, 'Etude clinique sur la maladie qui a reçu le nom de cirrhose du foie,' *Archives générales de médecine*, 4th series, xxix and xxx (1852); and Ad. Gubler, *Théorie de la cirrhose* (thèse d'agrégation, 1853).
5. For an amusing and instructive analysis of the French liver, see Lynn Payer, *Medicine and Culture. Varieties of Treatment in the United States, England, West Germany, and France* (London: Penguin Books, 1988), 56–61.
6. Jean-Charles Sournia, *Ces maladies qu'on fabrique – la médecine gaspillée* (Paris: Seuil, 1977), 11.
7. See Erwin H. Ackerknecht, *A short history of medicine* (Baltimore: The Johns Hopkins University Press, 1982), 164.
8. Cited in Valeer Desmet, 'Liver cirrhosis: evolving aspects of an old problem,' in B. Clément and A. Guillouzo, (eds), *Cellular and Molecular aspects of Cirrhosis* (Colloque INSERM/John Libby Eurotext Ltd., vol. 216 , 1992), 2.
9. In the 1980s arguments were still going on about defining the disease, although morphological (macroscopical) and etiological classifications provided a basis for professional agreement, especially in etiology. Cirrhosis is 'now recognised as a late stage of the most diverse liver diseases of various causes. The detailed mechanisms of 'the progression from normal liver into cirrhosis remain unknown.' *Ibid.*, 3–4.
10. Charles Murchison, *Clinical Lectures on Diseases of the Liver, Jaundice and Abdominal Dropsy* (London: Longmans, 1868), 239. The lectures, given to students of the Middlesex Hospital, were dedicated to James Syme; the first four were also published in *The Lancet.*
11. Charles Murchison, *On Functional Derangements of the Liver* (London: Smith, Elder, 1879), 2d edn, 153–9. This work originated as the Croonian lectures delivered at the Royal College of Physicians in 1874.
12. Professor of hepatology and gastroenterology at the University of Bordeaux, Claude Béraud, *Le foie des Français* (Paris: Stock, 1983), 144, noted that wine is perhaps more toxic for the liver than other

alcoholic drinks because of the tannins and other chemical substances it contains.

13. *Ibid.*
14. E. Lancereaux, 'Etiologie de la cirrhose des buveurs,' *Bulletin de l'académie de médecine (hereinafter BAM)*, 3rd series, xxxviii (1897), 202–08. See Lancereaux, 'Alcoolisme' in the *Dictionnaire encyclopédique des sciences médicales* (Paris: P. Asselin, 1865), and *De l'alcoolisme* (Paris: Doin, 1878). The labels acute, chronic, acquired, and hereditary were attached to alcoholism. For analyses of French doctors and alcoholism, see ch. ii of Patricia E. Prestwich, *Drink and the Politics of Social Reform: Antialcoholism in France since 1870* (Palo Alto, CA: The Society for the Promotion of Science and Scholarship, 1988), and ch. vii of Jack D. Ellis, *The physician-legislators of France. Medicine and politics in the Third Republic* (Cambridge: Cambridge University Press, 1990). Lancereaux was the willing victim of a banquet given by 120 of his friends and former students in 1896, when he was promoted to the rank of Officier de la légion d'honneur and hailed by banquet rhetoricians as the 'principal ouvrier' of Claude Bernard, 'the beginner of scientific medicine.' Intriguing but vague reference was also made to 'le beau et le néfaste côté de sa carrière.' *Banquet offert à M. le docteur Lancereaux le 8 février 1896* (1896). See also Jean-Jacques Peumery, 'Etienne Lancereaux (1829-1910), sa vie, son oeuvre, ses découvertes scientifiques,' *Histoire des sciences médicales*, xxiii (1989), 279–84.
15. See Lancereaux, *Traité des maladies du foie et du pancréas* (Paris: Doin, 1899), figs. 7 and 8, 278.
16. Lancereaux described this slow process as 'la prolifération conjonctive qui détermine le retrait du foie, les granulations de sa surface et l'hydropisie.' See *Journal de médecine de Bordeaux* [hereinafter *JMBX*], 37 (1907), 421–3.
17. Alfred Riche (Ecole de pharmacie), 'La cirrhose des buveurs et le plâtrage,' *BAM*, xxxix (1898), 304–313. Riche gave an optimistically low estimate of the amount of potassium sulphate in the wine of the Midi: between one and one and one-half grams per litre.
18. See Marie-Claude Delahaye, *L'absinthe. Histoire de la fée verte* (Paris: Berger-Levrault, 1983).
19. *BAM*, xxxix (1898), 255–59.
20. J.-V. Laborde, 'La cirrhose des buveurs et le plâtrage des vins,' *BAM*, xxxviii (1897), 334–46.
21. *Gazette médical de Nantes* (11 Dec. 1897), reprinted in *Journal des connaissances médicales pratiques et de pharmacologie*, 66e année, 10e série, xvii, 15.

22. 'Sur un mémoire de M. le Dr [Louis] Roché (de Toucy) relatif à l'alcoolisme et à la cirrhose hépatique dans l'Yonne,' par M. Rendu, rapporteur, *BAM*, xxxix (1898), 255–59.
23. Alfred Riche, 'La cirrhose des buveurs et le plâtrage,' BAM, xxxix (1898), 304–14.
24. Magnus Huss, *Chronische Alkoholskrankheit oder 'Alkoholismus chronicus.' Eine Beitrag zur Kenntniss der Vergiftungs-Krankheiten, nach eigener und anderer Erfahung* (Stockholm: C. E. Fritze, 1849–51; translation by Gerhard van dem Busch, Leipzig: Engelmann, 1852). Vallin quoted from the *Traité pratique des maladies du foie* (translated by Drs. Louis Duménil and J. Pellagot, 1862; 3d edn, Baillière,1877) by Fr. Theodor Frerichs, editor of the *Zeitschrift für klinische Medizin* (1880-85); Charles Murchison translated Frerichs's treatise into English in 1861 for the New Sydenham Society.
25. Giacinto Viola, 'Recherches sur l'étiologie de la cirrhose hépatique à Padoue et à Venise,' *Archives générales de médecine*, Jan.-Fév. 1898.
26. P. Gentilini and M. U. Dianzani (eds), *Liver Cirrhosis* (Basel: Karger, 1984), vol. 8 of *Frontiers of Gastrointestinal Research*. Papers given in the meeting of the Italian Group of Hepatic Cirrhosis, June 6-8, 1983.
27. Jean Miquel, *Le bon vin hors de cause dans la pathogénie de la cirrhose atrophique de Laënnec* (Thèse pour le doctorat en médecine, Faculté mixte de médecine et de pharmacie de Toulouse, 1938), which got a friendly reception in the *Revue de viticulture*, 90 (1939), 76–77. DNA fingerprinting of vines by Carole P. Meredith (Univ. of California, Davis) has shown that many vines we thought to be non-hybrid are really hybrid: for example, the cabernet sauvignon. The pinot noir has been pure for 2000 years, but it is not clear what medical advantage this gives to burgundy. See the *Science Times* (*The New York Times*, 23 Nov. 1999), D1-2.
28. Salvatore P. Lucia, *A History of Wine as Therapy* (Philadelphia: Lippincott, 1963), 184.
29. Agnes Fay Morgan, 'Wine in the Normal Diet,' *Bulletin of the Society of Medical Friends of Wine*, v, no. 2 (1962). Morgan links up liver and heart disease: 'since blood B (Beta)-lipoproteins and cholesterol originate in the liver and since these blood constituents are generally believed to be significantly related to the march of atherosclerosis, liver changes are significant.'
30. Loeper, *Thérapeutique médicale*, reviewed in *Bulletin de l'organisation internationale du vin* (hereinafter *BIV*), no. 59 (1933), 151.
31. Brenda Maddox, *Nora. A Biography of Nora Joyce* (New York:

Penguin Books, 1988), 286.

32. Richard Ellmann, *James Joyce* (New York: Oxford University Press, 1983), 455.
33. Cornelius S. Ough, 'Chemicals Used in Making Wine,' *Chemical and Engineering News* (Jan. 5, 1987), 23–6. Widely consulted by governments and industry on winemaking, Ough was then professor of oenology and chairman of the department of viticulture and oenology at the Univ. of California at Davis.
34. Ough, *Chemical and Engineering News* (Jan. 5, 1987), 24.
35. A list of the oenological products permitted in France is given in Yves Renouil (ed.), *Dictionnaire du vin* (Bordeaux: Féret et fils, 1988), 1122; potassium ferrocyanide is classified as one of the 'auxiliaires technologiques' for treating iron *casse* in rosés and whites. The limiting conditions for these 'manipulations permises' are given in Bernard Blanchet, *Code du vin et textes viti-vinicoles français et communautaires* (Montpellier: Ed. de la Journée viticole, 1970), article 4, 12 ff. The treatment has to be carried out by a technician with a degree in oenology.
36. The basic documentation for the debate over potassium ferrocyanide is found in BAM, 114 (1935), 332, 333, 841–5, 847, and 115 (1936), 3, 159–60, 217–26. See also the rubric 'Les questions du jour' for an article by P. Fruictier, 'Le vin français sera-t-il collé au cyanure?,' *La Clinique*, xxxie année (Paris: Février 1936), 49–50.
37. Study by Chelle, Dubraquié, et Turbet published in the *Bulletin des travaux de la société de pharmacie de Bordeaux*, cited in the report by the commission (Tenon, secretary), 'Sur l'emploi du ferrocyanure de potassium pour la vinification,' *BAM*, 114 (1935), 842.
38. These customers would be 'les légions de détraqués du tube digestif, des reins, du coeur, des vaissaux et du système nerveux dont nous voyons la marée monter autour de nous.' Fruictier, *La Clinique* (Paris: Février 1936), 50.
39. M. Barthe, 'A propos de l'emploi du ferrocyanure de potassium pour le vinification,' *BAM*, 115 (1936), 159–60.
40. J.-L. Faure, *BAM*, 115 (1936), 221, and Barthe, *BAM*, 115 (1936),160.
41. Clifford A. Hampel and Gessner Hawley, 'Sulphur and compounds,' *The Encyclopaedia of Chemistry* (3d edn, New York: Van Nostrand, 1973); see also entries under sulphur in the Oxford *Concise Science Dictionary*.
42. M. A. Amerine and M. A. Joslyn, *Table Wines. The Technology of their Production* (Berkeley, CA: University of California Press, 1970), 2nd edn, 383; see also 401, 456.

43. G. Paturel, 'La question de l'acide sulfureux dans les vins,' *Annales agronomiques*, 27 (1901), 305–317. Paturel was director of the Station agronomique de Saône-et-Loire.
44. L. Hugounenq, 'Sur le dosage du sulfate de potasse dans les vins,' *Journal de pharmacie et de chimie*, 6th series, i (1895), 349–54.
45. The procedure for whites was spelled out in the *Schweizerische Wochenschrift für Chemie und Pharmacie* in October 1894, and restated in the *Revue de chimie analytique* . . ., ii (1894), 309–10, with reference to *Documents sur les falsifications des matières.* For red wines the procedure used by the municipal laboratory of Paris to find sulphurous acid in beer was acceptable to Paturel.
46. See Peynaud and Fourcade, 'Le sulfitage du vin,' BIV, 252 (1952), 110–120. This article deals with sweet wines in an attempt to introduce more precision and thereby reduce doses of sulphur.
47. Amerine and Joslyn, *op. cit.* (note 42), 408.
48. Pierre Simonis, *L'hygiène du vin d'Alsace* (Thèse présentée pour le doctorat en médecine, Université Louis Pasteur, Faculté de médecine, Strasbourg, 1977). See section on SO_2, 33–34: 'Répercussions nutritionnelles et physiopathologiques du SO_2.'
49. The *vignerons* of Ammerschwihr, who gave Simonis a 'very warm welcome,' were among the large number of wine producers to whom the thesis was dedicated.
50. K. C. Fuselgang, 'Recent Research on SO_2,' *Wines and Vines*, 70 (1989). Fuselgang, a winemaster, was also an adjunct professor of oenology at California State University, Fresno.
51. 'Food Safety Panel - Sulphur dioxide in Foods,' *Journal of the Science of Food and Agriculture*, 32 (1981), 1141–42, gives a summary of a paper by Enrica Quattrucci (Istituto nazionale della nutrizione, Rome): 'Potential intakes of sulphur dioxide - the European situation.'
52. Ough, *Chemical and Engineering News* (January 5, 1987), 22.

PART IV

THE RENAISSANCE OF WINE THERAPY IN TWENTIETH CENTURY FRENCH MEDICINE

7

Establishing the Scientific Basis of an Ancient Remedy

In 1907, when the crisis-stricken wine business was feeling rather unfriendly to the medical establishment, doctors in Bordeaux devoted fifteen pages of their *Journal de Médecine de Bordeaux* to the 'wine question' in medicine.[1] In fact, the question was several, but there was a major question for doctors, especially doctors in the faculty of medicine of the University of Bordeaux: is wine good or bad for the health of the drinker? Though wine had been of concern to the medical mind from time to time in the second half of the nineteenth century, it took a poor second place to alcohol, the star in the debate over the alcoholic treatment of disease. As analytical chemistry identified more and more potentially beneficial (or harmful) elements in wine, it became possible for doctors to focus more specifically on the role of wine in medicine and the effects of wine on the health of the drinker. In 1907 doctors had another reason for their intense discussion of wine. The wine business found the medical profession to be a convenient scapegoat to blame for a slump in the wine trade. This bizarre idea seems to have been inspired by the fact that a few French doctors were active in the anti-alcoholism crusade. True, the refutation of this accusation did not concern doctors as much as the role of wine in health and disease, but the accusation was taken seriously enough to be given a careful rebuttal.

Any statement on wine to a medical group provoked controversy. In 1907 Dr. J.-A. Doléris gave a talk to the Société de médecine de Paris on the nutritional value of wine. He gave the sensible advice that modern man should drink a *little* wine with his meals. This innocuous advice gave rise to an 'animated discussion,' led by a vocal if small medical group hostile to wine. Doctors were properly concerned with alcoholism in France and in particular with the physical and mental devastation blamed on the popular 'green fairy,' absinth. Wine was hardly an accidental victim of a general campaign, since it was the sole source of alcohol for millions of Frenchmen.

Still, it seemed to the defenders of wine that it was being erroneously included in the totally evil category of alcoholic drinks, when it was really much more than just a drink.

In February 1907 the *Journal de médecine de Bordeaux* took note of a nasty petition, sent to the French parliament by the wine merchants of the Syndicat du commerce des vins et spiritueux de Lyon, condemning the anti-alcoholic and therefore unpatriotic campaign being carried out by abstainers and supported by some doctors. News of this campaign must have been a surprise to the medical community, which was, as a whole, notoriously uninterested in fighting alcoholism, particularly *oenolisme* (alcoholism resulting from excessive wine-drinking). A survey by *Illustration*, based on a questionnaire sent out to 300 doctors, found that sixty four per cent of the 173 doctors replying were in favour of moderate wine drinking (less than one litre per day) for promoting health, twenty six per cent indifferent to the effect of moderate drinking on health, and ten per cent against wine drinking. Any minor anti-alcoholic action or propaganda gave rise to a *grande peur* on the part of wine producers, especially in a time of surpluses aggravated by poor sales. Doctors were accused of inventing an alcoholic peril that was never a reality in France; their case was allegedly based on a few wretches in large city hospitals who came from the crowded, anaemic population of cities, especially Paris. Lancereaux was caricatured to illustrate the incoherence of the medical pontiffs of the anti-alcoholic league: he failed to distinguish between drunks and alcoholics, and even saw wine as the chief cause of alcoholism.

The all too successful capitalistic monoculture in the Languedoc had succeeded in flooding France with enormous surpluses of mediocre wine. Economic crisis led to political protest, including a mini-revolution of winegrowers in the Midi.[2] Looking for a scapegoat, a few pro-wine politicians seized upon the anti-alcoholic doctor as an enemy of the people. In the Chamber Joseph Lasies upheld his reputation for surprising wit and originality by equating disease and doctor: 'Le véritable phylloxéra, c'est le médecin.'[3] The crisis over wine surpluses and low prices was soon over, but the fight over winedrinking went on. Alcoholism with the debate over its causes is one of the permanent features of modern French history.

It was not clear how the Third Republic could help its wine-producing supporters by punishing doctors, who were not slow in denouncing an absurd calumny of their wine-loving profession. Some cynics said that the doctors who denounced alcoholism were being paid by enterprises peddling mineral water and, in England, even tea and coffee. Emile Mauriac, zealous propagandist since the end of the century for the medicinal virtues of wine, was the leader of the pack of doctors dealing with hygiene and therapeutic issues related to wine.[4] His colleagues were grateful for this multiple strategy in defending wine, and they especially appreciated his attack on advocates of teetotalism. Mauriac enjoyed the reputation of being the first to unmask temperance societies, especially the more hypocritical English ones, nearly always subsidised by tea and coffee merchants. Virtue and profit were happy bedfellows in perfidious Albion. Indignation and envy seemed to be the chief ingredients of this attack.

Joseph Vergely, who gave the message for the defence in the Bordelais medical journal, noted that very few mineral water establishments were run by medical groups. But the mineral water doctors were as vigilant as the wine doctors in guarding their turf. When the sober Clemenceau, prime minister and a member of the medical fraternity, took the waters at Carlsbad, a consulting doctor at Vichy complained in a letter to the journal. Some doctors partly blamed the slackness in the wine trade on people's disgust with the large amount of fraudulent wine thrown on the market as a result of the phylloxera-generated shortage of natural wine. Others idly speculated that perhaps people were drinking so much mineral water because stomachs ruined by eau-de-vie and absinth needed a respite from alcohol. Medical theories could only be a minor factor in producing the crisis. Not enough stomachs were abstaining, it seems, for Vergely warned that the alcoholic peril, a historical novelty, did exist in the early-twentieth century. And France was the most alcoholic country in the world.

Mauriac's boast to have unmasked the opponents of wine drinking as spokesmen for other beverage industries was a dangerous strategy that could easily be turned against the pro-wine doctors. Even someone inclined to listen sympathetically to Mauriac's arguments might be surprised to find at the end of his work *Le vin au point de vue médical* (1903) a detachable last page with a notice to wine merchants and producers that they had the greatest interest in spreading the brochure at the special price of fifty centimes each if bought fifty at a time. A promising address was given: 115, rue de la Trésorie, Bordeaux. Like many of his colleagues, Mauriac believed that it was possible to avoid any problems by hewing to the scientific line.

In noting the diseases attributed to alcoholism, Vergely paid particular attention to the great killer of the working poor, phthisis or pulmonary tuberculosis (TB), whose positive correlation with alcoholism had become a medical cliché of the age. TB was, Roy Porter notes, 'the single worst disease cultivated by monster cities'; it was responsible for up to forty per cent of the deaths in Paris hospitals.[5] About 1900 the French death rate from TB was still 300 per 100,000 persons; by 1947 it had fallen to eighty, a decline of about seventy per cent (seventy eight per cent in Paris).[6] Nearly three quarters of the TB patients in cities were classified as alcoholics. Medical axioms abounded: 'L'alcool fait le lit de la tuberculose' (Landouzy); 'La phtisie se prend sur le zinc' (Georges Hayem). Fear of the debilitating genetic effect of TB on human breeding stock fed into the more ominous general worry about alcoholism's contribution to the degeneracy of the French race.[7] Not that Vergely blamed wine. Indeed, he hoped that wine consumption would be encouraged at the expense of more alcoholic drinks.

French commentators usually limited the role of wine drinking in the etiology of TB or denied that there was any link at all. In his medical thesis, L. Manaud argued that wine had to be abused for a long time to 'cause' TB, at least ten years for the wine-drinking sons of fathers with TB; this compared favourably with five years needed for aperitif-drinking sons. The only two wine-drinking TB-infected sons found by Manaud drank three and one-half to four litres of white wine daily. So wine was less harmful than aperitifs, even when wine was drunk in large quantities.[8]

Overfeeding had been one of the traditional medical treatments for TB. Dujardin-Baumetz prescribed ten eggs and 200 grams of raw meat daily. Debove stuffed patients with a probe, as if they were foie gras-producing geese. At Falkenstein, in 1895, the patients, encouraged by organ music, sat down at food-laden tables six times a day.[9] It must have been a relief to many patients when wine became a minor weapon in the battle against TB, even if wine was a potentially dangerous medicinal item. 'Every medication is a poison; every poison is a medication.' Advocating the usefulness of red wine in the diet of tubercular patients became one of the countermeasures taken by pro-wine doctors especially after the wide distribution, during the Exposition of 1900 in Paris, of the damaging brochure *Propagande contre la tuberculose*, which urged the proscription of all wine. Emile Mauriac argued that all persons suffering from chest diseases could get relief and comfort from a glass of *vin généreux*. The wine could even begin the healing process. Red bordeaux was as good as a magic mountain; the ideal was to have both.[10] A bit of medical literature supported Mauriac's case. In the TB sanatorium of Angicourt (Oise) Dr. Plicque got the best results from red wines rich in tannin, a substance widely regarded a having considerable curative properties. With its more than two grams of tannin per litre, red bordeaux was an ideal medicine in this case. Using Chomel's method of dividing up doses of wine for some dyspeptic patients (excluding those with acute gastritis), Plicque reported getting excellent results with 'completely natural wines' in treating TB. Mauriac found no reason to doubt the good news, especially when it was backed by references to the healer Plicque and the professorial authority of Professor Chaumel.[11]

In an introduction to the collection of articles on 'la question du vin' in the *Journal de médecine de Bordeaux*, Xavier Arnozan also thought it necessary to defend doctors against the commercial complaint that they were among the culprits responsible for a soft wine market. (The successor of Armand de Fleury in the *Chaire de thérapeutique* in the faculty of medicine at Bordeaux, Arnozan seems to have been immortalised in literature as Dr. Courrèges by François Mauriac in the novel *Désert de l'amour*, published in 1925.[12]) Arnozan noted that some doctors did have an influence in the development of this new world in which wine was banished from aristocratic and even bourgeois tables. Like the main body of the medical profession, Arnozan believed that for most people wine in moderation is a healthful drink — 'la plus saine, la plus hygiénique des boissons' was Pasteur's classic line.[13] The use of light, natural wine and the abuse of alcohol should not be confused; abuse was not a word that went well with wine.

'La question du vin' was organised under three rubrics promising more than they delivered. The issues dealt with fell into the categories of public health and therapeutics, the connection between a fall in wine consumption and the progress of alcoholism, and the positions of doctors and medical societies on the 'question.' One of the chief concerns of the journal in organising this medical defence of wine was to separate wine drinking from alcoholism. It was an essential part of the medical belief system that a wine drinker could be a drunkard without being an alcoholic. The proposition was not easy to demonstrate convincingly, but with a little science and much good will towards wine, doctors concocted a case that satisfied themselves and the wine business.

Xavier Arnozan defended the innocence of wine against the accusations of the anti-alcoholics by sketching a traditional and debatable profile of the superb health of the wine-loving and long-lived Médocains, who in drinking natural wine, often cut with water, suffered from less mental disease, less tuberculosis, and, except in the alcohol-consuming port of Pauillac, even less cirrhosis than much of France.[14] Not that doctors did not recognise the existence of a high incidence of alcoholism in France. Quite the contrary. But natural wine and the alcoholic drinks distilled from it were excluded from explanations of the etiology of alcoholism. It is not easy to understand this position without wondering about the ulterior motives of the actors.

Wine had long been included in the therapeutic repertoire of physicians because of its role in the treatment of 'the disease called man.' With the large-scale commercial distillation of alcohol in the nineteenth century and the advent of the psychic malaise called bourgeois civilisation, it became possible for man to drink himself into disease and to a cheaper and quicker death. Doctors noticed this aberrant behaviour and invented the disease of alcoholism. The question soon arose whether to include the consumption of wine in the etiology of alcoholism. Doctors could not agree any more than anyone else on an answer, especially in the case of moderate consumption of good natural wine. This liquid was a rare commodity that assumed a mythic status in medical discourse and provided an escape from difficult arguments in which opponents could always be accused of basing their case on the consumption of inferior or even artificial wine.

Frédéric Cayla, a staunch defender of wine drinking, was an alarmist on the devastating consequences of alcoholism. 'At present [1901] alcoholics are legion.' Diseases resulting from alcoholism were supposedly reaching a desperate level: arterioslerosis, softening of the brain, suicide, and assassination. Hospitals and insane asylums, though ten times more numerous than when before alcoholism struck, were inadequate to take care of its victims.[15] His explanation of this deterioration in the health of a large part of the population was the common one: the widespread consumption of cheap industrially produced alcohols — a term that did not generally include the 'natural' products of the wine industry.

Cayla expressed better than nearly anyone the medical myth of winedrinking. It goes like this. Before the invasion of France by industrial alcohol there were drunks (*ivrognes*) everywhere, and alcoholics were exceptional. One can be an inveterate drunkard without being an alcoholic, and of course an alcoholic is not necessarily a drunkard. In drinking natural wine to excess, one gets inebriated, drunk. 'On se grise, on s'enivre, on ne se saoule jamais.' (Subtleties are better expressed in a language with a large capacity for dealing with drinking.) Alcoholism comes all too easily from consuming two to three drinks of alcohols like bitters or absinth, or anything not derived from the grape. Cayla wondered why natural wine taken regularly as a *boisson hygiénique* does not produce any of the effects of alcohol on the organism. Why do drinkers of wine as well as those who consume liqueurs based on wine alcohol not become alcoholics?

Cayla, a professional with a heavy scientific baggage, gave an answer based upon a scientific distinction then accepted by many in the medical community. The Pasteurian microbiologist Emile Duclaux had stated that pure alcohol and wine alcohol are not identical, adding the inevitable corollary that moderate consumption of wine is without danger to the health of the drinker. He also noted that the human organism can easily accommodate itself to absorbing small quantities of toxic alcohols. This covering model accommodated Pasteur's discoveries of several non-ethanol elements in wine and Duclaux's own on-going work on higher alcohols while justifying moderate drinking of the superb *eaux-de-vie* produced in France.[16] But Cayla's basic argument was that natural wine contains only pure ethyl alcohol, whose effects are in no way comparable to those of industrial alcohols, which he identified as the so-called higher alcohols, those distilled from beets, potatoes, and cereals. This view ignored the argument over whether the ethyl alcohol produced from grapes is any different from that of other products and, after all, ethanol is the main product of both wine and liquor production. Ignoring the existence of traces of these higher alcohols in wine, Cayla declared that the so-called industrial alcohols (poisons producing convulsions, artificial tetanus, and narcotic effects) were not found in natural wine, whose power of intoxication came only from ethyl alcohol, the gentle poison, 'the least toxic of all alcohols.' (Here Cayla fell back on the authority of the laboratory research of a stable of well-cited researchers: Dujardin-Beaumetz and Audigé, Kinzell, Magnan, Marcé, Cadéac, Meunier, Laborde.)

The argument concerning the uniqueness of wine alcohol had been pretty much destroyed by A. Riche back in 1895. Riche rejected Lannelongue's ingenious explanation of alcoholism on the basis of two periods in the history of alcohol in France: before 1854-5, the period of acute non-dangerous alcoholism caused by natural *eaux-de-vie* or alcohols, and after, the period of chronic and dangerous alcoholism caused by industrial alcohols. The distinction was based on the works of the two-alcohol men, especially Dujardin-Beaumetz, Audigé, and Laborde. Riche thought the distinction to be a complete mistake based on simple coincidence. Riche found that apart from bouquet, natural alcohol is the same as industrial alcohol. What was different in the new France was the higher quantity of alcoholic drinks consumed. In addition to consuming about 118 litres of wine per year by 1894, an average Frenchman drank 4.56 litres of alcoholic beverages. (In 1830 he had drunk his wine with only 1.46 litres of *eaux-de-vie.*) This increased consumption was a distinguishing characteristic of industrial and urban development with a growth of personal wealth and increase in wages.[17]

It also seemed that the worker had an advantage in drinking low quality alcohol: the better the cognac, the more dangerous the drink. Daremberg had shown that rabbits died on being given an injection of high quality cognacs or other comparable alcohols, whereas rabbits injected with ordinary *eau-de-vie* just got dead drunk and recovered. The difference between alcohols of *haute marque* and cheaper ones was found to be that the former contain more aldehydes, higher alcohols, furfurol, and ethers, which gave them their distinction and made them deadlier. Since industrial alcohols contained significantly less of the chemical substances than the high quality natural alcohols, they were less dangerous. A more perverse and logical argument could hardly be imagined.[18] Its cogency and experimental basis did little to get it accepted.

In spite of the putative safety of wine alcohol, Cayla still limited daily doses of wine: one half a glass (100 grams) for people aged four to eighteen years; one-half a litre for a non-hardworking adult; a maximum of one litre for a sedentary person in good health; and two litres for workers. More or less, the standard medical recommendation, though we should remember that the wine was far less alcoholic that our wines.

Doctors in the Bordeaux area had to deal with issues specific to the Bordelais as well as with the questions about wine-drinking common to doctors everywhere. One of the most important questions for doctors in Bordeaux was how widespread was alcoholism in France's most important wine area? Joseph Vergely manipulated numbers to show easily that Bordeaux was still a relatively sober place in the early-twentieth century.[19] Wine consumption in Bordeaux was less than a *barrique* (about 200 litres) per person annually. Between 1875 and 1901 consumption fell from 229 to 198 litres. In the Hôpital Saint-André daily individual consumption fell in this period from 337 ml to 281 ml. But people were consuming more alcohol: from 1875 to 1900, the increase was from 1.66 to 4.52 litres per person annually. Between 1895 and 1905 beer drinking fell off by about thirty per cent, which must have partly accounted for a drop to 2.73 litres in the per capita annual consumption of alcohol by 1905. Wine consumption stayed roughly the same in this period. In the case of the patients of the Hôpital Saint-André wine could not be judged totally innocuous. Of the more than seventy per cent of the TB patients who were alcoholics, one fifth were winos, that is, people who drank daily at least three litres of wine containing ten degrees of alcohol. Half of these patients were also victims of absinth.

Not that there was no alcoholism in the Gironde. Far from it. But it was said to be mainly a disease of the quai workers, drinkers of absinth and aperitifs. Serious medical men declared that alcoholism did not exist among wine workers.[20] Nor did foremen and workers in wine warehouses become alcoholics even though they drank considerable amounts of wine over many years. These workers were hardly ever found in statistics on 'delirious alcoholics,' who were mostly a population of dockers and sailors, victims of bars serving alcohol rather than wine. Nowadays of course it is recognised that in the champagne industry, for example, alcoholism on the part of workers who drink the product they are producing is a real problem.

Few doctors did a better job of depicting the medical horrors of alcoholism while defending moderate wine consumption than Emmanuel Régis, professor of clinical psychiatry in the Bordeaux medical faculty and president of the anti-alcohol section of the Girondin committee of the Alliance d'hygiène sociale.[21] Régis' case against alcohol was based on a skilful use of figures from the mental asylums in the Gironde. Although delirious mental states caused by alcohol were very rare in the upper classes in Bordeaux, there was no shortage of alcoholics in overcrowded asylums. Asylums were overcrowded, at least in Paris, because of the large number of male alcoholics admitted.[22] Régis argued that 'true alcoholism, that is, cerebral alcoholism, violent, aggressive, and criminal, showed up in the Bordeaux region after the spread of phylloxera,' which temporarily reduced wine production. So the evolution of alcoholism was seen as parallel to the growth of bars where 'dangerous drinks' were consumed. With one drinking dive for every eighty people, Bordeaux came right after Paris in opportunities to get drunk. Régis claimed never to have seen an alcoholic who drank only wine.[23]

Yet Régis admitted that alcoholism, regarded as rare in the working class in the past, was growing considerably, even among women. At the Maison de Santé du Bouscat out of 641 men admitted between 1846 and 1903, six and one-half per cent were alcoholics compared with one-half per cent of the women. Out of

2724 men admitted between 1888 and 1903 to the Asile public d'aliénés hommes de Cadillac, fifteen per cent were alcoholics. And at the Asile public d'aliénées femmes de Château-Picon only 0.8 per cent of the 3136 women admitted were alcoholics. Dr. Pons, head doctor at Château-Picon, noted a recent increase in the number of women alcoholics. Régis found that in his psychiatric clinic at the Hôpital Saint-André de Bordeaux female alcoholics went from one out of 116 of patients admitted in 1902-04 to six out of seventy nine (8.28 per cent) in 1906-07. Most alarming were the figures on males for Saint-André, where Régis found that between 1902 (when he organised the clinic) and 1907 out of the 407 men admitted, 20.7 per cent were chronically delirious and forty to forty five per cent chronic alcoholics — 'an enormous figure.'

Out of the alarm about alcoholism came reassurance about wine. Only one of the eighty four delirious male alcoholics was a wine warehouse worker. Twenty six of this sub-group were quai workers. Régis always tried to learn the type of alcohol drunk by his alcoholic patients. His observation that alcoholics often drank other alcohols in addition to wine lent some credibility to his general argument on the safety of moderate consumption of wine alone. White wine consumed without food was more likely to be the culprit than red wine; and several *petits blancs* could be particularly damaging for people who loaded up with other alcohols.

Many wine-friendly commentators always observed that alcoholism was a northern disease, found outside wine-producing regions, with heavy boozers pullulating in Brittany, Normandy, and the Nord. Even doctors incapable of imagining a sober south did not disagree with this view. In Paris over sixty six per cent of alcoholics came from the provinces; most came from Normandy, Brittany, departments of the north and the east, the centre, and other regions having a substantial immigration to Paris. The most dangerous occupations were in the food business, which accounted for nearly sixteen per cent of Parisian alcoholics, construction (nearly thirteen per cent), transportation (over eleven per cent), and commerce (over ten per cent).[24]

Even in France only the rare doctor denied that heavy wine-drinking eventually produces pathological disorders in the drinker's body. Lancereaux was probably the leading voice — one is tempted to exaggerate by calling him a *vox clamantis* — preaching the dangers of *oenolisme*, or acute intoxication by wine. He now welcomed the opportunity to refute certain opinions that had been attributed to him. In a way he was a friend of wine, and the *Journal de médecine de*

Bordeaux was happy to publish his critical appreciation of wine.[25] Since 1865 he had been advising Americans who came to discuss alcoholism with him to plant vines. He claimed to be one of the first to put wine in the category of *boissons hygiéniques*.

Lancereaux now seemed enlightened enough to accept the popular axiom that drunks are not necessarily alcoholics. He also agreed with his colleagues that wine drunk without food seems to do most damage, producing digestive problems (including gastritis and copious diarrhoea with pronounced malnutrition) and nervous problems such as lack of sensitivity, trembling, and delirium. The drinker of *eau-de-vie* and the person suffering from chronic *oenolisme* has the same disorders of the nervous system: delirium tremens, inability to sleep, bad dreams, startled awakenings, and loss of sensitivity in the extremities of lower body members. Workers who drink white wine without eating, usually in the morning, often suffer from cirrhosis of the liver. Over the preceding forty years Lancereaux had opened up 300 victims of cirrhosis who had drunk from two to five litres daily over a shortened lifespan. If they were wine drinkers, these people would mostly likely have been Parisian workers who had drunk too much of the plastered wines of the Midi rather than doctors who had drunk (in moderation) the wines of Burgundy. Lancereaux confessed that he had been slow to recognise that the disorders resulting from an excess of wine came came from adulteration and from foreign substances added to wine for preservation and transport. Lancereaux's excessively optimistic view was that adulteration can be easily avoided and other substances used for preservation; most of the problems arising from wine consumption seemed to be easily solvable.[26] The inclusion of Lancereaux in this Bordelais medical discussion of wine drinking ensured that the affair would not appear to be an attempt to downplay the dangers of drinking in order to placate the wine business. A friendly enemy could provide a useful worst case scenario that was not so bad after all.

A few doctors were not convinced by the new arguments. And Théodore Simon was less impressed than were the Bordelais doctors by the pro-wine theses coming out of medical faculties, including Paris. In 1906-07 he used the journal *La clinique* to subject two representative works to sceptical scrutiny. 'L'alcool est à la mode aujourd'hui en pathologie, hier c'était l'alcool en thérapeutique.'[27] Using a questionnaire he sent to doctors in the Armagnac area, Ducuron-Tucot had done a study of alcoholism exonerating wine as well as *eau-de-vie* distilled from wine if the liqueur were not 'abused.'[28] Simon found the recommendation to drink wine regularly a little vague, reminiscent of the anecdotes told about wine-abusing geezers still full of vim and vigour. It was easy enough for Ducuron-Tucot to criticise laboratory experiments on animals that did not distinguish between types of alcohol and to point out that wine-producing areas were not the areas suffering most from alcoholism. Blaming industrial chemistry for alcoholism had become popular in wine-supporting circles, but as Simon noted, it did not explain the descriptions of delirium tremens in works that had appeared before the drinks using industrial alcohol became available. Even if one admitted the rarity of delirium, what advantage could there possibly be in regularly consuming *eau-de-vie*? Since the doctor should be guided by the maxim of *primum no nocere*, Simon would have preferred a discussion on the innocuity of good quality water, which should be recommended for daily consumption, leaving alcohol to be prescribed, like morphine, for precise symptoms.[29] There was a danger in water drinking, however. Several scientific gurus, including the redoutable Armand Gautier, argued that water drinkers were more exposed to appendicitis, entero-colitis, and typhoid fever. Simon thought that there were greater dangers in wine drinking. Unlike the defenders of wine drinking, Simon drew attention to the fact that wine made the liver less able to counteract or destroy poisons and the body less resistant to different infections, including tuberculosis and pneumonia.

In waxing ironic on the bacteriocidal power of wine, especially in the case of making water safe to drink, Simon was questioning the importance of a major new claim of pro-wine doctors. Wine had been given a dual Pasteurian allure in the argument that it was a germ-killing agent whose efficacy had been experimentally demonstrated. Research done by Sabrazès, *professeur agrégé* in the faculty of medicine in Bordeaux, and Marcandier was published in the *Annales de l'Institut Pasteur*, an outlet that gave added scientific authority to both article and authors.

The medical pro-wine forces in the Bordelais probably felt a sense of relief when, in 1907, the Société de médecine de Paris released its commission's six-part report on wine and public health.[30] The report was generally favourable to moderate wine consumption, a conclusion not totally unexpected since it was strong drink rather than wine than was on trial. Given the national angst of French elites over widespread alcoholism and opium addition, wine drinking seemed a minor problem. True, some doctors had said nasty things about wine. And they were duly reported in the *Journal de médecine de Bordeaux*, though balanced by counter dogmas praising the medical virtues of wines.

Godefroy Bardet, advocate of *climatothérapie* and water cures, was among doctors most hostile to alcohol and suspicious of wine drinking, but even he admitted wine's possible therapeutic uses. He reminded the Société de médecine de Paris of a discussion that had been stimulated in the Société de thérapeutique when Henri Triboulet had presented a remarkable report denouncing both alcohol and wine. 'Alcohol cannot be considered a true food; it is a stimulating drug, capable of rendering services, but above all a medication and a dangerous toxic agent.' Triboulet, who viewed the use of wine as an old habit that nothing could justify scientifically, continued to say bad things about alcohol and doctors who did not condemn its consumption in any form.[31] Régis, described by Doléris as a stubborn water drinker, wanted scientific proof of the utility of wine drinking that would corroborate clinical observations. He learned instead Louis Izou had discovered that eighty per cent of wine drinkers in Martillac (Aveyron) showed signs of arteriosclerosis at the age of thirty five. Fortunately, later commentators were able to explain the lesions of these drinkers to the satisfaction of the pro-wine doctors by pointing out that the drinkers of Martillac were great consumers of charcuterie and meat, which could be blamed rather than wine or alcohol. And even Régis allowed adults to drink wine moderately. Still, it was a bad scene that Bardet had resurrected.

The three members of the commission, including Paul Dignat as secretary, saw the four conclusions of their report approved unanimously by the Société de médecine de Paris. Their first conclusion was that well-cellared good wine is a useful drink for regular use, even for children of second age, provided that a number of conditions are met: the wine must not exceed nine or ten per cent alcohol by volume; the wine must not be too old; the daily dose must not exceed an average of sixty centilitres; and the wine must be cut with water. For daily consumption, red is preferable to white wine, and the red should not be too acid or rich in bouquets. (The report ignored the model of the *grand vin* consecrated in gastronomy, which generations of favourable propaganda in its favour have accustomed us to see as highly desirable; indeed, the Société implied that such wine was a danger to the health of the drinker.) Secondly, since no system of certificate of origin and of sale existed to give an absolute guarantee of the qualities of the wine, the Société thought that given the importance of assuring the hygienic qualities of the wine being consumed, it was desirable that the seller give the buyer an analysis indicating the chief characteristics of the wine: degree of alcohol, tannin content, level of acidity, and potassium content. Thirdly, the Société believed that the social dangers arising from the consumption of distilled products were so great that it was desirable that serious restrictive measures, even prohibitive measures, be taken concerning the manufacture or sale of alcohol. Last, like most scientific groups, the Société called for more research. Biologists should take up 'the wine question' and do research on the effect of wine on nutrition and the functions of the organism. Not a bad report card for either wine or medicine.

The report's second section, dealing with adulteration of natural wines and with artificial wines, was less comforting for the pro-wine forces.[32] A lot of wines on the market did not contain the elements possessing the medicinal properties for which doctors recommended wine and, worse, some contained harmful substances. Wine fraud has a long history as a medical problem. Louis Hébert had warned, in his section on drinks in the *New Dictionary of Practical Medicine and Surgery* (1866), that 'few substances are as subject to fraud as wines.'[33] Not only were wines watered, flavoured and coloured with harmless natural substances, and cut with inferior wines (*gros vins*), but they sometimes had dangerous substances added, of which the most notorious was litharge or lead monoxide to mask the bitterness of soured wines. In the end, the doctor was dependent on the wine taster to judge the quality and authenticity of the wine and on the chemist to detect dangerous substances. Only the lucky drinker who found and could pay for pure wine would be able to benefit from a helpful stimulation of digestive functions. Such a wine was more likely to be bordeaux than burgundy, it seemed. Hébert thought that 'true gourmets, the true connoisseurs, rated the *crus du haut Médoc* of Bordeaux most highly, even placing them ahead of the great burgundies of corresponding quality.'[34] This opinion, typical of much of the nineteenth century, reflected serious problems of quality control in putting good burgundy on the market.[35]

The flood of artificial wines of all sorts on the market during the shortages of the latter part of the nineteenth century led to the rigorous application of analytical chemistry in detecting adulteration.[36] In 1877 Armand Gautier, professor of chemistry in the Paris medical faculty, brought out the first edition of his classic work on the adulteration of wines. The book was so successful and useful, and so much new research had been done on the subject, not least by Gautier himself, that he completely revised the work for the third edition in 1884.[37] With such a fine work circulating on all the tricks of the wine trade and how to detect them easily, it might be thought that the problems would be soon solved. No doubt there was eventually much less adulterated wine on the market, but adulteration continued and became more difficult to detect as experts in adulteration perfected their skills in chemical creation, though by the 1930s a great deal of the illegal manipulation of wine consisted in the using dangerous additives to give the pure product a longer shelf life.[38] Additives were fewer and easier to detect in the early-twentieth century.

The defence of wine mounted in 1907 by the *Journal de médecine de Bordeaux* included a laudatory presentation of the work of Emile Mauriac, widely admired by his fellow doctors as a vigorous enemy of the anti-alcoholic forces and a stout medico-scientific defender of the therapeutic powers of red bordeaux. And by 1907 his publisher was able to advertise him as an Inspecteur générale honoraire de la salubrité. Applying the general therapeutic dogma to wine, Mauriac drew on the latest oenological research 'to establish the precise composition' of wine as 'a complex liquid containing very useful elements' for the treatment of diseases. Tannin, abundant in red bordeaux, was considered to be the most important of these elements. Several acid salts, including ferrous, copper, and calcium sulphates added to wine's medicinal value. Mauriac's presentation of the chemical composition of wine was a standard oenological exercise in analytical chemistry organised according to the categories of volatile components or elements, dry extract, mixed components, and mineral salts. For medical purposes it was also important to classify wines according to their content in phosphoric acid and potassium. This chemical analysis was an overture to Mauriac's chief aim, the establishment of the therapeutic properties of wine, a subject that was, he believed, not yet dealt with as it deserved to be.

Contemporary classics in therapeutics grudgingly gave wine a few vague lines in their big treatises but typically treated wine as alcohol instead of taking into account the substances (iron, tannin, glycerine, lime, potassium, phosphorus, tartar, acids, and ethers) that gave wine its therapeutic properties more than did the alcohol it contained. The physiological properties of these substances were known to doctors. Mauriac argued that they are much more easily assimilated into the organism if given in wine rather than in pharmaceutical preparations, and their intimacy with other substances reinforces their power of action. This action could be compared to the marvellous curative effects produced by certain substances in natural mineral waters of complex composition that pharmaceutical doses ten to twenty times stronger are powerless to produce. Mauriac summed up by declaring the existence of a wine therapy (*vinothérapie*) comparable to hydrotherapy. Mauriac turned out to be a prophet: a new kind of *vinothérapie* is the latest rage in wine country, though the price of 3550 francs for a few days of wallowing in luxury even at Smith Haut-Lafitte might not be covered by medical insurance, even if the benefits of bathing in fresh presscake and massages with grape seed oil might seem worth every centime.[39]

Mauriac's line of reasoning had been at the heart of chemotherapy since the latter part of the nineteenth century and particularly since Paul Ehrlich had developed his 'side-chain theory' in the process of searching for 'magic bullets that seek their target of their accord.' This plan of anchoring a toxin molecule to the side chains (later called receptors) of a cell for which it had a chemical attraction was similar to Emil Fischer's concept of 'lock and key.'[40] In Mauriac's more general therapeutic scheme wine was the ideal delivery system for substances with curative properties.

Perhaps inspired by the work of Plicque and of Chomel, Mauriac studied the indications and counter-indications of the chief kinds of wines in different illnesses before giving his clinically coloured advice. He was especially interested in the hygienic and physiological aspects: the favourable effects of wine on the secretion of acid in the stomach and its anti-microbial action on the germs of cholera and typhoid fever with a consequent prophylactic value in these diseases. Mauriac also studied wine's nutritional value. Persons used to drinking wine eat more when they stop drinking but seem to get less nutrition than they did from less food while drinking. (The not so subtle implication here is that wine is a food.)

Red bordeaux, with its triple function of drink, food, and remedy, really worked wonders in patients recovering from acute illnesses or cachetic states. 'La médication de choix.' It was good for aiding patients who had been weakened by the 'eruptive fever' of typhoid, malaria, diphteria, scarletina, and smallpox. Anemic, chlorotic, and neurasthenic patients needed old wines of the Médoc, especially those of Saint-Emilion and the Graves, both wines rich in iron, phosphoric acid, and potassium. Suffers from syphilis could also benefit from these wines, which, according to Mauriac, counter the 'déglobulisation' of the blood that accompanies the disease.[41]

In presenting the therapeutic indications of wine, Mauriac used the traditional division based on colour. And white wines got short shrift. Riche had argued that whites contain products that go to the brain, affect the spinal cord and act on the entire nervous system. The popular expression for this stagger-inducing phenomena of whites was 'ils cassent les jambes.' Carles believed that the alcohol in whites is absorbed quickly because of the absence of the moderating effect of tannin found in red wines. Consequently, white wine congests and overworks the nervous system, sharply stimulating the kidneys, getting the drinker overexcited, and, if drunk daily, even hastening the onset of delirium tremens – a condition Mauriac optimistically classified as rare for red wine drinkers. White wines were certainly not for women and children except in small amounts. And neither were they for regular male consumption, especially without eating.[42]

In a revised version of his wine therapy several years later, Mauriac gave white wines a more friendly analysis, which emphasised their stimulating and diuretic qualities, mostly due to ethers, especially 'acetic ether,' and other volatile substances not yet identified. A later study showed that the most diuretic wines are Anjou, Muscadet, and Gros Plant.[43] Whites of weak acidity and low alcohol became recognised as good for patients with stomach illnesses such as excessive acidity with dyspepsia, pyrosis, and gastralgic pains. Obesity, liver disease, and problems with the bile ducts called for whites, whose diuretic properties made them useful in all illnesses where diuresis was used in healing. Following Dujardin and Beaumetz, Mauriac stated that the carbonic acid in champagne soothes and deadens the stomach's mucous membrane, thus making it useful in treating cholera, vomiting, including 'nervous vomiting' in pregnancy, irritation of the peritoneum, and in countering the exhaustion accompanying heavy haemorrhaging.[44]

Sauternes were classified as tonic but also stimulating. High in alcohol, Sauternes could be prescribed for patients convalescing from a serious illness or patients needing a *coup de fouet* following a strong fever, serious haemorrhaging, or great fatigue. A help to digestion at the end of a meal, Sauternes 'send a shaft of gaiety into the soul.' But sweet white wines and *vins de liqueur* were not recommended for cancer patients. Research by Freund and Bencke had found an excess of sugar and glycogen in the blood of these patients. So Mauriac leaped to the conclusion that they would be better off if all sugar elements were eliminated from their diet. Otherwise *vins de liqueur*, grudgingly recognised as better than absinth, were considered of some use in promoting digestion, if drunk ten to fifteen minutes before the meal, for they could stimulate the gastric mucous membrane and cause an influx of pepsin and hydrochloric acid. Most diseases of the nervous system and of the heart and aorta required the doctor to prohibit the big (*généreux*) white wines, champagne, and *vins de liqueur*.[45]

Mauriac's work was a perfectly respectable defence of wine by a doctor who had solid publications on other subjects. His book drew selectively on much scientific work but it was resolutely clinical, intended to give the practitioner another weapon in the battle against disease. Bordelais doctors had to recognise that any argument from Bordeaux in favour of wines, even if it exuded the aromas of recent research, might be regarded sceptically by the profession on a national level. A collective opinion of a powerful medical group would be more convincing, especially if it contained some big names in medicine, and this was exactly what the Bordelais doctors got when the Société de médecine de Paris gave its answer to 'the wine question.'

In 1909 Armand Gautier gave wine drinking a boost in the new journal *L'Hygiène* with an article establishing a scientific basis for the hygienic superiority of wine over beer and cider. His argument can be summed up briefly but fairly. Though man can abstain from drinking alcoholic beverages, he has always sought them. 'They satisfy a real need, that of finding a stimulant permitting a momentary effort superior to the ordinary one.' Of all alcoholic drinks, wine is the best value for money. Beer and cider are 'cold drinks,' that is they do not 'adequately stimulate the stomach and body strength, thus leading the unsatisfied consumer to drink alcohol after or between meals.' Since wine is able to satisfy man's thirst for alcohol, wine country generally escapes alcoholism. Beer is fattening and coarsening and leads to more drinking; cider is often mixed with perry, an irritant of the nervous centres. Gautier therefore considered wine to be the best 'boisson hygiénique.'[46]

During World War I everyone could express hostility towards non-wine cultures while disguising the opinion as science or scholarship with the approbation of at least one national intellectual elite. Discussions about wine consumption provided an excellent occasion to denounce dull, brutal, beer-drinking Germans. In 1916 the old anti-feminist promoter of scientific medicine Charles Fiessinger (1857-1942) gave an amusing if contested speech to the French academy of medicine.[47] Many of his pro-wine arguments were common in the medical community. The Academy provided a generally sympathetic audience for a pro-wine speech: it approved of the wine ration of three-quarters of a litre for French soldiers fighting Germany, a formidable foe in spite of beer being its national drink — presumably the brutality resulting from non-wine alcohol was an advantage in war. The difficulty with the anti-beer argument was that France also had its beer drinkers, like the valiant population of the Nord. In an ironic reply to Fiessinger, Georges Linossier, expert on the digestive system and its diseases and a believer in the therapeutic powers of mineral waters, did not fail to point this out, as well as to point out the absurdity of attributing the German mentality to beer consumption.[48] No one mentioned France's ally, the British, champion beer drinkers until a considerable inter-war drop in consumption. Nor did Fiessinger remember his fellow wine-drinking Catholics in southern Germany. The truth is that no counter argument would convince the pro-wine forces, who in peacetime would simply accuse the Nord and any non-wine drinker of contributing to alcoholism.

Fiessinger believed that personality disorders could be explained by the way in which mental traits and individualism are formed by internal secretions operating in concert with the organisation of the brain. He believed that wine positively influences the key to life, that is the internal secretions that regulate many vital functions. Medicine was reduced to oenophilism teaching by examples, and though the danger of *oenolisme* was not ignored, it was not viewed by pro-wine doctors as a problem in France. A parable illustrated the value of wine in psychiatric therapy. About twenty years before (c. 1895), a doctor in Divonne-les-Bains, where a large casino helped banish psychosomatic problems, was expecting the arrival of a desperate Parisian neurasthenic for a thermal cure. The patient never arrived. On the way he stopped to see his uncle, a winegrower in Burgundy, who was indignant at the idea of a water cure, vastly inferior to a daily bottle of Beaune. The patient stayed with his uncle for a month, less time than required for the thermal therapy, and returned to his business completely cured. Dr. Fiessinger explained to his fellow doctors that the wine had stimulated good internal secretions in the patient and re-established his nutritional equilibrium. His stomach, lulled into a less excitable state by an abrupt change of habits and environment, willingly tolerated the wine. Fiessinger's speech aroused the sceptical scorn of the teetotalers. Georges Linossier asked for the details of the physiological research on which Fiessinger based his opinion that internal secretions are favourably influenced by wine. And could he demonstrate the functioning of these secretions in the working of the brain? No.

Maurice de Fleury, who had treated a great number of neurasthenics, said that he had tried the wine treatment but found that his patients were cured quicker and better if they drank only water. This was not a problem, according to de Fleury, because the bourgeoisie, like their sons fighting the Germans, were water drinkers. So they joined the notorious French water drinkers, so few in number that it was easy for medical literature to give some of its valuable space to list them. Not many doctors were as bold as Legendre, who posted his anti-alcoholic principles in his ward at the Tenon hospital, in the twentieth arrondissement of Paris.[49]

Only a few hundred out of France's thousands of doctors (12,000 to 15,000 in 1900) supported anti-alcoholic activity of any sort, and some doctors did oppose the use of wine because they saw little difference between it and other types of alcoholic drinks. Serious interest in alcoholism as a disease was a quasi-monopoly of the psychiatrists.[50] But some research was done showing that wine could have negative effects on the human organism, even if it did not get any coverage in the publications that were so quick to report the research showing the beneficial effects of moderate wine drinking.

In his widely-used text *Les grands symptômes neurasthéniques*, de Fleury warned that alcohol harms the nervous person even if absorbed in its most diluted form. Some doctors assumed that beer, cider, and watered wine were acceptable. But de Fleury would not allow his patients any white wine or even bordeaux cut (presumably with Evian, Thonon, or Alet) to two or three times its volume. He believed that drinks low in alcohol increase stomach acidity by secondary fermentation, causing excessive flatulence with ballooning of the belly. In fact, a glass or two of low-alcohol beer (*petite bière*) or cider would disturb the digestion more than alcohol of ninety degrees. Nor did de Fleury believe that mineral waters were particularly suited for consumption by neurasthenics. True, the waters of Vals, Pouges, and Vichy could help greatly if a neurasthenic patient had dyspepsic problems. It was also a considerable medical advantage that the big stations, especially Vichy, had some top doctors on tap.[51]

All of the favourable medical propaganda in favour of wine did not bring about closure in the debate. Far from it. After World War I, the whole debate was replayed, *mutatis mutandis*. Nearly thirty years after Mauriac's pro-wine offensive, Georges Portmann, medical professor and dean at the faculty of medicine in Bordeaux and Girondin senator, was able to make a comparison between the anti-wine movement of the turn of the century and that of the 1920s. An important difference was the domination of the post-war market by natural wine as a result of the post-phylloxera reconstitution of the vineyards and laws against fraud and adulteration. When real wine is cheap there is not much profit in faking. Like Mauriac earlier, Portmann argued that the battle against the anti-wine forces had had to be fought on scientific grounds. Unlike Mauriac, Portmann and his colleague, Dr. Dougnac, another doughty defender of wine, were members of a dwindling band of doctors preaching the virtues of *vinothérapie* to an overwhelmingly indifferent profession. Doctors were increasingly inclined to see wine, at one end of the scale, as an item of importance in their religion of *haute gastronomie* and, at the other end, as just another alcoholic drink rather than an important tool in the practice of medicine. It made little difference that wine therapy was based on the latest research and the scientific case impressively technical. With no formal input into educational machines for producing doctors and pharmacists, wine could not become part of the medical curriculum and could not achieve prescribed-drug status. Nor could doctors have much interest in prescribing such a non-exotic product, no matter how much oenology grew in scientific status.

Notes

1. 'Le vin au point de vue de l'hygiène générale et de la thérapeutique,' *Journal de médecine de Bordeaux* (hereinafter *JMBX*), 37 (15 septembre 1907), 581–95.
2. See Leo A. Loubère, *The Red and the White. A History of Wine in France and Italy in the Nineteenth Century* (New York: State University of New York Press, 1978), ch. 12, 'Era of Crises.'
3. Joseph Lasies (1862-1927) began his political career in 1898 as deputy for the arrondissement of Condom. After 1914 he was a deputy for Paris.
4. Among Emile Mauriac's works on wine were *La défense du vin et la lutte contre l'alcoolisme* (Paris: Doin, 1901); *La lutte contre l'alcoolisme par la propagation du vin* (communication at the Congrès de l'association française pour l'avancement des sciences, section d'hygiène, Montauban, 1902); *Le vin au point de vue médical. Sa composition chimique, ses propriétés thérapeutiques, ses indications et ses contre-indications dans le traitement des maladies* (Paris: Doin, 1903); *Les vins de Bordeaux, leurs qualités hygiéniques et curatives* (Bordeaux: Féret et fils, 1907). A versatile faculty man, Mauriac published on urban ambulances and rabies (including Pasteur's treatment) as well as on issues in public health — e.g., poisoning attributed to salted cod: *La question des morues rouges, étude d'hygiène alimentaire* (Bordeaux: Gounouilhou, 1886) found that, contrary to rumor, the red-coloured fish were safe for consumption.

5. Roy Porter, *The Greatest Benefit to Mankind. A Medical History of Humanity* (London: HarperCollins, 1997), 401–2. See David S. Barnes, *The Making of a Social Disease. Tuberculosis in Nineteenth-Century France* (Berkeley, CA: University of California Press, 1995).
6. P. Savy, *Traité de thérapeutique clinique* (Paris: Masson, 1940), 261.
7. See Robert A. Nye, *Crime, Madness, and Politics in Modern France. The Medical Concept of National Decline* (Princeton: Princeton University Press, 1984).
8. L. Manaud, *Recherches nouvelles sur les rapports de l'alcoolisme et de la tuberculose* (Medical thesis, Bordeaux, 1906-07), reported in *JMBX*, 37 (15 septembre 1907), 591.
9. P. Salvy, *op. cit.* (note 6), 252.
10. At the International Sanatorium Berghof, Hans Castorp and Joachim Ziemssen drank the second-growth Gruaud Larose (Saint Julien) with their first meal there. Maria Mancini cigars reinforced the bourgeois atmosphere. See Thomas Mann, *Der Zauberberg* (Frankfurt-am-Main: S. Fischer, 1924).
11. August-François Chomel, successor to Laënnec in the *Chaire de clinique médicale de la Charité* was an authority on fevers and digestive diseases and other things. By 1863 his *Eléments de pathologie générale* (Paris: Masson, 1817) was in its 5th edn. His *Leçons de clinique médicale* (Paris: Baillière, 3 vols.) came out in 1834-40 and *Des dyspepsies* in 1857. In an article in the *Presse médicale* in 1899 Plicque recalled and approved of Chomel's opionion on wine as eupeptic. In 1902 Plicque, then head doctor at the Sanatorium antituberculeux d'Angicourt, put forward his defence of giving TB patients divided doses of red wine according to Chomel's method. See Mauriac, *Le vin au point de vue médical*, (note 4), 15–17.
12. See the 'Leçon d'ouverture du cours de thérapeutique' of Le docteur X. Arnozan: *Soignons-nous les malades mieux qu'autrefois?* (Bordeaux: Gounouilhou, 1893). Citing medical applications of discoveries in microbiology and progress in organic chemistry, Arnozan gave a clear positive answer to this question (can we cure the sick better than in the past?).
13. Louis Pasteur, *Etudes sur le vin* (2d edn, Imprimerie Impériale, 1873), 53.
14. Xavier Arnozan, 'L'alcool et le vin devant la médecine,' in *JMBX*, 37 (15 septembre 1907).
15. Dr. F. Cayla, *Le vin, le buveur de vin et le buveur d'alcool, les eaux-de-vie et les liqueurs* (Bordeaux: Gounouilhou, 1901). A work of seventy pages. Like many of the doctors who defended wine, Cayla had a solid medical reputation based on work unrelated to alcoholism, including

infant cholera, diet, consumption of liquids, meals in dyspepsia cases, and smoking.

16. E. Duclaux, 'Etudes sur les vins,' *Annales de chimie et de physique* (1874), and 'Sur la recherche des alcools de degré supérieur,' *Annales de l'Institut Pasteur*, ii (1888), 489–93. Note that the AIP article is about the discovery of 'high degree alcohols' in liquids — the difference in the alcohols was seen as in terms of their strength or degree.
17. 'L'accroissement de la fortune publique, l'augmentation des salaires ont suscité le goût et l'abus des jouissances; le luxe sous toutes ses formes a envahi la bourgeoisie, et l'amour de la boisson tout spécialement l'ouvrier des villes.' A. Riche, 'La loi sur les boissons alcooliques, l'alcoolisme,' *Journal de pharmacie et de chimie*, ii (1895), 309–18, 355–72, 405–23, etc.
18. *Ibid.*, 370–1, 411.
19. Dr. Vergely, 'L'alcoolisme à Bordeaux en 1905,' JMBX, 37 (15 septembre 1907), 594, and *Quelques chiffres sur l'alcool et l'alcoolisme à Bordeaux* (Bordeaux: Gounouilhou, 1902).
20. One of Emmanuel Régis's students, Dr. Moulinié showed this in his medical thesis *Les dégustateurs en Gironde et l'alcoolisme professionnel* (Bordeaux: Faculté de Médecine, 1887).
21. E. Régis, 'Le vin et l'alcoolisme,' *JMBX*, 37 (15 septembre 1907), 591, which draws on Régis, 'L'antialcoolisme à Bordeaux,' *Annales de l'alliance d'hygiène sociale* (août 1903), and L. Dréneau, *Contribution à l'étude du délire alcoolique, d'après cinquante-quatre observations prises à la clinique psychiatrique de l'hôpital Saint-André* (medical thesis, Bordeaux, 1905).
22. Patricia E. Prestwich, 'Drinkers, Drunkards, and Degenerates: The Alcoholic Population of a Parisian Asylum, 1867-1914,' in Jack S. Blocker Jr. and Cheryl Krasnick Warsh (eds), *The Changing Face of Drink: Substance, Imagery, and Behaviour* (Ottawa: Social History Inc., 1997), 119; see especially note 19 on Sainte-Anne.
23. E. Régis, *Précis de psychiatrie* (6th edn, Paris: Doin, 1923), 588.
24. R. Benon, 'L'alcoolisme à Paris,' *Annales d'hygiène et de médecine légale* (0ctober 1910), summarized in *Le Journal de médecine de Paris* (1908), 388. According to C. Curtel, 'Le vin et l'alcoolisme,' *L'Oenophile*, 6e année (1899), 324–6, the departments in which most alcohol was consumed (figures are for litres per person annually) were the Seine-Inférieure — 15.88, Calvados — 15.12, Eure — 12.14, Somme — 11.77, Oise — 10.64; the departments in which the least wine was drunk were Eure — 22, Seine-Inférieure — 21, Somme — 19, Morbihan — 18, Ille-et-Villaine — 17, Calvados — 14, etc.

Viticultural departments were calculated to have usually an average annual consumption per person of less than two litres of alcohol.

25. Lancereaux, 'Sur les désordres pathologiques causés par l'abus prolongé du vin,' *JMBX*, 37 (15 septembre 1907), 421 ff.
26. *Ibid.*, 593.
27. Th. Simon, 'Psychiatrie,' *La clinique*, no. 44 (2 Novembre 1906), 716.
28. Ducuron-Tucot, *L'alcoolisme en Armagnac. Contribution à l'étude du rôle du vin naturel et de son alcool dans la genèse de la folie alcoolique* (Thèse de Bordeaux, Faculté de Médecine, 1906), reviewed by Th. Simon in *La clinique*, no. 44 (2 novembre 1906), 716.
29. Simon gave an even more sceptical review to the excessively pro-wine thesis by Louis Izou, *La défense du vin dans la lutte antialcoolique* (Thèse de Paris, 1907): *La clinique*, no. 31 (2 août 1907), 493.
30. The report ('Le vin au point de vue de l'hygiène,' rapport du Dr. Dignat à la Société de médecine de Paris) and its discussion in the Société de médecine de Paris can be found in Dr. J.-A. Doléris, *Le vin et les médecins: le pour et le contre* (Paris: Vigot, 1907; 1931), part I, ch. II. A great defender of the benefits of wine-drinking, Doléris, former president of the Académie de médecine was president of the Chambre d'agriculture de Basses Pyrénées and a member of the council of the Société des viticulteurs de France et d'ampélographie. With doctors Dignat and Roeser, he was a member of the commission of the Société de médecine de Paris, which drew up the report.
31. *JMBX*, 37 (15 septembre 1907), 182.
32. The report was divided into sections: first, wine in general and its usual composition; second, wine fraud and artificial wines; third, the physiological effects of wine; fourth, wine in *alimentation*; fifth, wine in therapy; sixth, wine and the issue of alcoholism.
33. Louis Hébert, 'boissons,' *Nouveau Dictionnaire de Médecine et de chirurgie pratiques, v* (Paris: Baillière, 1866), 327–76.
34. *Ibid.*, 345–7.
35. See Harry W. Paul, *Science, Vine, and Wine in Modern France* (Cambridge: Cambridge University Press, 1996), ch. 8.
36. See Harry W. Paul, *The Rise of the French Science Empire* (Cambridge: Cambridge University Press, 1985), 211–20.
37. E. J. Armand Gautier, *La sophistication des vins - coloration artificielle et mouillage - moyens pratiques de reconnaître la fraude* (1877); *La sophistication des vins - méthodes analytiques et procédés pour reconnaître les fraudes* (Paris: Baillière, 1884) 3d edn, completely revised. Gautier continued in his teaching position at the faculty of medicine in Paris, where he was also the head of the laboratory of biological chemistry. By 1884 he was a member of the Académie de médecine, a member

of the Conseil d'hygiène et de salubrité de la Seine, and a member of the Comité consultatif des laboratoires municipaux et départementaux. By the 1890s Gautier had become one of the few international authorities to whom one appealed for arbitration when experts differed, especially when lawsuits and great profits were involved, as in the case in which van Houten's famous cocoa was identified in France as an adulterated product. See the article on Gautier by Mary Jo Nye in C. C. Gillispie (ed), *Dictionary of Scientific biography* (New York: Scribner, 1970-80; hereinafter DSB), and Ernest Lebon, *Armand Gautier — biographie, bibliographie analytique des écrits* (Paris: Gauthiers-Villars, 1912).

38. By the 1930s a larger number of these 'antiseptics' were available to tempt the unscrupulous winemaker or merchant. Most popular were benzoic, salicyclic, and bromacetic acids, formalin, and fluorides, as well as new organic substances. See Florentin et Munsch (Laboratoire municipal de chimie de la ville de Paris), 'Sur la recherche des antiseptiques bromés dans les matières alimentaires, en particulier dans les vins et les jus de raisins ou de fruits, BIV, no. 95 (1936), 33–4.
39. Claudia Courtois, 'Des propriétaires bordelais se lancent dans la 'vinothérapie',' *Le Monde* (11 Sept. 1998).
40. See Claude Dolman, 'Paul Erlich,' in DSB, iv, 295–305.
41. Mauriac, *Le vin au point de vue médical,* (note 4), 14–15.
42. *Ibid.*, 26–7.
43. Albert Vincent, *De certaines réactions du rein à nos vins blancs régionaux* (Thèse Doct. Méd., Paris, 1931).
44. Mauriac, *Le vin au point de vue médical,* (note 4), 20–1, 27. He excludes the use of wine in cases where the mucous membrance is *hyperesthésiée* or where contact with any stimulating liquid gives pain, and in cases of stomach cancer or ulcers.
45. *Ibid.*, 21–2, 26–7.
46. Armand Gautier, 'Faut-il boire du vin? Faut-il préférer la bière ou le cidre?,' *L'Hygiène*, 1re année, no. 1 (1909), and *Revue de viticulture*, 32 (1909), 701–06.
47. Charles Fiessinger, 'Le vin au point de vue psychologique,' *Bulletin de l'Académie de Médecine*, 80e année, 3e série, LXXV (1916), 141–47. Fiessinger finished his medical studies at Nancy with a thesis on *L'évacuation* des *éléments sulfurés par l'urine*, practiced medicine in the East of France until 1901, when he came to Paris to collaborate with Huchard as editor of the *Journal des practiciens.* Fiessinger was a well-known member of the numerous tribe of literary doctors. *La thérapeutique des vieux maîtres* (Paris: Société des Éditions Scientifiques, 2d edn, 1897) enjoyed what Fiessinger called 'quelques

entrées de faveur dans le monde littéraire.' Among his works: *Erreurs sociales et maladies morales* (Perrin, 1904); *Les conflits de la science et des idées modernes* (Paris: Perrin, 1905); *Science et spiritualisme: la valeur de la science, l'âme et Dieu, le matérialisme, la psychologie du catholicisme* (Perrin, 1907). In *Les conflits*, 69, Fiessinger notes that the association of fellow Catholic doctors increased from seven members in 1884 to over 800 by 1905. See also *Travaux scientifiques du Dr Charles Fiessinger* (Nantua: A. Arène, 1891). As for women doctors: 'Ces confrères en jupons ... la femme doctoresse est une de ces herbes folles qui ont envahi la flore de la société moderne ... par sa forme d'intelligence, une femme est incapable de soigner les malades....'

48. See Georges Linossier, *Traitement des dyspepsies par les eaux minérales* (extract of *Traité des maladies de l'estomac*, par le Dr Maurice Soupault avec la collaboration de MM. H. Hartmann, G. Linossier, etc., Baillière, 1906). Linossier taught chemistry at the faculty of medicine in Lyon between 1877 and 1899. See the article by Hallion in BAM, no. 41 (1923), 414–20. See also *Exposé des titres et travaux scientifiques du Dr G. Linossier* (Valence: J. Céas et fils, 1891). The term *dyspepsie* can be traced to Jean de Borris, or Vogel, in the sixteenth century; it only survives in medical French in the discourse of diagnostic elimination — e.g., 'dyspepsie flatulente,' — where functional problems occur without a discoverable organic lesion.
49. *La chronique médicale*, 7e année, no. 1 (Jan. 1, 1900), 21, lists Clemenceau, Magnan, Lancereaux, Legendre, Chevreul, and even the aged Victor Hugo among 'illustres buveurs d'eau.'
50. See Patricia E. Prestwich, *Drink and the Politics of Social Reform: Antialcoholism in France Since 1870* (Palo Alto, CA: The Society for the Promotion of Science and Scholarship, 1988), ch. 2.
51. Maurice de Fleury, *Les grands symptômes neurasthéniques — pathogénie et traitement* (Paris: Alcan, 1901), 2d rev. edn, 166, 364, 387–88.

8

New Support from Animal Models and Ionic Theory

If wine had any medical future in the early part of the twentieth century, it had to be in preventive medicine and nutrition, neither of which was then very high on most people's lists of medical priorities. This potential was implicitly recognised a generation later by J.-F.-N. Dougnac's medical thesis, which was turned into a successful book on wine therapy in 1935.[1] Since the early-nineteenth century ordinary chemical analysis had considerably expanded the knowledge of the composition of wine. Like Mauriac in his much shorter earlier work, Dougnac began his book by presenting the chemical composition of wine, but by the 1930s scientific knowledge about wine had been extended from presentation exclusively according to the rules of analytical chemistry to organisation under the rubric of the 'physico-chemical point of view.' Discovery of the B and C vitamins led to optimistic promotional claims for wine based on its small but highly utilisable amounts of these substances. When new scientific knowledge was integrated into the argument that wine promotes the well-being of the human organism, we find radioactivity, pH, and ions among the impressive novelties introduced by pro-wine writers. Alcohol, acids, tannin and other elements of wine were now explained in a discourse based on their biochemical properties. The problem was that this discourse could be applied to many other nutritional solids and liquids which, being non-alcoholic, did not give rise to the problems associated with wine. But promoters of wine as a source of vitamins were in no mood to listen to the warning of an older defender of wine, J.-A. Doléris, who argued that there was no need to introduce a new doctrine into the issue. Putting an optimistic spin on the outcome of the squabble of 1907, Doléris insisted that the health benefits of wine drinking had already been adequately demonstrated.

Dougnac integrated into his work all of the old arguments dressed up in new scientific garb. After the traditional Kyrie, he proceeded to a physico-chemical analysis of the composition of wine. This operation now required a trinitarian scheme beginning with the physiological action of wine on the body, then passing on to the health-promoting action of wine, and finally enumerating its therapeutic properties. Dougnac's physiological analysis assumed that wine is a food, analysable in the same scientific code as food, and that it facilitates the digestive process. Experiments done *in vitro* confirmed the assumptions about the action of wine *in vivo*. Whether it was the functioning of the liver, the circulation of the blood, the blood itself, the respiratory system, the kidneys, the endocrinal system, metabolism, the nervous system, muscular tone, or intellectual power, wine had beneficial effects that could be proved by hard scientific evidence. In wine-drinking countries men are better fighters and women are more beautiful and graceful: the ultimate tribal gifts Bacchus could bestow.

The case for wine in medicine had now evolved or perhaps hardened into a paradigmatic presentation emphasising favourable hygienic and therapeutic evidence. In addition to the traditional line concerning wine's antiseptic and anti-toxic properties, doctors began to present, in constructing their case, statistical arguments based on mortality and longevity. The increasing prevalence of cancer led some ingenious thinkers to discover a correlation between lower cancer rates and the substantial presence of magnesium oxide in the soil of food-producing areas. Low amounts of magnesium in industrially produced foods could then be suspected as a factor in the etiology of cancer. Drinking 'physiological doses' of wine could supply the organism with elements, including magnesium, needed in the body's battle against 'the attacks of cancerous viruses.' Wine-drinking nations were found to have lower rates of cancer than 'dry nations.' It was obvious to Dougnac that the moderate wine drinker lived longer and was healthier and happier. The quantitative part of the argument was clinched by comparing the rates of longevity in the departments of the Gironde and Calvados, with wine drinking Girondins outliving the calva tipplers. The qualitative part was left to the imagination of the reader, who, being as intelligent as the author, would easily recognise that there was more of *la dolce vita* in the Médoc than in Normandy.

Dougnac followed scientific convention in beginning the final section of his book 'Wine from a therapeutic point of view' with a historical survey of favourable medical opinion on wine ranging from the Hippocratic school to the *Ecole bordelaise*, including Pierre Mauriac, brother of François and a member of the medical faculty in Bordeaux. Even Ibn Sina or Avicenna (980-1037) could be harnessed to the cause because of his recommendation of an occasional binge. After commenting on the general use of wine in therapy, where its panacea value seemed to rival that of aspirin, Dougnac went through a list of illnesses grouped in traditional medical categories and drew upon the latest research to make specific recommendations in diseases of the respiratory system, the digestion, the liver, and the circulation. Nor did he ignore nutritional deficiencies. And he did not forget children's diseases. Catch-all sections swept in the uses of medicinal wines, external uses of wine, and cases in which wine should not be given, including limitations on the administration of white wines. It was evident that wine-prescribing doctors needed to know the physiological and therapeutic effects of different wines as well as they knew the effects of the drugs they prescribed daily.

Back in 1904, at the second Congrès des médecins amis des vins de France, Max Eylaud had proposed that a *Codex oenothérapique* be prepared. This direction had also been indicated by the *Lancet* commission of 1888. Eylaud now led the way by listing the indications for administering bordeaux so that doctors who knew little or nothing about the therapeutic properties of wines could easily learn to prescribe them. It was not a bad strategic move to elevate wine to an official therapeutic status, which wine's defenders thought that wine once had and should have again.

Some of the general issues debated in discussions of 'la question du vin' had lost nothing of their national significance by the late-1920s, when wine seemed threatened by the aggressive, even imperialistic moral crusade embodied in the American prohibition movement. Matters were made worse by the continuing existence of a surplus of wine in an economy where there was a strong risk of less wine being consumed by the post-war generation than in the belle époque. Wine was a dull drug for Europeans after the events of 1914-1919. Although some of the old basic questions of the early-1900s were still being asked, it seemed to many doctors and experts on food that scientists had now answered these questions satisfactorily.

So it was perfectly respectable in 1928 for J. Alquier to give a lecture on the 'Valeur biologique et hygiénique du vin' in the course on therapeutics at the faculty of medicine in Paris.[2] Of course the lecture was only part of the complementary courses on 'the therapeutic value of food.' Maurice Loeper, a leading medical professor, one of whose interests was the healing power of food, encouraged the Société scientifique d'hygiène alimentaire et d'alimentation rationnelle de l'homme to collaborate with the faculty on the lectures.[3] These lectures illustrated the healthy cooperation of leading agricultural politicians and bureaucrats with medical and agronomic researchers. All these interests came together at the top in the bureau and council of the Society with representatives from the faculty of medicine, the Collège de France, hospitals, the Institut Pasteur, and the Institut national agronomique.[4]

The role of wine in nutrition had been solidly established as a subject of general medical interest in France by 1874, when the ecumenical *Gazette des hôpitaux* published an article on the subject by Apollinaire Bouchardat, medical professor, Burgundian vineyard owner, and wine-tasting expert.[5] Bouchardat's argument flaunted the latest terminology and concepts provided by chemical analyses of wine.[6] The difficulty he faced, like other wine advocates, was how to show that wine has nutritional advantages over alcohol. His argument started by noting the importance of the happy association of alcohol with wine, a liquid of marked acidity. The acids moderate the destructive energy of alcohol in the body's economy, thereby reducing its effect on the nervous system. Acids exist in a free state or as salts with a very pronounced acid reaction. The density of wine being close to water, the body absorbs wine less rapidly than *eau-de-vie*, thus reducing the dangers of alcohol by spreading the process over a longer time. Of course Bouchardat admitted that alcohol plays the principal role in the physiological and hygienic action of wine.

Wine has traditionally been given a great advantage over alcohol alone because of the complex constitution of wine, with many substances that have significant effects on the body. Cream of tartar, succinic acid, and glycerine possibly add to the medicinal value of wine. Even the bouquet can be mustered as a nutritional recruit because of the positive influence exerted by very small quantities of sapid substances on nutrition. P.-P. Carles attributed to bouquet a valuable role of 'excito-moteur' and stimulant of digestive functions.[7] Tannin, with its important moderating effect on alcohol, and colouring matter were held to re-energise the digestion. Because of its tannin, red wine did not disturb the nervous system as much as white wine with an equal amount of alcohol or especially as much as *eau-de-vie*. Mixing with gastric juice in the stomach, wine did not require the intervention of digestive ferments to facilitate absorption and serve the purpose of nutrition. This was believed to explain the utility of wine in pyretic or fever-producing diseases.

In 1907 Xavier Arnozan had based his general therapeutic recommendation of bordeaux for sick people on 'facts established clinically by Charles Richet in a famous case of gastronomy.' Wine deserved its reputation as a eupeptic agent because once ingested in the stomach it activates the production of hydrochloric acid. Arnozan calmed the anxiety of people who knew that alcohol precipitates the digestive ferments (pepsin, pancreatine, etc.), which might be harmed by the acid: its degree of dilution in the wine would render its harmless for the ferments. Arnozan also praised the universal moderate use of bordeaux.[8]

Emile Mauriac had said much the same thing a few years before but with a less impressive scientific backup: as a eupeptic agent, red bordeaux activates the digestion to a physiological state. Peasants knew as much as doctors about this. Wine as an aperitif had a firm basis in rural areas where the juices were set flowing by *chabrot* (*chabrol*), a mixture of bouillon and wine consumed at the beginning of the meal at the time of eating *la soupe*. Mauriac believed that its moderate level of alcohol, weak acidity, and relative richness in iron, potassium, and phosphoric acid gave bordeaux its tonic and reconstituting power, without the effect of exciting or fatiguing the stomach. In stomach illnesses where the gastric juice is too rich in hydrochloric acid, the patient had to avoid wines too rich in acid and tannin, and stick to a light white wine of feeble acidity. Persons with a weak digestion were advised to drink red bordeaux to restore the stomach's peptic function.[9]

One of the results of the creation of a Pasteurian model of wine as a living liquid was the elaboration of an analogy between the complex organic materials that are part of the composition of wine and those of the human organism. Bouchardat thought that the nature of these wine materials explains the restorative action of wine in individuals exhausted by anaemia and deficient nutrition. In a discussion of the bases (meaning alkalis in pre-Arrhenius chemical lingo) in wine, he noted that they were those usually found in living organisms. So wine could be used to supply deficiencies of important nutritional elements – potassium, for example – in the body. It was an ingenious if not entirely new argument celebrating the chemical virtues of wine.

In his lectures in 1928 Alquier did his best to uphold the cause of the 'boisson hygiénique nationale,' whose economic importance can be seen in the fact that the average annual per capita consumption of wine was 162 litres in 1912, though a Parisian guzzled an annual average of 207 litres. Reflecting a new trend in thinking about drinking, Alquier believed that wine was an indispensable source of calories for the French population, supplying between seven and ten per cent of its caloric intake. The French diet had changed considerably over the nineteenth century, as can be seen from the following table.[10]

Foodstuffs	1832	1862	1892	1912
wheat (kg)	**248**	**280**	**353**	**322**
potatoes (kg)	**116**	**234**	**349**	**369**
sugar (kg)	**2**	**6.5**	**12**	**17**
wine (litres)	**65**	**94**	**97**	**168**
beer (litres)	**9**	**19**	**24**	**32**
alcohols (litres)	**1**	**2**	**4.5**	**4**
tea (grams)	**5**	**8**	**17**	**32**
coffee (kg)	**0.310**	**1**	**1.9**	**2.8**
cocoa (gr)	**10**	**120**	**400**	**700**
meat (kg)	**–**	**26**	**41**	**51**
daily calories	**1645**	**2255**	**3073**	**3160**

Like the consumption of sugar and meat, that of wine also increased. Alcohol consumption was higher than indicated because more than 100,000 hectolitres produced by private distillers (*bouilleurs de cru)* for family consumption were not included in official figures. Average annual per capita consumption of alcohol as various *eaux-de-vie* rose from one litre in 1832 to four and one half litres in 1892, a scandalous peak, falling gradually to two and a quarter litres by 1920, with lower consumption during the first world war.

The eating and drinking habits of Parisians differed from those of the average Frenchman. The average annual consumption by these two statistical abstractions for 1912-13 is shown in the following table.

Foodstuffs	Parisian	Frenchman
wheat (kg)	**193**	**232**
potatoes (kg)	**60**	**369**
meat (kg)	**70**	**50**
wine (litres)	**207**	**168**

The daily consumption of a Parisian in 1912-13 can be detailed further.

Foodstuffs	
wheat (gr)	**369**
potatoes (gr)	**165**
meats (gr)	**192**

poultry and game (gr)	**29**
fish (gr)	**6.8**
eggs (gr)	**29**
hard cheese (gr)	**9**
butter, oil, fat (gr)	**40.7**
milk (litres)	**0.36**
wine (litres)	**0.56**
cider (litres)	**0.02**
eau-de-vie (litres)	**0.012**
calories	**2500**

A large number of French people continued to drink mediocre wine or worse and eat the nutritionally deficient white baguette. Some doctors saw the working class as the great victim of this 'modern bread,' whose near simultaneous arrival with industrial alcohol caused it to be assigned major blame for alcoholism.[11] It became the task of science to show that wine was good for people if two important conditions were fulfilled: it had to be natural wine of good quality and consumption had to be moderate and limited to mealtimes. Only quality wine has *saveur* and bouquet; the consumer had to appreciate the bouquet if it were to have a stimulating effect on his appetite. According to Alquier, an increasingly large number of consumers knew little about good wine and cared even less. The public's taste had been corrupted by too much standardised wine, *vins de coupage.* Meanwhile pro-wine forces could still take comfort in the fact that the world's growing number of wine drinkers enjoyed a big majority over the non-alcoholic drinkers: 600 million drank wine, 500 million drank tea, and fifty million drank chocolate. Feeling on the defensive in France, the pro-wine forces needed the cold comfort of figures of fantasy.

It had become common to argue that wine is a remedy and a food. It was not easy to establish either claim according to scientific criteria that would ensure widespread medical acceptance. That task was carried out by the relatively new discipline of *hygiène alimentaire* or food science. And French doctors were quick to integrate the results of the new experiments into their case for moderate wine consumption. Alquier noted that information on the therapeutic properties of wine was always a little too vague to be convincing. To be scientifically convincing in answering therapeutic questions is difficult, but even Alquier was encouraged by the experiments showing the bacteriocidal power of wine, at least in laboratories if not in stomachs. Many issues important in the practice of medicine could be settled by solid science. The nutritional value of a food can be established by a chemist, who identifies its useful or harmful ingredients, a physicist, who determines its caloric value, and a physiologist, who studies the successive transformations of the food after ingestion and measures its useful physiological effect. An economist can be called on to establish the comparative costs of the nutritional values of foodstuffs. It was this total approach to judging food value that Alquier applied to wine, drawing on his own work as well as that of fellow experts.

In the late-1920s the first and most obvious scientific thing to be done with wine was to provide a complete chemical analysis of it. The complexity of wine, with its hundreds of elements, was well on the way to becoming the banal subject it is today. Alquier concocted a four-page table listing wine's organic and mineral components: volatile and non-volatile alcohols and acids, ethers and aldehydes, organic salts, tannic and colouring matter, a range of sugars, and a separate category of numerous mineral elements, including the physiologically significant calcium, phosphorus, potassium, and magnesium. Most analyses of wine were done to detect fraud, a process that concentrated on a few elements and those only superficially. 'Much remains to be done in order to penetrate the mysteries of the equilibrium of the different elements and food factors of wine, an equilibrium on which depends its quality, its organoleptic and even nutritional properties.' So knowledge of 'the intimate chemistry of wine' not only satisfied the *libido sciendi*, it promised useful, even profitable results. Unfortunately, Alquier noted, courses in oenology were rare and laboratories studying the composition of wine were even rarer.

Knowledge leads to problems and worries. It was hard enough to incorporate wine's substantial dose of ethyl alcohol into the idea of a healthy diet, but it was more difficult to justify ingesting higher or secondary alcohols of considerable toxicity. Some dogs were poisoned to make this information a scientifically acceptable part of physiological knowledge. But experiments on luckier dogs and on pigs showed the relative innocuousness of wine alcohols, which was compared with the toxicity of alcohol distilled from beets, corn, and other non-grape sources. The digestive tract of the pig was accepted as close to that of humans; indeed, human and porcine organs were assumed to be similar enough for reaching conclusions on the one by research on the other. Thirty months of consumption of alcohol distilled from potatoes and grains produced congestion and inflammation in the pig's digestive tract, liver, and lungs, with degeneration of the large vessels, especially the aorta. In the end Alquier was able to show, with experimental props to spare, that public health had nothing to fear from moderate consumption of wine even with its sulphur dioxide, yeast residues, and copper and arsenic traces derived from viticultural fungicides and insecticides.

It was all very well to give an impressive chemical anatomy of wine, but one of the questions that medical men wanted answered dealt with the important biological consequences of ingesting these wine substances. Alquier himself hammered home the importance of minerals in human nutrition. A comparative table of the mineral content of various foods showed the value of wine as a source of phosphorus, calcium, magnesium, potassium, and iron. But a keen reader of the numbers in the table might conclude that prunes were a better source of minerals than wine. Alquier was particularly keen on the importance of phosphorus, the basis of some medically popular organic compounds, though there was no proof that they fixed any phosphorus in living tissue. The trick was to stimulate tissues into receptivity for it and that was best done by a person's consuming foods like wine and molasses, rich in organic acids and salts as well as potassium compounds. (Alquier had done experiments on feeding different diets to forty horses over a period of fifty three months to determine the effect of a diet rich in molasses.) Here was a way to achieve a significant and durable retention of phosphorus. And to promote the consumption of wine.

The processes of digestion and assimilation produce goodly amounts of acids, which are partly regulated by different food intakes. Alquier thought that the excessively acid modern diet, especially in cities, could be countered by wine, which, in the dialectical economy of the body, becomes an alkaline resource when its organic acids are destroyed by oxidation, leaving different kinds of carbonates. 'Wine helps to keep the blood alkaline.' Without using the term, Alquier was talking about 'acid-base regulation,' a 'system of physico-chemical processes' to kept the hydrogen ion concentration of the blood at 'a constant level of pH 7.4,' the normal limit.[12] Thus according to this ingenious argument, wine has its role in preventing acidosis, 'any condition in which the hydrogen ion concentration of blood and body tissues is increased, that is the pH is lowered.'[13] The stability of the 'reactions of the living internal milieu' was linked in this scheme to the excretion of purines, especially uric acid, from the system. Unlike most foods of animal origin, except milk, wine and fruit have the advantage of forming only traces of uric acid.

Alquier's arguments show that the animal model with its implications for humans had become an essential part of medically-related biological research. In research on wine consumption the animal model had socio-economic as well as medical uses. When guinea pigs were fed an amount of wine that is the equivalent of two to two and one-half litres of wine at nine degrees of alcohol for a human of seventy kilos, they gained more weight, had more offspring per litter, and lived longer than the control group. The implications for the French nation were obvious. Experiments comparing the productivity of wine-fed horses with teetotalling horses showed agriculture and industry an easy way to increase equine productivity. The lesson was meant to be applied to workers. A healthy temperate worker would experience a favourable effect on his muscular activity if he drank wine. 'Le coup de fouet du verre de vin': the stimulation of wine for the worker could be compared to the effect of the judicious use of the whip on the horse.

Experiments probing the practical food value of meat, eggs, and wine showed the comparative caloric value of these foods and the force that could be derived from them as measured on the dynamometer. Examination of urine and faeces gave the coefficients of digestibility of important foods, not excluding wine. Blood analysis measured haemoglobin and the number of red blood cells to show that wine improved the consumer's blood. 'Le vin est un reconstituant.' These claims were made exclusively for wine, excluding other alcoholic drinks. Alcohol was accepted here as a medicine but not as a food that increases the consumer's capacity for work. Wine was beneficial, but pure alcohol was badly tolerated by the organism, whose addiction to it masked its dangers and toxicity.

One of the most scientifically impressive medical defenses of wine was undertaken in 1934 by Louis Genevois, biochemist at the University of Bordeaux, who employed the latest ionic artillery to shoot down teetotallers and critics of wine consumption.[14] Genevois even emanated an aura of specifically medical authority, for he had worked in the laboratory of Otto Meyerhof, one of world's leading physiologists. Genevois was chiefly responsible for the introduction of ionic theory into university oenology in Bordeaux. In his pro-wine arguments Genevois drew upon the work of Klinke, Heubner, Aubel, and Mauriac. His ionic defence covered five points in 'the objective appreciation of wine.' Chemically, wine is an acid drink, with a pH of 2.7 to 3.2, as determined by the proportions of tartaric acid and potassium bitartrate, but it is physiologically alkaline because the different organic acids it contains are easily burned by the tissues of the organism. This is especially true of the tartaric, malic, and acetic acids. Genevois' argument took an ingenious turn at this point. Acids like citric and lactic acid are normal constituents in human fluids and tissues, most of which have the same nature as wine. The similarities are not coincidences. Wine represents a living tissue, evident in their sharing the common characteristic of being, organic salts of potassium – calcium accumulates only in membranes, bones, etc., and in their having mineral or inorganic cations (positively charged ions) in the same proportions. 'Sodium, potassium, and chloride ions are the chief electrolytic components of cells and body fluids.'[15] From the ionic viewpoint muscle tissue and white wine are practically the same, though wine has more calcium (among its many minerals) than tissue. The common ration of a litre of wine per day supplies half or one third of the cations the tissues of the organism needs in minerals, except for the ones wine is deficient in – phosphorus, sulphur, and calcium.

The ionic gospel furnished another unusual medical defence of wine, namely, the osmotic pressure of wine in the stomach.[16] Wine contains about 200 to 300 osmotically active milli-molecules, which, having an osmotic pressure lower than blood serum, pass naturally from the stomach into the bloodstream. 'Wine thus tends to dilute the blood quickly ... [and] is a liquid very suitable for quenching thirst without dangerously upsetting the organism's water equilibrium.' The custom of serving a sequence of wines going from dry whites at the beginning of the meal to *vins sucrés* like Sauternes at the end is physiologically correct, for wines must be drunk in the order of increasing osmotic pressures, thus facilitating the process of digestion. (Presumably the classic combination of Sauternes and foie gras at the beginning of a meal is physiologically unwise in spite of the succulent satisfaction it gives.)

Yet another clever ionic defence of drinking wine with meals was based on the idea that its acidity facilitates the peptic stage of digestion. After the enzyme ptyalin in the saliva has converted insoluble starch (carbohydrates) into soluble sugar and the enzymes of the stomach have done their work on the food (including proteins and fats), leaving it permeated with hydrochloric acid, the enzyme pepsin catalyses the breakdown of the proteins so that the product, after being abused by other enzymes, can pass through a membrane.[17] Wine, the eupeptic drink.

Genevois was a firm believer in the French central drinking dogma that wine is different from all other drinks, including beer, cider, and fruit juice. Wine has a higher real acidity, that is a lower pH, which is one of its most remarkable qualities. And there was more good news: wine is the drink whose acidity is closest to that of gastric juice. Wine helps reduce the pH of albuminoids (meat) to a level at which pepsin can operate, a case of reducing the pH from 4.7-4.9 to about 4, the level at which pepsin attacks. Above pH 3 the attack on meat is slow. Use of lemons, vinegar, and wine in cooking have the result of lowering the pH and thus making digestion easier, whereas beer is no good because it has a pH of 4 to 5. Wine is the only drink to accompany meat or fish without forcing the stomach to work harder. But wine is no good with feculents like bread, whose digestion is carried out by the saliva and the pancreatic juice in a neutral environment. (Pancreatic juice really has three different enzymes, which act on proteins, fats, and carbohydrates respectively.) Genevois did have a good word for beer: it is better than wine for quenching thirst because it has less acidity, which is of no use without food. And he also declared beer ('the drink for thirst') to be more nourishing than wine. Genevois did not seem eager to join the camp of those who extolled the food value of wine.

Genevois' main purpose was to show how wine differs from an alcoholic solution. From a physiological viewpoint, alcohol is not the most interesting element in wine. Why is wine different from other alcoholic liquids? It is the content of a living cell, relatively untransformed by fermentation. It contains elements essential to cellular life, nearly in the same proportions that they are found in the cells of our organism. The traditional analogy with blood springs to mind. It is also the only drink whose acidity and osmotic pressure permit an easy digestion of proteins. All of this was known vaguely for centuries in culinary practice but only in the 1920s and 1930s did ionic theory and total analyses of the properties of enzymes furnish the scientific evidence showing that Hippocrates, Rabelais, Pasteur, and other great men of western civilisation were right on the beneficial effects of wine drinking.

The position taken by Genevois agreed in some respects with research done in Lucie Randoin's laboratory of physiology in the Centre de recherches sur l'alimentation.[18] Randoin recognised that fermentation, in addition to being a process of preserving liquids and easily alterable nutritious substances, also fulfilled another powerful human need, the desire for alcohol, for an excitant. A potentially dangerous desire. So hygienists, doctors, and physiologists had been concerned for a century – Randoin was writing in 1930 – with the value of wine as an energy food and especially with the question of whether it is innocuous or toxic. In 1924 and in 1927 she had carried out experiments on guinea pigs, pigeons, and white rats to see what amounts of vitamins B and C wine supplies and how toxic it is. The question of what effect fermentation has on the juice of fresh grapes was not easy to answer because of the small quantities of vitamins in wine. She abandoned her efforts in 1924 and began again in 1927 only because of the cooperation of E. M. Paillard, a winegrower (champagne) at Vitry-le-François in the Marne, who was interested in her work. Her research confirmed the knowledge that there is little C in wine, lots less than in fresh grape juice, which, like grapes, is an excellent food with substantial amounts of B and C. The fermented juice is a new liquid – a quite different view from that of ionic theory à la Genevois – with somewhat different nutritional substances and, terribly important, with alcohol, whose favourable action depends on the quantity ingested. Once the optimum quantity of alcohol is exceeded, it has a toxic action, and its toxicity increases with the quantity consumed. A daily dose of one to 1.2 grams per kg of weight is not toxic; indeed, it has a tonic effect. Only the abuse is harmful. To the delight of researcher and winegrower, research once again supported the moderate consumption of wine.

In the flurry of research on vitamins in the inter-war period the French participated only in a minor way, and they regretted that American laboratories, which were doing much of this work in the prohibitionist period, did so little on grapes and wine. French scientists looked in envy across the Atlantic at well-equipped physiological laboratories in agricultural stations and universities: Lafayette Mendel's laboratory with 600 white rats to experiment on at the Yale Medical School and McCollum with his army of rats at Johns Hopkins. Vitamins became a key subject of medical research but wine necessarily had little role in it. This was soon reflected in the new books on therapy. Gabriel Florence's *La thérapeutique moderne* (1930) had a chapter on vitamins but nothing on wine. And French researchers – Gabriel Bertrand, for example – found that investigating the intervention of elements like zinc in key biological phenomena, including reproduction, was the way to work in the prevailing paradigm of the international physiological community.[19]

Medical history often unfolds in the ironic mode. The most logical and rigorous scientific case for a standard therapy is established shortly before it disappears in a puff of paradigm collapse. Two of the best known and most vigorous medical defenders of wine, Georges Portmann and Max Eylaud, prepared in 1936 a summary of the physiological and therapeutical uses of wine, published by Editions Namain in the *Repertory of new Treatments.* Every claim was supported by reference to an appropriate medical authority known for research on wine in medicine or for the use of wine in practice. Portmann and Eylaud employed general categories to deal with the physiological effects of wine as well as its use in therapy, including specific doses in certain cases.[20] A brief analysis of the *Repertory* gives a good idea of the state of the art of wine therapy in the 1930s.

Wine as an excipient. Portmann and Eylaud thought that wine was being used more and more in preparations listed in the *Codex*. Perhaps there was some room for optimism in France, but elsewhere wine was being eliminated from official therapeutic lists. The new medicine would leave little role for wine, even in France, where the *Codex* listed only seven wines in 1965. In 1936 Portmann was keen on replacing foreign wines in the *Codex* with French wines having the same properties.

The value of wine in bioenergetics. A small dose of wine produces a positive effect. The output of the living machine was calculated to increase five to fifteen per cent, especially if the amount was taken in small doses throughout the work and the machine itself received a neuromuscular stimulus. The substitution of an equivalent amount of sugar lowered output. In 1949 R. J. Weissenbach (1885-1963), well known for his work on rheumatism and skin diseases, defended the role of wine in nutrition. What appealed to him was the fact that wine provides to the organism, in an active and assimilable physico-chemical form, not only usable calories but minerals, vitamins, various trace elements, organic matter, amino acids, etc. He followed Charles Richet's posology: in 24 hours one-half litre for intellectual workers and one litre (one and one half litres in rare cases) for manuel workers, to be drunk during meals. Wine without food is harmful. Women should drink two thirds of the male dose – not bad advice according to the latest research, which has shown that the female liver lacks the enzyme that enables the male to drink too much.[21]

Wine in feeding children. Different doctors suggested different amounts but at age four the child can start with about fifty grams mixed with water so as to benefit from the biochemical properties of wine and avoid taking a liking to strong alcoholic drinks later. (Weissenbach proscribed wine before the age of seven or eight years.)

Therapy for Children's diseases. Wine helps a child resist certain intestinal infections; it is an element in the defence against eruptive fevers. Wine contains antirachitic vitamins; this argument seems to have disappeared from pro-wine literature. It can be prescribed for children suffering from gastric or kidney diseases. (Wine is a cholalogue, an intestinal antiseptic, and a tonic. Wine is not generally allowed for patients suffering from serious kidney disease, especially acute nephritis. Nor for people afflicted with Bright's disease or with proteinuria – *les albuminuriques*, but by the early-twentieth century some doctors argued that these patients could drink wine. Mauriac allowed a moderate amount of red wine of low acidity and alcohol.[22]) In postoperatory care wine can be used instead of alcohol as the basis for medicines and even given to the three-year-old child.

Prophylactic role of wine. For someone who unintentionally consumed hemlock, wolf's bane, poisonous mushrooms, belladonna, strychnine, or digitalis, immediate consumption of wine was recommended to act against the effect of the poison. Wine was also good for snakes bites and other nasty toxic surprises like diphtheria. At that time white wine appeared to have more prophylactic power than red.

Longevity. People who drink wine live longer. Proof? In the Médoc there were 1.981 octogenarians per 100,000 inhabitants in 1921, whereas the average for France was 1.05. Although logic was applied with Ockhamite ruthlessness to anti-wine discourse, it played a very small role in the pro-wine arguments. Laubry and Lemant had argued that the moderate consumption of wine has no demonstrable bad effect on the cardiovascular system; so, according to Portmann and Eylaud, people with cardiovascular diseases can also drink wine without fear after consulting with a pro-wine physician on the type of wine and the amount. They did not dismiss the dangers of excessive consumption of wine and emphasised the importance of diet in heart disease. And who can deny their thesis on the importance of keeping the patient happy?[23]

Influence of wine on the activity of digestive ferments. The negative findings of Louis Hugounenq did not affect the generally favourable view of doctors on the role of wine in digestion. Portmann and Eylaud admitted that these recommendations were based on studies carried out *in vitro* but assumed that the results would be the same *in vivo.* In certain dyspeptic states resulting from gastric hypoacidity, wine should be prescribed because it assures a pH favourable to the action of the pepsin.

Wine and pulmonary tuberculosis. This bacterial killer of the working class had much to fear from wine – taken in small doses, which was precisely what workers were not likely to do. As a tonic it is superior to alcohol because of its tannins, glycerine, mineral salts, oxygen, and especially its vitamins. It has a good effect on respiratory passages and improves the psychic state of the patient.

Glycemic equilibrium. The ingestion of wine does not disturb the mechanisms regulating the constancy of glycemic equilibrium. Professor Corsy of the faculty of medicine of Marseille established that the diabetic whose diet is being supervised by a physician can drink daily up to three quarters of a litre of wine, about one gram of alcohol per kilo of body weight. Heavily alcoholic wines and wines with sugar are excluded.[24]

Malaria. 500 to 700 grams of pure wine help the victim regain lost weight. Wine reinforces the action of quinine. Certain cases of tertian malaria treated only with wine have been cured in ten days.

Typhoid fever. Certain patients treated with wine for a short period show no typhoid bacilli in their stools.

Colibacillosis. Drinkers of water are more susceptible than wine drinkers to urinary system infections from E. coli. It is useful to prescribe white wine as a preventive because of its acidifying action.

Gonorrhoea. Medical professors and urologists agreed that wine with meals helps boost patient morale and increases the body's resistance.

Physiological properties of wine. Apart from the banal furnishing of calories, the stimulation of digestive juices, and providing tonic effect from organic matter and minerals, the most interesting item for Portamann and Eylaud in this category was the radioactivity present in the potassium salts.

Beneficial effect of the radioactivity of French wines. Weak radioactivity used to be much talked about as a beneficial property of mineral waters; medical friends of wine wanted to draw attention to the fact that wine was also radioactive. Indeed, it could be as radioactive as certain famous thermal waters. The waters of forty springs at Bagnères-de-Luchon varied between 0.5 and 41.5 millimicrocuries. Patients and doctors could therefore enjoy the benefits of radioactivity without wine. In August 1920 Freud, 'pretty well worn out,' wrote to Ernest Jones from Bad Gastein, that he was 'waiting for the beneficial effects of radioactive water and delicious air.'[25] The weak natural radioactivity of young wines was believed to activate gastric, pancreatic, autolytic, and anti-toxic ferments. It can also act as a sedative. Wines ranged from 0.06 mmc to 0.80 mmc, with white wines being more radioactive but more variable than reds.[26]

Psychiatry. In France the treatment of alcoholism was chiefly the domain of the psychiatrist. Statistics were always cited to show that alcoholism was rare in the wine-drinking populations. This curious idea led to advocacy of treatment by paradox. Doctors were authorised to recommend wine as a means of fighting alcoholism. Popular medicine had also fought alcoholism with wine but the wine often had a repulsive item added.

Champagne and post-operatory care. Portmann and Eylaud noted that the prudent use of good wine exercises a beneficial effect on recovery by stimulating vital organs as well as helping in urination and elimination. Champagne was widely prescribed because it suppresses vomiting and gives a great boost to morale. (Any carbonated beverage may have similar somatic results but the discriminating mind prefers champagne.)

The *Codex* of 1884, like most of the official literature on the medical use of wine, ignored *vins mousseux*, sparkling wines. Since champagne, along with its lower-class relatives, is a recent invention in the history of wine, with its large scale commercialisation taking place in the second half of the nineteenth century, it is not surprising that its definite entrance into traditional therapy came so late. By 1900 medical opinion was turning strongly in favour of giving champagne an important place in therapy because of its soporific influence and its soothing effect on the mucous membrane of the stomach. In 1902 a doctor from Bordeaux praised it at the meeting of the French association for the advancement of science.[27] Iced champagne was used to treat all sorts of fevers, cholera, and cholera-like infectious diseases. Iced champagne in repeated small doses was recommended for treating persistent vomiting resulting from an irritated peritoneum, pregnancy, or a purely nervous condition. Champagne was also reputed to reduce stupidity because of its stimulating and cerebral action: the intellectual power of wine is raised to a maximum by the carbonic acid. Good geriatric medicine too: old people in a state of dangerous debilitation have a vigorous reaction to champagne, which can even bring one back from a close encounter with death as a result of trauma or great loss of blood. The dying Keynes was right to have regretted not to have drunk more champagne. Miracles with wine did not end in Reims with the death of Saint Rémi in 530. And champagne quite reasonably continues to be, at least in theory, the beverage used in hospitals to speed patients' recovery from surgery, or at least to give them a cheery perspective on their pain.[28]

White Wine, including Sauternes. Research unfavourable to wine, especially red, was not popular. Louis Hugounenq (an expert on urea) of the medical faculty in Lyon did an experimental study of the effect of wine on the digestion. He found that the action of pepsin – later discovered to be an enzyme secreted by the cells lining the interior of the vertebrate stomach – is not so effective in breaking down proteins after the ingestion of doses of alcohol much smaller than were then (about 1890) believed to have a therapeutic effect. Cream of tartar hinders digestion but free tartaric acid speeds it up. This argument could not help sell much wine because there is, as Berthelot pointed out, little or no free tartaric acid as such in wine, where it exists rather in the guise of potassium bitartrate or cream of tartar.[29] Since Hugounenq found that wines rich in tannins slow digestion considerably, he argued that white wines are better than red for digestion. Hugounenq worried that late-nineteenth red wines coloured with substances derived from coal tar would, even in small doses put a strong brake on peptic digestion because the colours transform albuminoid substances into products digested with great difficulty. So much for the claim made by some authors that the colours are innocuous because they are non-toxic. Hugounenq advertised this finding as an important result showing that he was doing practical research relevant to the important contemporary problems posed by the illegal concoction and sale of artificial wines. And further mysteries remained to be cleared up. Certain full-bodied wines with a strong and characteristic bouquet seemed to have a harmful effect on the digestion, but its cause was hard to establish. This essentially negative critique of wine seemed to undo all the good that had been done to promote wine drinking as an integral part of eating since St. Paul gave his favourable opinion. Neither the research nor the researcher, well known though he later became, got inserted into the medically generated literature on wine and health.[30]

Hugounenq's conclusions favourable to dry white wine clashed with popular wisdom as well as with medical opinion. In his pamphlet *Le vin au point de vue médical* (1903) Emile Mauriac had still been conventionally hard on white wines. Given the former poor reputation of Bordeaux's dry whites – 'sulphurous and mawkish' according to David Peppercorn – this view is not surprising. (Nowadays of course Bordeaux makes excellent dry white wine.) The older generation of wine defenders were suspicious of white wine, though they gave it a minor therapeutic role. Portmann and Eylaud led an effort to ensure that white wines, especially Sauternes, enjoyed their role in therapy. The popularity of sweet wines may have increased in medicine as that of sugar decreased, though sugar had been more a medical nostrum of the English than of the French. And Eylaud recommended that anyone suffering from melancholia could cheer up with the high alcohol and sugar of Sauternes. A Girondin, Eylaud had been practising for ten years at Langon, a port on the

Garonne in the Sauternes region, when he did an analysis of the famous white to signal its medicinal possibilities. (When absent from his beloved Grand Véfour, the former Girondin Raymond Oliver found that nothing could console him like a glass of Sauternes.) The wine's high glycerine content helps the functioning of the gall bladder and makes it useful in treating some liver conditions. Its residual sugars are higher in levulose or fructose than in glucose, and its dry extract indicates a standard range of trace items like potassium salts. Specific medical uses of such elements were hard to pinpoint in the 1930s. 'Dry' Sauternes were recommended for asthenics and melancholics; sweet Sauternes for those who needed a tonic or those who needed energy after illness or shock from trauma or bleeding.[31]

Delaunay and Portmann, signaling their pedigrees as professors of the faculty of medicine of Bordeaux, emphasised the complete agreement between clinical observation and experiment for the treatment of diseases in which the organism needs heat. If the longtime listing of wine in the *Codex* and in different pharmacopoeias was not convincing to certain doubting minds, they could derive satisfaction from the therapeutic guidance furnished by numerous theses in medicine and pharmacy, especially at Bordeaux, and from the authoritative pronouncements by professors of the stature of Bouchardat and Arnozan. Mauriac summed up in a simple dogma. 'Le vin est véritablement le remède héroique.' Better even than all the valuable medicinal tonics. 'A la fois boisson, aliment et remède, le vin constitue la médication de choix.' And defenders of the healthful effects of wine never tired of recalling the guinea pigs of professor L. Roos of the oenological Station of the Hérault. Given wine instead of water, these happy animals weighed 12.9% more than a control group after five months of indulgence. In Bordeaux Mauriac and Aubert showed that Médoc-guzzling rabbits did just as well as the guinea pigs did on the *crus* of the Languedoc.

The medical defence of wine could be summed up in 1930 in terms of its physiology: wine is antiseptic – Charles Richet, *fils*, recommended white wine with oysters; a fermented drink, wine contains vitamins; and wine is mildly radioactive – this was viewed more positively in the age of man's brief love affair with radioactivity. And, in addition, wine stimulates the flow of digestive juices, thus helping digestion and nutrition. Victor Pachon, occupant of the chair of physiology in Bordeaux, gave a scientific gloss to the Pauline argument in favour of a little wine for the stomach's sake. Pasteur had got it right again: 'le vin est une boisson hygiénique.'[32]

Wine was viewed as more than a good food and medicine, preventative as well as curative. It was an essential ingredient of civilisation, as necessary to bourgeois comfort as fertile wives, art, literature, dogs, and comfortable slippers. Professors Delaunay and Portmann cleverly ended their austerely clinical and experimental defence of wine with a quotation on wine as an essential ingredient of civilisation. Professor Starling, one of their favourite voices of authority, summed up, sounding more convincing in French than in English.

> *Le vin, avec le principal repas, après le travail quotidien, fait partie des bienfaits de la civilisation de même que le vêtement propre, les fleurs sur la table, une pièce chaude et une compagnie sympathique. Il représente une part du confort que recherche l'homme civilisé pour rendre son repas meilleur et mieux se remettre des fatigues du jour.*[33]

Like the practice of medicine itself, wine therapy seemed to be an activity carried out on male turf. Yet by the 1930s it was not unusual to find medical practice and mentality changing. In one sense it could be argued that women were naturally closer to wine than were men. Indeed, it has been suggested by that one of the reasons grapes and their juice appealed to doctors and patients as a therapeutic agent is because of the resemblance of grape juice to the milk produced by the human female. The analogy between grape juice and milk was viewed as science, not symbol, insofar as the two can be separated. Some doctors compared the action of grape juice with that of a 'living serum,' while others discoursed gravely on the juice as a sort of plant milk strongly resembling human milk. The chemical composition of the grape pulp and must approximates, *grosso modo*, the analysis of human milk in terms of water, sugar, nitrogenous matter, and mineral substances.[34] This curiosity of nature gave some nutritional advantage to women. According to Maurice Loeper, women could derive special benefits from taking a grape cure, without medication or dieting. More *vinothérapie*. In addition to helping women avoid constipation and migraines, two traditional complaints of the pampered bourgeoise, the grape cure kept the body young and lissome and even produced a bewitching complexion.[35] Few mineral water cures could promise as much.

One of the areas of medicine conspicuously absent from the Portmann-Eylaud repertory was that of female diseases and women's health care. Apart from traditional areas like psychiatry, urology, gynaecology, and obstetrics, women were spared medical scrutiny; indeed, until recently women have not usually been chosen specifically as medical research subjects. Doctors do seem to have pinpointed bourgeois women as especially subject to constipation and to invasion by *E. coli* bacteria, which produce urinary tract and bladder infections, both classic aliments of urban civilisation.[36] It was clear by the 1930s that attention had to be given to the medical uses of wine for specifically female diseases and to the general issue of the role of the wife-mother in preventive medicine through management of the household, where female power had its centre. However, wine had generally been an item of male choice, at least until the arrival of the supermarket with the inclusion of wine buying in the housewife's shopping routine.

Wine appeared to be a subject of exclusively male monopoly.

> There is a father, Noah; a god, Bacchus, who himself had a nursing father, Silenus; there is nothing feminine in his genealology. Worse, wine, a precious liqueur made for gods, heroes, men, and even the dead ... long remained forbidden for women and children. Women filled the cups that passed far from their lips. They could no more claim a glass of wine than a soul. Times have changed. Persevering feminism demands its fair share of liquor. I say fair share in order to reassure you on the limited nature of our claims.[37]

This was the opening of a talk given in 1936 at the end of the Congrès des médecins amis des vins de France, just before the doctors went off to an evening of drinking wines from the excellent cellar of a Bordelais colleague. The topic was 'woman and wine,' more specifically 'wine in the feminine aesthetic'; the speaker was Dr. Poudensan, who had a degree (1922) from the faculty of medicine of the University of Bordeaux. The president of the congress introduced her in the language of the *femmes savantes*, the proper way for the 1930s: 'Notre consoeur, Mlle Poudensan, doctoresse.' But Dr. Poudensan did not say anything to alarm her colleagues, friends of wine. (No mention, for example, of the frenzied female companions (Maenads or Bacchantes) of Dionysus or Bacchus who in oenophilic ecstasy ate their meat in bloody shreds torn from the fresh carcass they killed.) Quite to the contrary. Rejecting the idea that the so-called crimes of wine should be put under the empire of pathology, she went on to defend the physiological need for a moderate consumption of wine.

Begin with the young woman – 'la femme en son printemps' – afflicted with the burdens of puberty, a budding knowledge of the erotic science of modesty, and a family solicitous about her health or, nearly as bad, a penny-pinching boarding school headmistress. Both guardians deny her wine, though the young woman needs a daily ration of wine for both nutrition and general hygiene. Doctors and doctoresses believed not only in the value of vitamins, minerals, and trace elements in wine, but also in its power to stimulate – gently, of course, in the female case – the intellectual qualities of the student. Dr. Dougnac, indefatigable in his quest for the physical and mental virtues of wine, had carried out a survey of about 20,000 girls in the Bordelais region to confirm his suspicion that the best students drink wine. Wine does not lessen individual intelligence; it increases that of the race. Like her wine-loving colleagues, Poudensan believed that the weight of a vast body of empirical evidence, supported by the authority of professors and practitioners, had established an irrefutable case in favour of the beneficial effects of moderate wine consumption.

One of the more interesting parts of Poudensan's speech dealt with the growing alcoholism of women as a result of their having moved to cities and to jobs vacated by males during the great war. The health of males was being ravaged by alcoholic drinks and cocktails in drinking dives, visited between meals, while rural women had increased their consumption of wine. Wine has good nutritive value and increases muscular strength, thus making it possible to force more work out of the human machine; so women who do heavy work should drink more wine than other workers do. Since women were engaging in traditionally male sports, the regular use of wine was a good thing for these amazons, infinitely preferable to the frequent doping by alcohols like cognac to achieve better performance. The working woman and the sportswoman need moderate amounts of wine, which also saves them from the evils of strong drink. The daughters become mothers. And wine for the pregnant woman should not be proscribed but prescribed: up to 0.60 litres at ten degrees of alcohol daily with meals. Preferably red wine, which helps fight against the demineralisation and decalcification common in pregnancy. Vomiting calls for *vins mousseux*, champagne if the woman is lucky. And wine can play its usual happy role in fighting the bacterial infections to which the pregnant woman is subject. No fear of the fetal alcohol syndrome here.

As in the Portmann-Eylaud repertory, there was no mention of what we now worry about in the consumption of alcohol by pregnant women, damage to the fetus; it is debatable, of course, whether there is a valid medical research basis for the American bureaucratic construct of the fetal alcohol syndrome.[38] R. J. Weissenbach recommended sugared wine for diabetics after their primary insulin treatment, and Poudensac thought that this was useful to know in the treatment of diabetic precoma that could happen unexpectedly in pregnant women. Inclusion of wine in the diabetic diet, based on clinical observation until the twentieth century, was experimentally justified by work done at the Institute of Diet and Nutrition in Rome, especially in the 1930s and in the United States in the 1950s. Wine with a meal produces a lower sugar level in the blood; the fructose in the wine is metabolised more rapidly than glucose. The sugar in wine is mostly levulose (*d*-fructose). It is stereoisomeric with glucose; both are optically active, but most naturally occurring glucose is dextrorotatory whereas fructose is levorotatory. Conclusion: wine 'may contribute significantly to adequate control of carbohydrate metabolism.'[39] Poudensan thought that drinking wine benefits mother and baby through the period of lactation. In fact, she believed that science had shown the advantages that a woman can derive from wine during all her 'physiological life.'

Poudensan's medical model was based on a very wide knowledge of the available research literature in wine therapy, or at least on the knowledge, contrary to the opinion of a number of doctors, that wine does not adversely affect certain diseases. In the treatment of adolescent dermatological problems, so important to young women, doctors and families often agreed to banish wine. On what grounds? Dermatologists needed to explain. Wine had been forbidden for persons suffering from rheumatism until Weissenbach showed that its moderate use was therapeutically beneficial. This positive approach to wine seemed important for women's health because they were threatened by more diseases than men. Bad health, which nearly always has external manifestations, was more threatening to women than before and at a time when physical attraction was being demanded just as much as robustness and recognised abilities. In domestic, professional, and social life the growing importance of the feminine aesthetic was clear. Moderate consumption of wine had a positive role to play here. Poudensan took note of the complaints of the modern husband, forced to support a nervous and peevish wife lacking in charm and emotional equilibrium. The tensions of being working woman and wife-mother were already clear to the medical profession, or at least to the women who had penetrated the male medical bastion in France.

At least on the home front Poudensan had some advice for women, though males would not necessarily like it. The mistress of the house should take charge of wine. Given the view that wine should be an integral part of meals, this made a lot of sense. Nor should women avoid conversation on wine. And drink it? Only to the point of reaching 'the euphoria that makes the heart indulgent, the mind sparkling, the imagination lively, sensibility more refined, the soul more poetic.' There was much in the old medicine that we could have kept with profit. Poudensan ended cleverly with an intimation of feminine wiles and power that might have given any Freudians present a suspicion that the speaker was a phallic mother who finally delivered herself of her belief in castration. And what was the contemporary significance of recalling that in the procession for the feast of Bacchus, some celebrants carried phallic representations? 'Feminine art, which creates a hospitable and elegant table, prepares and increases the pleasure of wine tasting. The only thing left for the male, enlightened by the sad history of Judith and Holofernes, is to defend himself against this form of seduction.' Not an easy task, we might say, for 'smelling the perfumes of spring, the young woman [becomes] sharply aware of her destiny.'[40] Love and pregnancy, with the male reduced to a genetic footnote and the fertilizer of her ovum. He consoles himself with Dionysian myths and tries to hog the wine supply.

Notes

1. Jean-François-Napoléon Dougnac, *Le vin au points de vue physico-chimique, physiologique, hygiénique, et thérapeutique*, with a preface by M. le professeur Portmann (Bordeaux: Delmas 1933).
2. J. Alquier, 'Valeur biologique et hygiénique du vin,' *Bulletin de la société scientifique d'hygiène alimentaire*, xvii (1929), 115–59. This article is a development of the 'Leçon annexe au cours de thérapeutique faite à la faculté de médecine' on Dec. 15, 1928. Alquier, agronomic engineer, general secretary of the Société scientifique d'hygiène alimentaire et d'alimentation rationnelle de l'homme, was the head of the Laboratoire de recherche et station d'expérimentation sur l'alimentation du bétail (Ministry of agriculture: Institut des recherches agronomiques, Station centrale de recherches sur l'alimentation de la Société scientifique d'hygiène alimentaire ....). Lucie Randoin's Laboratoire de physiologie du centre de recherches sur l'alimentation was also under this ministerial umbrella. Her lecture to the faculty was on irradiated food.
3. For an example of collaboration between Alquier and Loeper, see their article 'La valeur alimentaire du vin,' in *Progrès médical*, no. 40 (1929), 1637, and 'L'action physiologique et thérapeutique du vin,' in *ibid.*, no. 42, 1725.
4. The Société scientifique d'hygiène alimentaire was founded in 1904,

following the international congress of hygiene and demography at Brussels in 1903. Among the founders were Berthelot, Brouardel, d'Arsonval, Gautier, Emile Levasseur, and Chautard. In 1909 the administrative council included Dr. Henri de Rothschild, Roux (head of the Institut Pasteur), and the founding president of the Société, Dr. Henri Ricard, senator of the Côte-d'Or and the minister of commerce. Recognised as having public utility in 1904, it could receive governmental funds. The Pleiad of scientists making up the society had as its aim the study and popularization of the best methods of feeding man scientifically and economically as well as the determination of the rules of food hygiene, to which the members would finally give their social application. The high social scope of the work was evident in such interests of the society as food contamination and adulteration and the connection between nutrition and disease in cities. It published a *Bulletin*, called a *Revue* between 1904 and 1910.

5. Apollinaire Bouchardat, 'Rôle du vin dans la nutrition,' *Lancette française. Gazette des hôpitaux civils et militaires,* no. 131 (Nov. 12, 1874), 1042–43.
6. Bouchardat provided a table of the average composition of a red wine on page 473 of an article entitled 'Sur les vins de France,' *Journal de chimie médicale, de pharmacie et de toxicologie,* fourth series, viii (1862), 471–3.
7. Pierre-Paulin Carles, *Journal de médecine de Bordeaux* (*JMBX*), 37 (1907), 584–5. Carles, professeur agrégé de la faculté de médecine et de pharmacie de Bordeaux, was a well-known writer on oenological and viticultural topics. One of his areas of expertise was the bouquet of wines; see 'Le bouquet naturel des vins et des eaux-de-vie,' *Bulletin des travaux de la société de pharmacie de Bordeaux* (août 1896), also published as a twenty-page pamphlet by Féret et fils in 1897.
8. Xavier Arnozan, JMBX, 37 (1907), 587-8.
9. Emile Mauriac, *Le vin au point de vue médical* (Paris: Doin, 1903), 12, 14.
10. Sources for tables are R. Legendre, 'La nourriture de la France,' *Bulletin de la société scientifique d'hygiène alimentaire,* xi (1923), 169, 170, 176, and Alquier, *loc. cit.* (note 2), xvii (1929), 120–1.
11. Dr. Montennis, 'L'hérésie du pain blanc et son remède,' *Bulletin de thérapeutique* (1913) summarized in *Bulletin de la société scientifique d'hygiène alimentaire,* iv (1914-16), 667–68.
12. See *Van Nostrand's Scientific Encyclopedia* (4th edn, Princeton, N.J.: Van Nostrand, 1968), 15.
13. John Walton and others (eds), *The Oxford Medical Companion*

(Oxford: Oxford University Press, 1994), 3.

14. L. Genevois, 'Rôle physiologique des éléments ionisables du vin,' *Annales de la Brasserie ...*, xxxii (1934), 7–9, 23–26.
15. Potassium is an 'essential element' for living organisms, meaning that it is required for normal growth, development, and maintenance. 'Major elements' are calcium, phosphorus, potassium, sodium, chlorine, sulphur, and magnesium. 'Trace elements,' which are present in lower concentrations, include iron, manganese, zinc, copper, iodine, cobalt, and selenium. *Concise Science Dictionary* (Oxford and New York: Oxford University Press, 1987), 250. See also 'parenchyma' in Abercrombie *et al*, *The Penguin Dictionary of Biology* (London: Penguin, 1981), 221.
16. Osmotic pressure became a standard item in physiology. See, e.g., Ernest Starling, *Principles of Human Physiology* (London: Churchill, 1912), 59 and 64–5. Starling says that the expression 'osmotic water attraction' is more correct than 'osmotic pressure.'
17. See Kenneth Walker, *Human Physiology* (London: Penguin Books, 1956), chapter II, 'The Digestive System.'
18. See Lucie Randoin (Directrice du Laboratoire de physiologie du Centre de recherches sur l'alimentation, Institute des recherches agronomiques et Société scientifique d'hygiène alimentaire), 'Recherches sur la valeur alimentaire des jus de raisins frais et du vin au point de vue de leur teneur en vitamines,' *Revue de viticulture*, lxxii (1930), 381–89, 421–27. Randoin had been working on wine and nutrition for a long time: see, e.g., her article with Dr. Portier on 'Les boissons fermentées et les idées nouvelles sur la nutrition,' *Bulletin de la Société scientifique d'hygiène alimentaire*, x (1922) 345–55. Alquier's article in the *Bulletin de la Société scientifique d'hygiène alimentaire*, xvii (1929), summarizes Randoin's findings on vitamins.
19. See *Notice sur les travaux scientifiques de Georges Schaeffer* (Paris: Impr. Maretheux et Pactat, 1931), professor of physiology at Hautes Etudes and then at the faculty of medicine in Strasbourg. He translated Jacques Loeb into French in 1908: *La dynamique des phénomènes de la vie.*
20. 'Extrait des fiches médicales (Répertoire des traitements nouveaux),' presented in the *Bulletin de l'organisation internationale du vin* (hereinafter *BIV*), no. 96 (1936), 30–33, by Georges Portmann and Max Eylaud, 'Le vin en physiologie et thérapeutique humaines.'
21. Dr. R. J. Weissenbach (Médecin des Hôpitaux de Paris and president of the Comité de Paris et de l'Ile-de-France de l'Association des Médecins Amis des Vins), 'Le vin dans l'alimentation,' *BIV*, no. 225 (1949), 45–48. See also the VIIe Congrès international de la vigne et

du vin (CIVV), IIIe section on oenology, 'Thème B: Valeur alimentaire et hygiénique du vin. Etude biologique des effets du vin dans l'alimentation,' BIV, no. 274 (1953), 68 ff. When Weissenbach, who had been writing friendly things about the therapeutic uses of wine and grape juice since 1932, retired in 1951, Georges Portmann praised Weissenbach's 'series of magnificent works' on wine in medicine. See *Hommage au docteur R. J. Weissenbach* (1951), 21–3.

22. Mauriac, *op. cit.* (note 9), 19, 26–7. Mauriac cites the authority of Senator in Berlin, who allowed red wine cut with alkaline water, and of Lépine in Lyon, who did not approve of an exclusive milk diet for *les brightiques.*
23. Charles Laubry et J. Lemant, 'Le vin dans les affections cardio-vasculaires,' *BIV*, no. 139 (1940), 80–92.
24. Prof. Corsy, 'Le diabète, le vin et les gens du monde,' *BIV*, no. 137 (1939), 100–107.
25. Peter Gay, *Freud. A life for our time* (New York: Norton, 1988), 403.
26. Jean Schmitt, *Etude oenologique, médicale et philosophique du vin et particulièrement du vin du Languedoc* (Paris: Faculté de Médecine, 1949), 52. Citing A. Nodon and G. Cuvier, 'Recherches sur la radioactivité des vins,' *Comptes rendus de l'Académie des sciences*, 187 (22 Oct. 1928), Alquier, in the *Bulletin de la Société scientifique d'hygiène alimentaire*, xvii (1929), 188, gave slightly different figures. In disagreement with Portmann and Eylaud, Schmitt observes that wine seems to remain radioacive indefinitely.
27. Dr. Maurice, paper given on Aug. 11, 1902, cited in C. Moreau-Bérillon, *Au pays du Champagne: le vignoble, le vin* (Reims: L. Michaud, 1922), 106.
28. Adrien Berget, *Les vins de France. Histoire, géographie et statistique du vignoble français. Manuel du consommateur pour la connaissance, le choix et l'achat des vins naturels* (Paris: Alcan, 1900), 22–3. The volume was published by Alcan in its Bibliothèque utile. 22–23. Berget took his medical typology of wines from the work of the hygienist Dujardin-Beaumetz, *L'hygiène alimentaire*, (1887).
29. See Mauriac, *op. cit.* (note 9), 12.
30. Louis Hugounenq, *Exposé des titres scientifiques* (Lyon: Association Typographique, 1890).
31. M. le docteur Eylaud, 'Le vin de Sauternes et les médecins,' *BIV*, 2e CIVV (1929), 117–120. Eylaud was a noted scribbler, among whose works are *Dans les vignes* (Bordeaux: Delmas, 1934); and *Montesquieu vigneron de France* (Bordeaux: Féret, 1949).
32. H. Delaunay et G. Portmann, 'Défense médicale et physiologie du vin,' *BIV*, no. 28 (1930), 50–56.

33. *Ibid.*, 56. Ernest Henry Starling (1866-1927) was a household name because of a letter-preface he wrote to Mary Carmichael Stopes, *Married Love* (London: G. P. Putnam's Sons, 1920), 8th edn.
34. M. le Dr Maria Rosa, 'Le rôle physiologique du vin et du raisin dans le métabolisme humain,' *La Journée vinicole* (Montpellier), nos. dated 26, 27, 28 Sept. 1944.
35. Léon Douarche, 'La valeur alimentaire, hygiénique et thérapeutique du vin et du raisin,' lecture at the Salon des Arts ménagers, Grand Palais, 2 Feb. 1932, *BIV*, no. 58 (1933), 97–102.
36. 'La constipation est une maladie de civilisés qui se produit par suite de mauvaises habitudes, d'erreurs alimentaires, par la sédentarité; ... d'une fréquence extrême dans les villes....' Victor Pauchet et H. Gaehlinger, *La constipation* (2d edn, Paris: Doin, 1933), 3.
37. M.-J.-G. Poudensan, 'La femme et le vin. Le vin dans l'esthétique féminin,' *BIV*, i (1937), 144.
38. See Wells Shoemaker, 'How researchers 'sold' the fetal alcohol syndrome,' *Wines and Vines* (April 1990), 16–19, and Per-Henrik Masson, 'New Study Finds Pregnant Women Can Imbibe Safely,' *The Wine Spectator* (Aug. 31, 1991) a report on the study by F. Forrest and others, 'Reported social alcohol consumption during pregnancy and infants' development at 18 months,' *British Medical Journal*, 303 (1991), 303: 22–6. The study in the *BMJ* recommended a limit of a drink a day.
39. Claudia Balboni, cited in Lucia *A History of Wine as Therapy* (Philadelphia: Lippincott, 1963), 192–193.
40. Alain Corbin, *The Foul and the Fragrant. Odor and the French Social Imagination* (Cambridge, Mass.: Harvard University Press, 1986), 200.

9

The Civilisation of Wine and the Organisation of Doctors

Some doctors thought that the French character was identified with their model of wine therapy and the wide range of secondary effects associated with the culture of wine drinking. The views expressed by Charles Fiessinger, one of the well known Parisian doctors of the belle epoque, were only a mild caricature of what many doctors believed.[1] Moderate wine consumers were thin because their systems burned up waste products quickly, ensuring that, unlike beer drinkers, they did not suffer from thick flesh as well as dull minds. No better lubricant than wine for the metabolic pathways. 'Les buveurs du vin sont gais, maigres, agiles, prime-sautiers.' The quintessential Frenchman before the arrival of the *malbouffe américaine.* Doctors also believed that wine stimulated sexual functions and perhaps indirectly through the sexual glands stimulated the rest of the endocrine system of glands. Wine helped the thyroid gland, for example. It also benefited the bronchial tube, the nervous system, and the arteries, where it could sometimes break up a 'yellow plaque.' And wine stimulated thought by activating associations of ideas. The attributes of the individual, fixed by their passage through generations, ended by constituting the characteristics of the race. For Fiessinger, the Frenchman as a type and his creative genius had become part of the fight over wine consumption.

Doctors took the idea of a positive correlation between wine and cultural character quite seriously. Fiessinger noted that in the early middle ages an original art developed in the Champagne, Burgundy, and the Ile-de-France, all wine country. He plundered the work of art historian Emile Mâle to argue that the art of Normandy and Brittany was based on the originality of others. And there was always Greece, land of art and wine, where the mythic medical father Hippocrates drank wine until he died at a hundred. To deviate from such wisdom might be dangerous. Balzac, like Voltaire and Fontenelle, was an insatiable coffee drinker, but his great vice was that he drank water, not wine. His punishment: obesity, easy exhaustion, and death at the age of fifty-one. It was easy enough to point out that several well-known medical works actually argued the reverse of what Fiessinger claimed: Tissot, *De la santé des gens de lettres* (1759), Riant, *Hygiène du cabinet de travail*, and Réveillé and Carrière, *Hygiène de l'esprit*. And Georges Linossier, ever sceptical, refused to credit the beauties of *Phèdre* to the account of Racine's wine merchant.[2]

The medical praise of wine was soon reflected in general works. Wine's elevated medical status even gave rise to popular works exclusively devoted to its healthful effects. Adrien Berget, an adviser to the society of winegrowers of France, undertook the ambitious task of giving the public an oenological education with a book on the wines of France that was advertised as a manual for consumers of 'natural wines.' The author gave himself authority with the title of 'professor agrégé de l'Université.'[3] Berget undertook to show that wine is not a harmful element in the human diet but an item with natural stimulating and tonic properties, a necessary stimulant for the working man. Following Munk and Ewald, he recommended a glass of wine as a good stimulant for the heart and the circulation. But wine was recommended only for those healthy enough to take it, unless prescribed by a doctor, and even then it had to be diluted with water to reduce the alcohol to between four and six degrees. And if one were not convinced by the moderns, a useful ploy could be to declare that the Hippocratic corpus recommended the moderate consumption of wine.The medical case for wine, now increasingly based on the latest experimental science, also had roots in the empiricism of the finest antique minds.

Berget had a cozy arrangement as adviser to the Société des viticulteurs de France. Though his *Vins de France* (1900) appeared as volume 123 of a series of the famous publisher Alcan (a quasi-official pedagogical voice of the Third Republic), his ambitious aim of delivering 'the oenological education of the public' falls clearly into the category of special pleading by an interested party. While this was accepted as perfectly legal and ethical bourgeois behaviour for individuals or commercial organisations, it was somewhat difficult for public authorities to promote the consumption of wine without accepting the idea that wine drinking is an essential part of the French way of life. Political encouragement of wine production led to political encouragement of wine consumption, particularly during the difficult years of surpluses between the two world wars.[4] True, it was difficult to see the bad effects of wine consumption in France, especially with the medical profession split on the issue, but there was excessive pro-wine enthusiasm in certain ministries. This blatant propaganda in school and army in favour of wine as a food was a continuation of an old policy that had often been camouflaged as promotion of hygiene and nutrition.

One of the most active propagandists for wine drinking in twentieth-century France was Raymond Brunet, agricultural engineer, chauvinist gastronome, oenophile, editor in chief of the *Revue de viticulture*, and a *propriétaire-viticulteur*. The second edition of Brunet's book on *La valeur alimentaire et hygiénique du vin* came out on the eve of the first world war, just in time to assure the *poilus* (infantrymen) that the general *pinard* (wine) would ensure that they would prevail against the *boches* (Huns). Intimately associated with literature, religion, and music, wine was offered as a food, the most healthful of drinks, a remedy for diseases, a weapon against alcoholism, and the sensible way of avoiding water. 'L'eau est une mauvaise boisson.' Tea was worse than water, as one could see from looking at the extent of decadence in England, symbolised by the frigid old maid.[5] (In this piece of anglophobia, Brunet ignored the fact that tea was the drink of major areas of the French empire.)

Wine is the French national drink, said Barthes.[6] This myth is undamaged by the fact that only a small proportion of the French population drinks wine. Civilisations have to be defended against the barbarians, who destroy it by transforming it. The perceived danger was that a new France would no longer be a wine drinking culture. To head off such a danger, the defenders of cultural values had to organise. Since the late nineteenth century few groups had been better at organising than doctors, and so it is not surprising that one of the distinguishing features of the medical defence of wine in the twentieth century was the organisation of pro-wine physicians to promote the moderate consumption of wine in the interests of preventive medicine and therapy.

The wine industry began mobilising for the hostile new world in the 1920s, when an economic downturn in sales quickly followed a short period of postwar prosperity. The vineyards producing quality wines (*les vignobles de crus*) were hit first.[7] The world of buyers had been transformed with the disappearance of three empires: it appeared that the aristocratic sippers of champagne and *grands crus* had been replaced by the lower class swiggers of vodka, beer, and even water. Wine lobbyists, led by France, organised on an international scale, as if they had an intimation of the greater disasters of falling consumption and over-production lying ahead in the 1930s. The Office international du vin (OIV) came into existence in l924. In 1933 the French congress of the Médecins amis des vins de France held its first meeting, where original works with inevitably friendly conclusions were presented on many of the classic topics of medical research relating to wine.[8] Hundreds of French doctors who believed in the therapeutic properties of wine were alarmed by attacks on wine drinking from the forces of anti-alcoholism. Wine producers generously supported medical efforts to justify moderate wine drinking.

In 1935 this vino-medical organisation became openly international. Its published proceedings provided vital information on the medical debate over drinking and on the alliances that doctors formed with politicians and producers to ensure the triumph of their ideas and the defeat of the militant teetotallers. The French organisation was in contact with The Physicians' Wine Appreciation Society in San Francisco. An emphasis on wine as preventive medicine emerged. Some of the work done by Lucie Randoin, well-known for her research on vitamins, appeared in medical publications favourable to moderate wine consumption. Much of the research done by Agnes Fay Morgan at the University of California (Berkeley) was comparable to that done by Randoin. The whole debate over wine drinking came to focus on the specific issue of nutrition within a general context of human mental and physical well-being.

Wine interests were dealt a hard blow when the United States included wine in its prohibition amendment of 1920. Nature punished the barbarians by providing four fine Bordeaux vintages in the 1920s, especially the great one of 1929. In the depression of the 1930s the woes of the hungry proletariat were matched by those of a thirsty bourgeoisie that could not afford its usual *crus*. Wine sales were further depressed by the fact that many French peasants, more interested in purse than palate, were producing their own wine from hybrid vines they had planted on returning from the front in 1919. And then French wine producers were the victims of an all too successful colonialism in Algeria, which produced twenty two million hectolitres of wine in 1934 to add to France's seventy eight million. Although French consumption was high – an annual per capita consumption of 136 litres, higher than the 103 litres consumed in 1904 – there was a large wine lake left for politicians to worry about and winegrowers to grumble about. Nature helped for three years when Bordeaux was hit seriously by mildew in 1930-32, but the Midi was in full over-production. 'Le vin est une richesse de la France.'[9] And sometimes an economic nuisance.

Doctors frankly recognised the more urgent necessity of publicising the hygienic and therapeutic value of wine because of the threat to production from the prohibitionist campaign, felt even in France. So two medical men, Loeper and Alquier, well known for their work promoting wine consumption, thought it relevant to begin their defence of wine with a reference to the quarrel between prohibitionists and wine-drinking enthusiasts. Truth was assumed to lie somewhere between the extremes, though 'everyone agreed' that a moderate amount of natural wine never hurt anyone. Their next step was to give a production figure and a value to the product: sixty million quintals (one quintal is 100 kg), worth over a billion francs. They noted that the increase in annual wine consumption, starting in the early-nineteenth century, reached the figure of 169 litres per person in the 1920s, before dropping to just over 130 litres in the 1930s. Loeper and Alquier employed the popular argument of a calorie count: a litre of wine delivers 730 calories, equal to a litre of milk, a kilo of potatoes, or a half-pound of bread. 'Wine is therefore a food.'[10]

Scientists make the same point today in a slightly different language. 'The role of ethanol in human health and nutrition is complex. Ethanol is a macronutrient energy source, capable of providing calories for all of the essential biological activities of the human organism: replication, function and maintenance of individual cells; energy for physical work; and thermogenesis.' Ethanol differs from other energy sources in not having a storage form and in freely diffusing across plasma membranes without requiring protein-mediated transport.[11] And of course it is dangerous to have too much of a good thing. Or to get addicted to this strange food.

It was easy for defenders of the value of the moderate consumption of wine to show that the authority of medical research and practice supported their position. During the *Semaine nationale du vin* in 1922 Jacques Bertillon, head of army medico-surgical statistics, put together some notes on the hygienic and food values of wine.[12] Publication by the Association nationale d'expansion économique gave a nice illustration of the cooperation of doctors, businessmen, and bureaucrats, with the blessing of politicians, in the promotion of wine drinking. In 1922 H. H. Richard, the former minister of agriculture, who was, oddly enough, an agricultural engineer rather than a lawyer, became the president of the Semaine nationale du vin.[13] To support the cause, the living and the dead (Gautier, Roux, Duclaux, Brouardel, Proust, Bouchardat) were summoned from the citadels of research and the bastions of establishment science: the Institute Pasteur, the faculties of medicine, the Academy of Medicine, and the Academy of Sciences. Pierre Lereboullet, general secretary of the Association des médecins de France, summed up the case. 'Le bon vin français restera ce qu'il a toujours été: un aliment de premier ordre et, dans certains cas, un médicament précieux.'[14] So wine should be drunk to help the digestion, the nervous system, nutrition, and hygiene; wine would also provide general stimulation, body repair, and a cheerful outlook in sickness and in old age. More wine would mean less medicine, or so it seemed to the doctors who trumpeted approval of the elusive state of health found at the bottom of the wine bottle. If Bertillon had not managed to do anything else, he had effectively showed how the medical presence had become an important part of wine events.

In 1928 the OIV began publishing its monthly *Bulletin de l'organisation internationale du vin* (*BIV*). Up to 1939 the OIV office was strategically located next door to the Chamber of Deputies on the Place du Palais-Bourbon. The OIV, like most successful organisations, was closely allied to influential politicians and bureaucrats.The French presence was strong: Edouard Barthe, deputy from the Hérault, head of the viticultural group in the Chamber of Deputies, was president of the OIV steering committee, which also contained the French Directeur de l'Agriculture, and Maurice Sarraut, head of the viticultural group in the Senate. Other European viticultural countries had representatives, but only the regions of Bordeaux and Champagne were given separate representation. Algeria, Tunisia, and Morocco added to French strength.

The OIV carefully cultivated good relations with the medical profession, including opening the pages of its bulletin to doctors and giving some financial support for the discussion and diffusion of good news from medical-scientific research on wine. The *BIV* carried hundreds of pages of communications given by doctors at the meetings of their own special organisations for the protection of the good name of wine. In 1937 the OIV budgeted 225,000 francs for propaganda and a subsidy of 25,000 francs to its medical committee of wine-friendly doctors. Income of the OIV in 1938 was projected at 808,279 francs with expenses of 614,474 francs. Although not a fat cat, it could spend enough money to spread considerable propaganda.

In 1936 the OIV adopted more of the ritualistic behaviour characteristic of official and officious organisations. The OIV prize committee, presided over by senator and ex-minister Capus, decided to hand out diplomas to prize winners. A plaque was given to those whose ardent defence of wine was particularly meritorious. The first Grand Prix of the OIV was won by the Narbonne enologist, Lucien Sémichon, who was a defender of the virtues of *vins de pays.* This choice had a subtext of a medical recommendation for popular but pure table wine. Another prize winner in the oenophilic family was Raymond Brunet, editor of the *Moniteur Vinicole* and president of the Association des gastronomes régionalistes, author of many books defending wine, especially French wine. His book also had a silly and winning title – *Sa Majesté le vin de France.* Among other prizes awarded was one to the Confrérie des Chevaliers du Tastevin (Nuits-Saint-George) for its original propaganda in favour of the wines of Burgundy; the Grand Maître of the knights of the tasting graal was the big wine merchant and vineyard owner, Faiveley. The physician Emile Roudié was given a prize of 1000 francs for his lyric play *Bacchus.*[15] The Committee rewarded serious science and humanistic frivolity with equal joy. Any doctoral thesis on wine was awarded 1000 francs, which ensured that the Committee of the OIV would obtain forty copies of each thesis. Professor Doléris, obstetrician-gynaecologist, a former president of the Academy of medicine, defender of quality wine as a healthful drink, was given a prize of 1000 francs for his books on wine and doctors and on the wines of Béarn (Bourdieu's *pays*). Doléris's attacks on prohibition, especially at the anti-prohibitionist congress of Paris in 1925, had not been forgotten.[16]

By 1938 the sum of 50,000 francs was being divided in equal amounts for prizes in the areas of general propaganda, oenology and 'technicité viti-vinicole,' doctoral theses, publications by hygienist doctors as well as for a general work defending wine. There were other prizes, including one up to 100,000 francs, offered by Greece, for the person who succeeded in producing from grape must an inverted sugar that could be used to replace sucrose in chaptalisation. Les Amis de Pierre Viala established a prize for his former students or disciples whose works were inspired by his oenological gospel. In 1937 Moreau and Vinet of Angers won the Viala prize for the totality of their viticultural and oenological works.

Medical propaganda enjoyed a special place in the general campaign carried on by the OIV in favour of wine and other 'products of the vine.' In 1936 the OIV sent to the three ministeries of national education, agriculture, and public health copies of three resolutions passed at the meeting in Lausanne of the 'first international medical congress for the defence of wine and grapes.'

The congress called for a campaign of public education in schools to discriminate between the use of wine and of alcohol and to expose the harmful results of both alcoholism and the abuse of wine (*vinisme*), all according to the teachings of the International Medical Committee for the Scientific Study of Wine and Grapes. The second resolution called for a general campaign, with committee help, to establish the food and health value of wine and grapes for all classes and also to spread a warning concerning the effects of *vinisme* and alcoholism on social diseases like TB, VD, madness, and pauperism. Last, the anti-alcoholic forces were appeased: institutes of agronomy, schools of agriculture, and unions connected with viticulture and viniculture were encouraged to use their influence in starting a campaign to improve the growing of table grapes and to encourage the medico-hygienic use of grape juice. Even here, however, the wine supporters entered a special plea for the use of medicinal wines specially fermented and sold with guarantees of type, origin, and purity. The Comité médical international pour l'étude scientifique du vin et du raisin believed that the well, the sick, and the dying could all profit from the modest consumption of wine.[17]

Organisations promoting the moderate consumption of wine cooperated formally and often worked for the same aims through interlocking structures and overlapping memberships. Barthe presided over both the OIV and the Comité national de propagande. Any international event could provide the occasion to promote the connection between medicine and wine. When in 1935 the Ligue Belge des amis du vin gave a banquet for the gastronomic forces of the international exposition in Brussels it was presided over by Dr. René Beckers. By the late-1930s, a significant and well financed structure of medical support existed, especially in France, to promote wine drinking and, above all, to counter the attacks on wine drinking from the anti-alcoholic forces, which now included some big guns in the medical profession. Since the anti-wine doctors encouraged the consumption of grapes and grape juice, they were at least on economically sound ground even if their Hippocratic *Grundrisse* were shaky.

The idea of encouraging the formal organisation of doctors who approved the consumption of wine was embodied in a motion passed at the second international conference of vine and wine in Barcelona in 1932. The Comité médical international pour l'étude scientifique du vin et du raisin was founded the next year at the third meeting of the congress in Rome. This neutral designation of the wine-doctors as a committee took place when the society became a serious international (chiefly European) organisation because foreigners pointed out to the French that the literal translation of 'Médecins amis du vin' into other languages created a phrase meaning doctors who like wine too much, a society of drunks. So the charming title of 'Médecins amis du vin' was changed into the cumbersome but safe International medical committee for the scientific study of wine and grape. The creation of the Société des médecins amis du vin had been encouraged and helped by some of the best known of numerous French wine organisations: Amis des vins de France, Association de propagande pour le vin, Syndicat des Côtes du Rhône, and Comité de propagande pour le vin de Champagne. Support by the ministries of agriculture, national education, and public health was channelled through the two organisations presided over by Barthe. Three provincial medical committees – Girondin (Bordeaux), Méridional (Toulouse, Montpellier, Béziers), and Sud-Ouest (Nîmes) – were soon born; others for Burgundy, the Champagne, Anjou-Touraine, and the Lyonnais were not long in sprouting. And the organisation started its own modest *Bulletin* for the spread of the news about the healthful and therapeutic benefits of wine.[18] Annual assemblies met at restaurants in Paris: the Rôtisserie Périgourdine in 1936 and Lapérouse in 1937. Expenses for the national committee in 1937 amounted to 25,000 francs and the subvention of the fourth national congress, in Alger, was 60,000 francs.

Who were the main men behind the organisation of the Médecins amis des vins de France (MAVF)? The two most important were doctors Max Eylaud, who operated out of his base in Bordeaux, and Georges Portmann, eternal professor in the faculty at Bordeaux and senator for the Gironde. Portmann created the doctor-deputy inter-parliamentary group, whose president was the minister Chauveau. Professor Paul-Marie-Maurice Boulet of Montpellier also belonged to this special category of *médecin-député*. The society's propaganda campaign got a big boost when, with the support of the *ministre des postes* (Jardillier), the P.T.T. (post office and communications) aired the sessions of its meeting over radio. Governments gave similar public support in all viticultural countries where doctors organised. At the meeting in Béziers Gaston Doumergue, former president of the Republic and then prime minister, was the president of honour of the congress (1934). The Comité d'honneur et de patronage included political heavyweights like Herriot and Tardieu, as well as other ministers, senators, and provincial politicians. The doctors of Burgundy formed a sub-group, the Comité médical Bourguignon. Highly important for the general society was the strong support given by Charles Fiessenger, advertised as a member of the Académie de médecine and the editor of the *Journal des practiciens*, which stretched out its tentacles to the general population of doctors as the scientific organ of the pro-wine doctors. He was able to publish all the scientific articles on wine studied from a medical point of view. Fiessinger was also a member of the society's 'Office of the central committee.' Students, quick to spot power, soon started doing medical theses on both grape and wine.

What was the aim of the organisation of doctors as friends of wine? At the first congress in Bordeaux agreement was reached on the ambitious goal of showing scientifically the nutritional, hygienic, prophylactic, and therapeutic values of wine and its role in the human economy. Not forgotten either was the national economy as related to the social and economic role of the doctor, both in France and its colonies. A sop was thrown to teetotallers. The society would be equally interested in showing the medical value of grape cures, whether in special grape cure stations or at home. Back in 1881 *La Médecine populaire*, an illustrated weekly, had attempted to stimulate some French interest in grape cures, but 'wine in capsules' did not lure many patients. Germany and Switzerland were much more open to the grape gospel on the treatment of boulimia, loss of appetite, insomnia, lethargy, diarrhoea, constipation, and other common afflictions of civilisation. Though Germans were described as 'fanatiques de *la cure au raisin*' the French admitted that it was a respectable therapy with the proper historical references: Pliny, Galen, and Dioscorides had given the grape an important role as medicinal food. Dr. Félix Bremond, the author of the article in *La Médecine populaire*, thought that grape therapy did have a limited medical value, though not as the panacea advertised by such stations as Durkheim, Glesweiler, Beingen, Kreusnach, Grüneberg (all in Germany), Vevey, Veytaux, and Montreux (Switzerland).[19] The OIV orchestrated a national campaign to encourage people to eat more grapes, which took on all the virtues that oat bran recently had for the American consumer. But the pro-grape propaganda was not successful in establishing a large enough grape-consuming community to compensate growers for their losses in the wine market. Their goal was given a more economic statement when the Comité médical international pour l'étude scientifique du vin et du raisin met in Rome in 1937. The basic aim did not change, but two significant new emphases appeared: studying the problem of the consumption of normal wine, which did not exclude a consideration of wine alcoholism, and giving the grape equal status with wine, rather than relegating it to a therapeutic coda. At the conference in Dijon, after the welcome by the head of the Ecole de Médecine, Portmann elaborated the program of the pro-wine doctors' organisation.

In the beginning Eylaud and Portmann had been disappointed and discouraged by condescending smiles and sarcasm as they travelled around France promoting the good cause of wine drinking. Portmann claimed that they were downright sickened in seeing people attempt to promote prohibition by destroying the good reputation of French wine on scientific and humanitarian grounds. The guiding idea of the two pilgrims was to counteract the scientifically-based anti-wine campaign by re-establishing the truth and showing the detractors of the national drink that they were wrong. Not that the anti-wine lobby was easy to win over from its false and dangerous doctrine that the consumption of wine and alcoholism are the same thing. According to Portmann, the first Congrès national des médecins amis du vin was a strictly scientific tribune, independent of all commercial or economic considerations, where the prohibitionist doctrine could be confronted with serious arguments.

One of the arguments used repeatedly by the pro-wine group was the paradoxical one that encouraging the consumption of good wine is the best protection against alcoholism. Portmann believed that after the first world war people turned away from wine only to become addicted to the poison of alcohol. Such was the origin of drinking cocktails, whose invention Dr. A.-T. Malachowski blamed on Americans. A sad people who don't know how to eat, they invented it to give themselves artificial fun and the courage necessary to swallow their awful food. In the 1920s as in the 1990s, Americans provided ideal targets for Gallic barbs and even therapeutic attacks. Paul Ramain, the notorious cigarette-smoking, gourmand physician, told the story of the dried-out anaemic American woman whose oenophilic French physician raised her level of red blood cells with injections of red wine and distilled water, administered to her 'pudiques fesses.' The founding fathers of the pro-wine doctors' society – which included president Louis Dartigues, famous for his surgical skill in grafting testicles, and the honourary presidents Fiessinger and Paul Guéniot (100 years old) – all believed in the moderate consumption of wine as the best antidote to alcoholism.[20] Portmann believed that as defenders of public health, doctors have a professional duty to defend wine consumption. By 1934 over 1200 members agreed with Portmann. But the forces of prohibition were strong and the battle had to go on.

In 1936 the enemy also met, at an anti-alcohol congress in Strasbourg. One of the speakers, an intrepid defender of the grape and its unfermented juice, denounced wine and his Bacchic colleagues, who were failing in their duty as doctors and as men in recommending wine. After all, more than one third of the people treated in insane asylums owed their madness to an abuse of alcohol. Nonsense, replied Portmann. To make such a scurrilous attack on honest people like the pro-wine doctors indicated that the fellow was not worthy of the title doctor. Was not the best reply given by Emmanuel Régis, professor of psychiatry in Portmann's own faculty at Bordeaux – '*une des plus belles figures*' of contemporary psychiatry? 'Alcoholism in a region is in inverse ratio to the quantity of wine made and drunk there.' Régis prescribed wine for his patients but was in the fortunate situation of not needing the medicine himself. 'Je suis un buveur d'eau, boasted Régis, thus emulating the abstemious Freud, whose psychiatric hypotheses he had brought to the attention of his innocent fellow doctors.'[21]

Doctors are as notorious for their scribbling as for their love of good wine.[22] The doctor-writer was soon enrolled in the cause. A poetic competition was organised among the *médecins littérateurs* with the collaboration of a couple of literary societies. And Bacchus was offered much bad poetry. Doubts were cast on the literary virility of Swiss doctors for not joining with the French and for sticking to prose. There seems to have been general approval of the Buffonesque approach to the French language as a monument of civilisation. Gastronomy and wine together could be guaranteed to produce hieratic prose. An article by Eylaud on 'Le vin en gastronomie' in *La Journée vinicole* (22 août 1935) gave general advice wrapped in the high aesthetic literary line; the general secretary of MAVF had his priestly position to maintain. In the 1960s Eylaud became president of the Académie Montesquieu.

The first meeting of the wine-doctors at Bordeaux in 1933 showed that bourgeois support was more than literary. Some of the support came from the nobility, such as it is in France, but in form and function it was not distinguishable from that of the bourgeoisie. The doctors engaged in several days of educational activity: a morning tour of some of the great vineyards of Saint-Julien, Saint-Emilion, and Pomerol (châteaux Beychevelle, Ausone, Trotanoy), followed by an afternoon visit to warehouses of the leading merchants of Bordeaux, where lectures were given on how to compose a meal and to lay down a cave as well as on the art of drinking wine. A well-deserved reception was given by the chamber of commerce. Lunch at Château d'Yquem included seven wines, ending with Yquem 1929. ('M. Jacob, répresentant le propriétaire, M. le marquis de Lur-Saluces [a supporter of Action Française], leur fit les honneurs de ce cru unique au monde.') Among the nine wines on the table at Château Beychevelle were Châteaux Margaux 1928, Lafite 1928, and Beychevelle 1921. Châteaux Haut Brion and Latour were tasted at another meal. All these wines were given to the society by the proprietors, grateful for this powerful medico-scientific rehabilitation of wine. The Comité d'honneur et scientifique included some weighty men of science: Viala, Hughes, Semichon, and Ravaz.

Even the church got into the doctors' act. At the congress of Béziers there was a feast of grape and wine in the Cathédrale Saint-Nazaire with young Bitterrois and Bitterroises in Languedocien costume distributing grapes blessed by the higher powers. 'Sans le vin, pas de messe.' Members of other religious persuasions like materialism, even if they rejected the higher function of wine as the vehicle of the blood of Christ in the mass, must have been amused by this atavistic activity cementing the social bonds of the wine-loving community.[23]

The third congress of French wine-doctors met in Dijon in 1936; the fourth in Alger in 1937. Maurice Bourlier, president of the Confédération des vignerons algériens, presided over the last pre-war congress, held in Reims in September 1939.[24] The last meeting of the Comité médical international pour l'étude scientifique du vin et du raisin was held in Lisbon in 1937, and the committee did not meet again until 1957 in Bordeaux. Funding was on a solid basis in 1938 with support from the departmental committee for the promotion of Bordeaux wines. The general council of the Gironde appropriated 300,000 francs of departmental funds for the committee's activities in categories labelled medicine, tourism, the press, cinema, and radio; these funds were also used to pay hotel and restaurant bills. A big show was planned for the world's fair (1939) in New York. The committee singled out the medical campaign of Portmann and Eylaud as worthy of support.[25]

If the organisations of wine-doctors evolved in any one direction, perhaps it was toward becoming less humanist and more scientific in the experimental sense. This meant that people like Max Eylaud, recognised in 1936 by Portmann as the man who had thought up the idea of organising doctors to defend wine and as the indefatigable pilgrim-promoter of the French organisation, could be left on the periphery as embarrassing relics of another age. Or at least this is the impression one gets from a complaint by Eylaud to Portmann that he was completely left out of the plans for the meeting in 1961; worse, he had not been asked to give a talk on his book *Vin et santé* (1960, preface by Portmann). Studying alcohol-induced lesions on rat livers was what vinous medical science had become; prescribing wines to drink for people who had a tendency to get urinary tract infections was no longer where the action was. Of course books giving therapeutic advice on wine consumption are still moderately popular, as shown by Dr. Maury's classic *Soignez-vous par le vin.*

After World War II the old patterns of financing and international cooperation were restored, even improved. Eylaud was the eternal general secretary. Portmann, the well connected *Einheitsführer* (dean of the medical faculty in Bordeaux, mayor of Sainte-Eulalie, senator of the Gironde, member of the Conseil de la République), promoted this imperial expansion. By the 1960s the Association de propagande pour le vin, presided over by Dr. G. Bouys in Béziers, boasted of the membership of the Duc de Lévis-Mirepoix, winegrower and member of the Académie française, and Wladimir d'Ormesson, also an immortal, and, more significant, president of the ORTF (radio). The congress of 1957 was budgeted at one and a half million francs. Wine organisations were generous. The Conseil interprofessionnel des vins de Fitou-Corbières, hoping perhaps to acquire a little social prestige for their wines from medical support, sent Portmann a check for 50,000 francs. Other groups, such as Anjou, Touraine, Pays nantais, Côtes du Rhône, Côtes de Provence, and Bergerac, were not stingy. Regional organisations were rebuilt or established all over viticultural France. The 1957 congress saw the first delegation of French Canadian doctors, led by Samuel Letendre, a Montréal gynaecologist, globetrotter, and trencherman. By 1961 cooperation was established with the United States. Representatives of the Medical Research Wine Advisory Board and The Society of Medical Friends of Wine in California attended the 1961 conference in Bordeaux. In 1962 about thirty eight members of the New York based Physicians' Wine Appreciation Society visited French wine areas. The society's approximately 120 members were advised on wine purchases by Browne-Vintners. Groups proliferated in Miami Beach, Boston, Chicago and other places not lacking doctors interested in building wine cellars. The return of the United States to the civilisation of wine heralded a new era of medical support of moderate wine consumption as a defence against the ravages of alcoholism.

The pro-wine doctors believed that their common sense opinions would be proved right by science, and even by social science when the numbers came out right in surveys. In 1936 a survey of 4000 French doctors was undertaken by the Société des médecins amis des vins de France – the French were still using the good old name for themselves rather than the cumbersome committee cognomen. In 1937 the survey was extended to cover 22 countries. By the end of May 1937 the society had received 4686 replies, of which 956 (20.58%) were from non-drinking physicians. Even non-Pythagoreans will find a breakdown of the results to be of some interest.

Number	Percentage	Opinion
411	**8.77**	consider wine indispensable
3525	**75.22**	consider wine useful
425	**9.07**	consider wine harmful
2667	**56.9**	prescribe wine
491	**10.48**	forbid wine
973	**20.7**	tolerate wine consumption
1076	**22.95**	equate wine drinking and alcoholism
3473	**74.11**	do not equate the two
2592	**55.31**	believe it useful to have pro-wine medical propaganda
1852	**39.53**	do not want such propaganda

A significant number of replies was received from Bulgaria (336), Rumania (2314), Chile (93), Greece (96), Morocco (75), Tunisia (77), and Switzerland (58). By late 1937 the Greek medical establishment had surveyed 223 doctors, who were generally favourable to the moderate use of wine, though modern Greece is not a wine-drinking culture. The Greek higher council of hygiene appointed a commission of medical bureaucrats and professors to study various questions relating to alcohol consumption in Greece. Although the commission admitted that drinking a small quantity of wine with meals is good for healthy people because it stimulates the appetite, aids digestion, strengthens the organism, and creates an agreeable frame of mind, it pointed out that in certain pathological states the physician should prohibit all alcoholic drinks. The commission also recommended that a campaign be organised to encourage the consumption of grapes, raisins, and their non alcoholic products. Since alcoholism had recently risen, peasant distillation of poor quality alcohol in their home stills should be forbidden. And watering holes frequented by peasants and workers should be allowed to sell only beer and wine. This was good advice, generally ignored, which could have been equally valuable in the rest of Europe. In France only the authoritarian regime of Vichy dared attempt, with some success, to prevent Frenchmen from poisoning themselves by an excessive consumption of alcohol. But Pétain's collaboration with the anti-alcoholic axis of Hitler and Mussolini was only a brief period in the Bacchic history of France.

Notes

1. See note 47 in chapter 7. Fiessinger was also the author of *La thérapeutique en 20 médicaments* (Paris: Maloine, 1911; five editions; written with Huchard) as well as *20 régimes alimentaires* (Paris: Maloine, 1921; four editions). Information from *La presse médicale* (20 avril 1942).
2. Charles Fiessinger, 'Le vin au point de vue psychologique,' *Bulletin de l'académie de médecine, 80e année,* 3e série, lxxv (1916), 141–47.
3. Adrien Berget, *Les vins de France. Histoire, géographie et statistique du vignoble français. Manuel du consommateur pour la connaissance, le choix et l'achat des vins naturels* (Paris: Alcan, 1900).
4. Patricia E. Prestwich, *Drink and the Politics of Social Reform: Antialcoholism in France since 1870* (Palo Alto, CA: The Society for the Promotion of Science and Scholarship, 1988), 211–17.
5. Raymond Brunet, *La valeur alimentaire et hygiénique du vin* (Paris: Librairie Agricole de la Maison, 1914), 2d edn.
6. '... Savoir boire est une technique nationale qui sert à qualifier le Français, à prouver à la fois son pouvoir de performance, son contrôle et sa sociabilité. ... C'est le vin qui est national.' Roland Barthes, 'Le vin et le lait,' in *Mythologies* (Paris: Seuil, 1957), 74–7.
7. Marcel Lachiver, *Vins, vignes et vignerons. Histoire du vignoble français* (Paris: Fayard, 1988), 484–90.
8. Among these works were 'La valeur bioénérgétique du vin,' par M. Douarche (Directeur de l'Office international du vin); 'Les propriétés physiologiques du vin,' par M. le professeur agrégé Fabre; 'Le vin dans l'alimentation de l'enfant,' par M. le professeur Dieulafé; 'Les indications du vin dans le régime alimentaire des rhumatismes chroniques déformants progressifs,' par M. le docteur R.-J. Weissenbach, médecin des hôpitaux de Paris; and 'Le rôle phylactique du vin,' par M. le professeur René Cruchet. See *Journal de médecine de Bordeaux* (JMBX), 31 (30 nov. 1937), 817–42.

9. Maurice Loeper et J. Alquier, 'La valeur alimentaire et thérapeutique du vin,' *Bulletin de l'organisation internationale du vin*, no. 12 (1929), 11 and 13.
10. *Ibid.*
11. Linda F. Bisson, Christian E. Butzke, and Susan E. Ebeler, 'The Role of Moderate Ethanol Consumption in Health and human Nutrition,' *American Journal of Enology and Viticulture*, 46 (1995), 449–62: 449.
12. Jacques Bertillon, 'Notes remises...', *Semaine nationale du vin; Compte rendu des travaux* (1922), 42–49.
13. The *Compte rendu des travaux* (1922) carried an advertisement for the Plaza-Athénée: 'L'hôtel le plus élégant de Paris. Celui qui a conservé, intactes, les grandes traditions culinaires françaises. Et sert les meilleures années des meilleurs crus de France.'
14. *Semaine nationale du vin, op. cit.* (note 12), 46. Among Lereboullet's works are *Les cirrhoses biliaires* (Paris: Masson, 1902) and *La grippe: clinique, prophylaxie, traitement* (Paris: Baillière, 1926). He was one of the editors of the *Nouveau traité de médecine et de thérapeutique* (Paris: Masson, 1927).
15. Emile Roudié, *Bacchus, pièce héroïque en 3 actes* (Paris: J. L. Lejeune, 1937).
16. 'XIXe session de l'O.I.V.' (décembre 1936), Alençon, 16–19. Jacques-Amédée Doléris (1852-1938), elected member of the section of *accouchements* of the Académie de médecine in 1905. He and Jean Bouscatel were the anxious authors of *Hygiène et morale sociales, néo-malthusianisme, maternité et féminisme, éducation sexuelle* (Paris: Masson, 1918).
17. 'XIXe session de l'O.I.V.' (décembre 1936), Alençon, 19.
18. The *Bulletin* appeared three times a year between April 1936 (no. 1) and Jan. 1943 (no. 23). The editorial committee included some of the prominent medical defenders of wine: professors Portmann, Dieulafé, and Vires, doctors Ribot, Ozanon, Mouret, Malachowski, and Eylaud.
19. 'L'actualité médicale: le raisin,' *La médecine populaire*, no. 52 (15 Sept. 1881), 818–20.
20. Louis Dartigues (1869-1940) was an expert on the technique of grafting monkey's testicles on men by using Serge Voronoff's method. Among Paul Guéniot's claims to fame was his *Thérapeutique gynécologique* (Paris: Baillière, 2d edn, 1922).
21. Emmanuel Régis (1855-1918), influenced by his asssistant Hesnard, gave a modest boost to the spread of Freudian doctrine in France, though he recognised it only as a 'seductive but extremely

hypothetical system.' See entry on Régis in Pierre Morel, *Dictionnaire biographique de la psychiatrie* (Paris: Synthélabo, 1996).

22. On medicine and literature, including the doctor as writer of prose and poetry, there is a vast literature. See the journal *Literature and Medicine*; among interesting recent works is Charles M. Anderson, *Richard Selzer and the Rhetoric of Surgery* (1989), in the Medical Humanities series of Southern Illinois University Press.
23. See the chapter on wine and religion in Raymond Brunet, *La valeur alimentaire et hygiénique du vin.*
24. Bourlier's medical thesis was an *Etude sur le mimo-tanin; son action antiseptique en médecine et en chirurgie et plus spécialement dans les angines à fausses membranes* (Toulouse: Faculté de Médecine, 1896).
25. Archives départementales, Gironde, 7 M 206.

PART V

MEDICINE ON THE MOVING FRINGE – PREVENTION AND PARADOX

10

Wine Defences Against Bacteria, Heart Disease, and Cancer

There is still a trickle of literature on wine therapy, including several books extolling the therapeutic virtues of specific wines such as champagne and bordeaux.[1] A search of the *Index Medicus* for the 1980s and even into the early-1990s, when the 'French paradox' started generating medical interest, is likely to be a depressing experience for the believer in the beneficial effects of wine. There was little research reported, and most of the articles dealt with topics such as 'wine poisoning as a source of lead intoxication,' whether from containers for home-produced wine or, much less serious, the lead foil that used to adorn wine bottles. Red wine as a culprit capable of causing migraine was another funded subject of research. Historians of medicine have not been much more encouraging than medical researchers, for they frighten us with past epidemics of plumbism, whether the *colica Pictonum* (colic of Poitou) of the seventeenth century or the notorious saturnine gout of the Roman aristocracy. A friendly assessment of the beneficial effects of moderate consumption of wine can be found from time to time in newspapers and especially in wine magazines.[2]

Much of the traditional and experimental evidence in favour of the therapeutic use of wine was lovingly surveyed in *A History of Wine as Therapy* by Salvatore Lucia, Californian physician, researcher, and a member of the Society of Medical Friends of Wine. Published in 1963, Lucia's book drew on work done on 'the nutritive and protective powers of wine' up to the 1950s. He made it clear that the medical literature showed wine therapy to be just as solidly based on clinical observation and medical research as any other therapy. Nor was all the work done at institutions in wine areas. And some of the world's leading research institutions obtained positive results in testing wine therapy. The results were published in mainline journals. In fact, experiments on the physiological effects of ethyl alcohol and wine seem to have been standard if scarce items of experimentation since Claude Bernard did his work on alcohol and digestion.

1. Wine as a weapon in the war against bacteria

Human life is a footnote to bacterial action. The late-nineteenth century, strongly Pasteurian (or Kochian), was keenly aware of the pathogenic role of bacteria, a cause of disease and a killer. In the overkill society we know more about antibiotics than about bacteria and suffer from 'paranoid [antibacterial] delusions on a societal scale.'[3] Pigs, chicken, cattle and people are excessively protected from infections by being plugged into the system of mass-produced drugs. We complain of over-medication of man and beast, but the nineteenth century, plagued by bacterial diseases like TB, typhus, and cholera, would probably have preferred our predicament to theirs.

The beginning or origin of a practical knowledge of the antiseptic property of wine would be hard to date. Christ showed his familiarity with the use of wine in dressing wounds when he told the parable of the Samaritan traveller who poured oil and wine (*le baume samaritain*) on the man mugged and beaten up while on his way down from Jerusalem to Jericho. In the period between the acquisition of the knowledge that bacteria cause disease and the advent of sulphanilamide and penicillin, the healing powers of medicine were limited, even if doctors had certainly not, as Lewis Thomas morosely proclaimed, 'given up on therapy.'[4] In France there was a great deal of interest in and considerable research done on the bacteriocidal power of wine, which some enthusiasts believed to be a liquid weapon against several major pathogenic organisms. Emile Mauriac attributed the efficacy of wine in treating wounds, burns, and contusions to its acids, tannin, and alcohol. He described *gros rouge*, rich in tannin, as excellent for the local treatment of 'chronic catarrhs' of the vagina and the urethra. The aromatic wine listed in the *Codex* was always used successfully to clean nasty wounds and treat ulcers. Mauriac said that late in the nineteenth century he had seen people daubing the bodies of smallpox victims twice daily with red wine. Tens of thousands of people were still dying from smallpox in the late-nineteenth century.[5] Surgeons and accoucheurs could use wine if other antiseptics were not available; some country doctors had long used wine as a reliable antiseptic.[6]

Before anyone knew about bacteria, human powers of observation had led to the empirical knowledge that water could produce sickness and that mixing wine with the water several hours before consumption makes the water safer. Montaigne's doctor allowed him to drink water only when it was diluted with wine and left standing for several hours. The authority of the doctor distinguishes medical advice from folk wisdom. The traditional practice of drinking wine with oysters would presumably fall in the same category of empirically-based preventive medicine. In 1992 a report in the journal *Epidemiology* stated that one was less likely to catch Hepatitis A from eating contaminated oysters if one drank a beverage with a high alcohol concentration (over ten per cent), including wine, though not some cheap light rieslings. In addition to giving some protection against the viral pathogen, alcohol was previously shown to give protection against the bacteria *Shigella* (dysentery) and *Salmonella* (gastroenteritis and typhoid fever). But Florida and Louisiana gourmands who like to live dangerously should not eat too many raw oysters, for the risk of catching the two bacterial diseases increases with the amount of contaminated food eaten.[7]

When the microscope made it possible to identify specific pathogens of diseases, experiments could be designed to test the bacteriocidal action of wine on the leading killers of the nineteenth century. In 1879 Karl Josef Eberth discovered the bug causing typhoid fever; the typhoid bacillus now known as *Salmonella typhosa* used to be called *Eberthella typhosa.*[8] In 1892-93 Aloïs Pick of the institute of public health in Vienna tested the ability of the bacilli of typhoid and cholera to live in wine, both diluted and straight. Depending on the wine and on the amount of water with which it was diluted, the bug could take up to 24 hours to expire. Undiluted Vöslauer, an Austrian red wine of Bad Vöslau, was found to be potent enough to kill the bacillus in 15 minutes. Interesting if not practical news to announce during the cholera epidemic in Hamburg in 1892.[9] In spite of the passions of Pasteur and the so-called pasteurisation of France, French scientists seemed slow to pick up on this obviously fertile area of research, replete with rich pro-wine propagandistic opportunities.

The work done by Pick and that done by Taverni, who was at the institute of public health in Modena, eventually proved useful to doctors supporting a pro-wine position based on the sanitary properties of wine. Their research offered foreign confirmation of an argument of which some people might have been suspicious had the phenomenon, like N-rays, been limited to detection by French observational powers.[10] It also confirmed the probable truth of the story told by an old officer of the *chasseurs d'Afrique* (light cavalry), who had spent ten years in Algeria. Long subject to the country's endemic fevers as a result of drinking local water, the *chasseurs* found that the only remedy was a daily glass of warm wine or just a glass of *vin à la française*, that is, cold.[11] Research confirmed anecdotal evidence.

Pick's work was thoroughly verified by J. Sabrazès and A. Marcandier, both at Bordeaux.[12] They found that the length of time of survival of the bacteria was inversely proportional to the bacterial load introduced into the wine. White wine was a more effective killer than red wine, and champagne the champion of the whites in killing Eberth's bacillus. In working out their explanation of these curious phenomena, the bordelais scientists drew upon the work done by Shibasaburo Kitasato on the bacteriocidal power of acids. Pick's results were nearly the same for the formic, acetic, tartaric, and citric acids acids found in wine. Sabrazès and Mercandier believed that it is the hyperacidity of white wines, in particular their relatively high content of sulphurous acid (then thought to be the acid formed along with sulphuric acid when sulphur dioxide is dissolved in water) which give them their superior bacteriocidal power. The free or 'active' sulphur dioxide was found to be significantly antiseptic, rather than the part (most of it) which combines with organic matter like aldehydes and sugar in the wine; nor was it the part of the sulphur that oxidises to form sulphates, making the wine richer in potassium sulphate. Lamathe adhered to the isodynamic view that the metallic salts in wine explain its bacteriocidal power: 'Quand le métal part, le bacille rentre.'[13] A bottle of good wine contains about three grams of salts; so a bottle a day keeps the doctor away, at least until some alcohol-induced illness occurs.

The degree of alcohol was not found to affect the bacteriocidal power of wine. Some acidic wines could be considerably diluted with water before undergoing a reduction of their killing power. Temperature was also important. An old wine of Saint-Emilion was more antiseptic at thirty seven than at fifteen degrees centigrade. Equally important was the number of germs to be killed. Five drops of bouillon culture took five hours to be purified compared to two hours for two drops. And of course there was no guarantee that wine, especially diluted wine, would have any effect on germs already in the digestive tract. But researchers were certain that Eberth's bacillus died in a solution of equal parts of wine and water if they were mixed before consumption, six hours before for white and twelve hours for red.

Although no governmental policy was based on these findings, the practice of mixing water and wine before serving, common in collective restaurants and boarding houses, now had a basis in preventive medicine, even if its origins were in greed and a social desire for relative sobriety. These findings also gave a boost to the standard model French wine, sulphured to the maximum degree consistent with drinkability, and especially to the *vin de cru* of Bordeaux, further propped up in its pre-emininent position of a wine for the weak of stomach and of heart, which did not in any way detract from its appeal to the stout bourgeois. The results obtained by the Bordeaux scientists were confirmed by André Kling and Daniel Florentin of the municipal laboratory of Paris. The comforting and impractical conclusion was that even very polluted water could be made safe for human consumption by mixing it with wine.[14]

Wine, especially white wine, has a diuretic reputation, though the proverb about the pissing power of the wine of Montmartre ('*C'est du vin de Montmartre / Qui en boit pinte ... en pisse quatre!*') finds no echo in the elite literature of therapy. Arnau of Villanova stated that for medicinal purposes white wine is better than red: 'it is more subtle and more receptive to all the vapours of everything pressed into it. It carries the virtues of incorporated substances through all members, with delectation and in a natural way.' He also recommended wine passed through ground winter cherries as a remedy for urinary troubles. With this concoction he induced relief in a bloated cardinal who had not urinated in three days. Perhaps, as Lucia says, the medicine worked because of the benzaldehyde (benzenecarbaldehyde) in the cherries, which is also found in almond kernels. 'It drives out the urine immediately ... and extracts the sandy matter from the kidneys and bladder in great quantities....'[15] This knowledge seems not to have reached Bordeaux by the seventeenth century, for a faculty doctor used a cather to relieve Cardinal Richelieu during one of his trips to the southwest.

One of the commonest afflictions of civilisation is the UTI (urinary tract infection), which occurs when the ubiquitous bacteria *Escherichia coli* gets where it should not be. Nowadays the afflicted pay a visit to a urologist who, after delivering a warning on the risks of *fellatio*, prescribes ten days of tetracycline or Vibramycin. What did doctors do before drugs made them miracle workers? Some doctors found that wine had a favourable influence on killing the errant bacteria. Emile Mauriac did not recommend wine in cases of urethritis or acute cystitis, unless it was cut with an alkaline water such as Vichy-Célestins or Perles de Vals.[16] In a communication to the Société de Thérapeutique in 1928, Henri Gaehlinger and Auguste Bécart reported that acidifying agents disturb and often prevent the development of the bacteria.[17] Many urologists used ammonium chloride, first recommended by these two doctors, to treat chronic cases. Diet came under scrutiny: drinks like tea, coffee, and many mineral waters were suspect because of their alkaline influence; the only acidifying drink easily available seemed to be wine.

Gaehlinger and Bécart reported on a case that one of them had treated in 1932. The young owner of a big vineyard in Bordeaux, of necessity a professional drinker, got married and promised his wife that he would not drink any wine at all during one month every year and also give up meat. During his abstinence (from wine) he got a bad UTI with all the trimmings, including infected testicles; his urine was cloudy, loaded with bacteria, slightly alkaline, with a pH of 7 to 7.4.[18] He was put on a diet to produce more acid and thus a less alkaline urine. The diet included lots of meat, fish, and cheese; vegetables and fruits were not permitted. A little ammonium chloride and half a bottle of Bordeaux a day, soon increased to a bottle, gave him clear urine in three days. Two months later he came to the Institut Pasteur in Paris, where Professor Alexandre Besredka, a man who knew everything about germs, proclaimed him cured. No observations are given on the patient's liver or libido, both presumably in good condition in a young patient. As the infecting agent became better known, doctors were able to diagnose more males suffering from prostatitis. In women the disease was discovered to have often spread into the womb and the fallopian tubes. 'A healthy patient is an insufficiently diagnosed patient.'[19]

Urologists reported that well-off people had more UTIs than the working class. No doctor consulted could remember finding a drunk or a habitual drinker with a UTI. The most likely victim was a well-off woman who ate too many vegetables and fruits, was often constipated, and detested wine. Constipation, another common disease produced by the bad eating habits typical of urban life, was integrated into the bacterial empire because it could be aggravated by infection. The *grande bourgeoise*, often obsessed with dieting, ate poorly – often only a few sweetmeats daily – drank mineral water and tea, and avoided wine. Her diet produced an alkaline urine favourable to the development of bacteria. The labourer, who usually ate a bad diet full of meat products and often drank excessively, produced an acid urine in which bacteria rarely develop. Doctors thought that both diets were defective. They counselled the golden mean of traditional food with moderate consumption of wine. Among food items recommended to acidify urine were meat, fish, cheese, vegetables, rice, some flours, nuts, plums, and prunes.

Liquids that turned urine alkaline included tea, coffee, and many mineral waters; wine had the field of acid liquids pretty much to itself.[20] Cranberry juice was not a French option.

By the 1930s doctors knew that the injection of wine into veins or muscles was effective against infections because it brought about a rise in the white blood cell count. The injection could be made fairly safe by adjusting its pH level to about that of the normal level of the blood (7.4). The best security was achieved by diluting the wine in a 'physiological serum': five cc of wine in fifteen cc of serum for intravenous injections and five cc of wine in ninety five cc of serum for subcutaneous injections. The intramuscular injection was the preferred method when speed was not necessary.[21]

In the 1940s R. Schnerb (Inspecteur divisionnaire de la Santé), carried out a series of studies related to public health. One of his findings was that though the bacteriocidal power of red wine is not in the alcohol, it reinforces that power in the killing of pathogens such as *Eberthella typhosa* and *Salmonella paratyphi.* Scherb had been pushed in the direction of this type of research by the belief prevalent among the 'higher authorities' in 1939 that bacterial warfare was a possibility. What could be easier than to dump a microbial culture into a supply of drinking water or even a tank car of wine? So Schnerb and his colleagues quickly turned to the study of a counter weapon, red wine, which turned out to be 'an excellent defensive arm' against typhoid fever and other intestinal diseases of bacterial-water origin. Schnerb was pleased that studies carried out at the Hungarian ampelographical institute confirmed his findings. But the *Wehrmacht* carried out a *Blitzkrieg,* not a *Bakteriekrieg,* and the Germans drank the wine instead of contaminating it.[22]

A new direction in research on the bacteriocidal properties of wine was established in 1951, when Jean Lancepleine showed that the antiseptic power of white wine cannot be attributed to any of the elements, especially acids, which had been given the credit up to this point. Nor did he find that the pH factor is an explanation of that power except in the case of abnormally acid wines. He started with white wine and moved on to red wine, which he found to be very different in its chemical composition and a better antiseptic by the very nature of its being red. Lancepleine found the killer property in the anthocyanins (red pigments); this flavonoid is one of a group of naturally occurring phenolic compounds that give wines their colour and most of their flavour. Their anti-bacterial property develops with fermentation. The researchers who could not get plant anthocyanins to kill bacteria slowed acceptance of the work done at Bordeaux. In the best of circumstances, experiments are difficult to replicate, but some researchers seem not to try very hard to confirm other people's work. Later researchers did find plant tannins to be effective in inhibiting the growth of staphylococci cultures. Given the number of different pathogens and the complexity of wine, it was always possible that some clever researcher would find that some bug or other was inconvenienced by some element in wine. The bacteriocidal power of colouring matter in wine remained a fruitful line of research in the 1950s.[23]

The work done by Hélène Jensen was an important extension to red wine of the work that Lancepleine had done on the bacteriocidal power of white wine.[24] Experimenting on *E. coli*, bacterial slave of the microbiological laboratory (and our large intestines), she used a bacterial density or load of about 100 *E. coli* per cubic centimetre of water, which obtained a condition comparable to the natural condition of polluted water. Her results were therefore significant for food hygiene when she showed that polluted water is made drinkable by mixing it with wine. A wine that she decoloured with charcoal lost its killing power. The element in the colouring factors responsible for killing bacteria again turned out to be in the colour pigments of the red grapes.[25] This bacteriodical power, weak in young wines, turned out to be most effective when the wine was seven to ten years old; then after a long stable period, the power declined. The correlation between the antibacterial index and the age of wine results from the chemical transformations that take place in the aging process. By drawing upon microbiology and biochemistry Jensen gave an explanation of a puzzling phenomena, which had been given many previous explanations, some wrong, some partially correct. Like all good explanations in science, it left a good deal unexplained, in this case about the action of polyphenols (phenols) in wine.

It is easy to illustrate research findings favourable to wine therapy, or at least results that can be harnessed to promote it, in gastroenterology and cardiology, two major areas of modern medicine.[26] There is general agreement that wine must be taken in small or moderate amounts, and in the case of serious diseases it must be prescribed if not administered by a physician. First, the appetite: Pavlov's praise of wine as 'a psychic stomachicum' seems justified. Franz Goetzl's post-world war II research carried out organoleptic tests on the appetite-stimulating properties of dry red and white wines; in identifying the responsible constituents, he obtained similar results with solutions of tannic, tartaric, and acetic acids. Shortly after Goetzl's good news, Giorio Lolli and his colleagues did research comparing the diets of Italians and Italo-Americans that showed 'the possible value of wine in the control of obesity.'[27] A little wine facilitates digestion, beginning with the salivary stage, including the promotion of gastric secretion, and stomach motility, with an increase in the secretion of pancreatic juice. Solutions above twenty per cent alcohol and large amounts harm the digestive process. The 'inhibitory action of wine on proteolysis [the enzymic splitting of proteins] is neutralised by the increase in gastric flow.'[28] No doubt St. Paul should not replace St. Luke as the patron saint of physicians, but he deserves at least the status of joint veneration by gastroenterologists.

2. Heart disease

Throughout history many doctors have believed that the moderate consumption of alcohol has a beneficial effect on the cardiovascular system, though few now doubt that excessive drinking increases the probability of a heart attack. But what about the moderate consumption of wine, perhaps a quarter to a half a litre a day? A great deal of recent scientific work indicates that wine is good for the heart. This work covers a wide range of scientific approaches: ecological studies (correlation between different countries), prospective or cohort studies (of population groups), case control or directed experiments, and biochemical connection studies. It is interesting that much of this research has been published in *Lancet*, which thus continues its great nineteenth century tradition of publishing studies showing the medical importance of alcohol and wine. The following analysis will first consider the arguments based on experiments on the possible physiological effects of drinking on health and disease and then move on to the macro level of epidemological arguments apparently based on large, often ethnic groups.

In the 1950s work done by Agnes Fay Morgan and others confirmed the results of research published in 1919 by I. G. Koutateladze demonstrating that wine has an action different from alcohol as a cardiac restorative and vasodilator. Wine is low in sodium and high in potassium; so it is useful in the treatment of hypertensive and cardiac patients. The magnesium content of wine makes it valuable for the cardiovascular system. It is generally (though not universally) accepted that experiments on animals – given hieratic physiological status by the phrase *in vivo* – 'have shown that a cholesterol-rich diet will produce arteriosclerotic lesions in many species.' Does wine drinking prevent the lesions? Maybe. Morgan and her collaborators fed young rats and hamsters normal and cholesterol-rich diets accompanied by one of the following liquids: (1) water *ad libitum*, (2) restricted water, (3) a fifteen per cent alcohol solution, (4) dry red wine, and (5) dry white wine, both wines containing fifteen percent alcohol. The results showed less of an increase in serum cholesterol in both wine-fed groups. 'This illustrates the possible differences between the physiological effects of alcohol solutions and wines of the same alcoholic content.' Why? Possibly the effect of inhibiting or stimulating congeners, or the so-called by-products resulting from the making of wine and giving it its distinctive character.[29]

It is a lot easier to identify the important compounds in grapes, musts, and wines than to discover their effects on living organisms. Morgan listed the compounds in eight groups: amino acids and other nitrogenous compounds; carbohydrates; inorganic elements; acids; alcohols and aldehydes; tannins and colour pigments; vitamins; aromatic constituents, esters, enzymes. The careful Morgan offered little encouragement to those who hoped for an experimental proof that drinking wine satisfies at least part of the needs of the organism for certain elements. 'As far as is known the traces of inorganic elements have limited physiological value.' No concessions to the homeopathological fringe here, but her view predates research showing the importance of trace elements in life processes. She hoped that future research would show the nutritional value of 'the traces of many metallic ions as well as of anions such as the halogens, sulphites, sulphates, carbonates, and phosphates' and 'congeners of unknown but possibly large importance.' But there still remained what Morgan called 'the main questions concerning the metabolic value of wine in the daily diet.'

> 1) What is the range of occurrence of recognised nutrients in wines, namely amino acids, inorganic elements, vitamins and carbohydrates?
> (2) How do the kind of grape, vinification process and other factors affect these nutrients?
> (3) Are these nutrients fully utilisable in wines, and is their ratio of occurrence in the various wines of physiological significance?
> (4) Is the alcohol of wine indistinguishable from alcohol of other media in its physiological effects?

In 1962 Morgan recognised that much work had been done on these questions but that no conclusive answers had been given. 'The reason for our persisting uncertainty may perhaps be the presence of different congeners in every wine tested, even in those of supposedly identical origins.'[30] Morgan was an optimist concerning the possibility of answering these questions through experimentation, though she did not expect miracle cures and immortality – what people normally expect from modern medicine.

Work done in Italy in 1961 tried to show that wine prevents arterial degeneration. A more recent study of the intake of sixteen men found that red wine and, to a lesser extent, white wine increase 'the amount of high density lipoproteins (HDL) ... [which] help reduce the risk of heart disease and atherosclerosis.'[31] Tannins have also been recognised as having effects that may give protection against heart disease. All this supports a finding published in *Lancet* in 1979 associating wine consumption with low mortality from heart disease. A recent study indicates that one drink a day cuts the risk of a second heart attack by twenty to thirty per cent. Some people may have to support migraines to get this benefit, for the Toronto physician Michael Mather suspects that tannin in food triggers migraine headaches, which are often associated with red wine as well as with non-tannic items such as chocolate and cheese.)[32]

Wine has long been known to chemists and oenologists (sometimes overlapping professions) as a liquid loaded with flavonoid phenolics, also called phenols or polyphenols. The chemistry of phenolic compounds in wine has been studied carefully because they are effective antioxidants that enable wine to age while remaining drinkable and, according to some bourgeois taste models, even to improve in quality. So it may be that the same elements enable both man and wine to attain a seductive maturity or, as Andrew Waterhouse put it for wine, to age gracefully. (Though many people age well, few wines do.) Researchers trying to determine the medical effects of wine drinking have concentrated on the phenols, especially on resveratrol and the flavonoids. The four major classes of flavonoids provide lots of experimental material and fruit for speculation: flavonols, anthocyanins, catechins or flavanols, and oligomers [procyanidins] and polymers [tannins] of the catechins). Tea, onions, and apples are noted for their high levels of flavonols, which is good news because research has shown 'a direct correlation between reduced coronary heart disease (CHD) mortality in elderly men and dietary levels of flavonols....' University of Glasgow researchers found that Chilean red wines have the highest level of flavonols among wines. The high level of the antioxidant epigallocatechin gallate in green tea has led to slightly excessive claims for that mouth-puckering drink.[33] Wine has no monopoly on nutrients promoting health and longevity, though some publications tend to encourage that kind of blinkered thinking. Nor is it clear from this type of research that moderate wine drinking promotes health. One recent study failed to find any significantly increased flavonoid concentrations in human plasma after the ingestion of red wine, while another study found that a significant increase was insufficient to have any influence on ex vivo lipoprotein oxidation.[34]

Older clinical medicine necessarily limited itself to general pronouncements on the effects of different types of wine; often these ideas receive confirmation from contemporary medical research, whose aim is to test the ideas and to isolate the specific compounds with their physiological effects as well as to understand the mechanisms at work. In 1961 J. Masquelier (faculty of pharmacy, University of Bordeaux) researching the hypocholesterolemic action of wine, concluded that a number of polyphenols 'capable of reducing the cholesterol level in animals are present in red wines.' Work done by Cornell's plant scientists Siemann and Creasy, who first described the presence of resveratrol in wine, attributed the cholesterol-lowering power of red wine to 'one specific phenolic compound, the phytoalexin *trans*-resveratrol,' a sort of natural pesticide found in vines as well as in other plant *genera.* (Phytoalexins are the protective chemicals produced by plants when attacked by predator micro-organisms.) Probably because of different techniques used for making the two types of wine, red wine has a much higher level of resveratrol than white wine. Barry Gehm and colleagues at Northwestern University Medical School have shown that resveratrol is estrogenic, having a molecular structure similar to that of diethylstilbestrol, which might mean it has benefits with side effects, especially if given as a supplement.[35] There seems to be a similarity 'between ... decreased lipid deposition in rats' livers from resveratrol [orally administered to the lab rodents] and ... reduced serum lipid levels in humans drinking wine.'[36] Traditional Chinese and Japanese medicine uses dried, powdered Japanese Knotweed, in which the active ingredient is resveratrol, to treat a wide variety of ailments, including hyperlipemia and arteriosclerosis. (And then researchers at the University of Illinois found that resveratrol acts as an antioxidant to inhibit the beginning and the developmental process of cancer in mice. Talk about a panacea!) Red bordeaux has the highest level of resveratrol of thirty wines tested. But researchers at the University of Burgundy's wine institute have carried out research to show that the pinot noir grape, used to make red burgundy, is also an excellent producer of resveratrol, if it is attacked by grey rot and successfully resists the disease.[37] It is hard to know what to make of the therapeutic implications of all of these intriguing findings. Perhaps not too much. Waterhouse points out that wine has low levels of resveratrol and even if 'the levels needed *in vivo* may be different from those seen to be effective *in vitro* .. the likelihood that resveratrol from wine would have a physiological effect on a wine drinking population appears to be low.'[38] In this situation it pays to believe in the efficacy of homeopathic doses. Meanwhile the scientific enthusiasm for promoting the drinking of red wine has not abated.

Fortunately, there are more promising phenols in wine. Edwin Frankel and fellow researchers at the University of California at Davis found that the phenols quercetin, epicatechin, and resveratrol in grape skins work better than the alpha-tocopherol component of vitamin E (used as the experimental control) in preventing low-density lipoprotein from oxidising in the bloodstream and in slowing the formation of plaque in the arteries. Epicatechin and quercetin were the most potent. Had these laboratory sleuths found that the explanation for the French paradox was lurking in phenolic compounds? With good reason they thought so.[39] Another component in grape skin has been found to cause blood vessels to dilate, which increases blood flow in the arteries (if you have a good 'pump') and presumably reduces the risk of ischemic heart disease. The defenders of the virtues of alcohol also scored a minor triumph when a study showed that alcohol protects against the formation of blood clots by promoting a higher level of TPA (endogenous tissue-type plasminogen activator), an enzyme playing a role in the body's system of breaking down clots. In addition, alcohol was shown to increase the level of high density lipoprotein or HDL cholesterol, the 'good' stuff that prevents clogging of the arteries, which it does by helping clear the other major lipid fraction of human blood, low density lipoprotein or LDL cholesterol (the 'bad' stuff), and other lipids from the bloodstream).[40] The spirit of Arnau of Villanova must have been pleased at how powerful his ersatz elixir of life was turning out to be.

Late in 1996 Waterhouse emphasised that it had not been proven that phenolics reduce heart disease, though 'the theory that dietary phenolics can inhibit atherosclerosis has been widely accepted as a plausible explanation for wine's effects.' Nor can 'phenolics flush out the arteries,' any more than other frequently touted health foods and herbs, for 'plaque is an integral part of the arterial wall, not a residue' that can be reamed out like a pipe or even a prostate. And we don't know if phenolics reduce cholesterol though we assume that they prevent the oxidation of the 'bad' LDL cholesterol, thus slowing plaque development. Waterhouse has been able to console us with the information that chocolate contains phenols, which have the same effects as those in wine, whatever they might be. And if one is willing to disregard the rigorous code governing what not to eat when drinking red wine, one could benefit from the 'synergistic advantages' of a double dose of phenols. (One should eat chocolate made with cocoa butter, however; cocoa is rich in stearic acid and does not increase cholesterol levels like increasingly widespread cheaper substitutes do.)[41]

Research always finds a new substance or makes a discovery about an old substance that presents a new benefit or a new danger to organic life and leads to a new commercial game. The pro-wine people always have an advantage over other alcoholic drinks because they can claim any benefits found in alcohol consumption as well as those found only in wine.[42] Still nothing has been proved in a clinical sense. Waterhouse notes that 'data in the field of flavonoid absorption by humans are very sparse, though we have evidence for the partial absorption of catechin compared to the non-absorption of quercetin into the bloodstream. So we can only speculate on the direct effect of these compounds on the prevention of heart disease or reduction of CHD mortality.'[43] One of the serious studies of the French paradox took up the issue of the supposed beneficial effects of red wine's 'non-ethanol substances which act as antioxidants, or have effects on thrombosis,' only to conclude that 'these effects are small compared with the apparent effect of ethanol through an HDL-cholesterol pathway, and effects of ethanol on thrombotic factors such as platelet aggregation and fibrinogen.' (Fibrin is an insoluble protein in the blood providing the basic structure for the clot or thrombus.)[44] The tenacious hold of the therapeutic power of alcohol on the medical mind seems to be difficult to break, for there is always some new piece of evidence to tempt us into hope and belief.

Anti-alcoholics might protest that a flavonoid found in grapefruit or a dose of ascorbic acid (vitamin C) has the same effect. Fresh fruit, for example, provides a rich source of phenolic compounds; aerobically produced juice does not. Baptists and the Welch Grape Juice Company recommend drinking grape juice; and it is also true that many of the beneficial compounds found in wine or their equivalents are found in other products. Supporters of grape juice base their case on the work done by a research team led by John D. Folts, cardiovascular physiologist and director of the Coronary Thrombosis Laboratory at the University of Wisconsin. He used an animal model ('anesthetised open chest dogs ... with a flow probe on the stenosed and damaged circumflex coronary artery') to show that a high level of alcohol and a lower level of red wine 'caused significant platelet inhibition.' In the heroic tradition of self-experimentation, the researchers did experiments on their own blood after drinking red and white wines. White wine did poorly in the experiments. A platelet inhibiting effect was also found after grape juice was given to the dogs. Flavonoids were given the credit for the heart protection provided. Folts' work confirmed the results of the Zutphen study (805 middle-aged men observed for eight years) showing that 'the men who had the highest intake of flavonoids had the lowest risk of dying from a heart attack.'[45]

Lucie Randoin's research in the inter-war period had shown that vitamin C and B-complex vitamins are present in wine; though vinification destroys much of the C, nutritionally significant amounts of thiamin, riboflavin, pantothenic acid, pyridoxin, niacin, and folic acid survive in wine, especially port wines, which were wisely recommended by our ancestors for 'blood-building.'[46] At his Galamini institute in Fascist Rome, Baglioni had carried out similar research on vitamin B in wine as well as on topics such as the food value of lipids.[47] Recent research has shown the role of folate and vitamin B_6 in maintaining lower homocysteine levels in the blood and therefore in lowering the risk of CHD, among women at least.[48] The plant substance rutin, which vitamin manufacturers often include in their bioflavonoid capsules, is believed to make capillaries more resistant to haemorrhage and to be important in homeostasis.[49] Of course, other sources not burdened with the potential dangers of wine consumption can be used for nearly all substances found in wine. Or for that matter, there is always the vitamin counter at the health food store, even in France. Whether the body is able to make better physiological use of these elements administered in wine is still a question. Wine is just more fun. It has been the constant companion of *Homo ludens* since the disasterous experiment with apples in the Garden of Eden. It's comforting to know that science shows that moderate consumption may produce good physiological effects. Well, sort of; no molecular mechanism has been found yet.[50]

In recent years the media have been skillful in exploiting the debates in medical research about the effects of alcohol on the heart. The most famous media event for wine was the presentation by CBS television of the 'French paradox' by '60 Minutes,' on Nov. 17, 1991, with more coverage on Nov. 5, 1995. R. Curtis Ellison, Serge Renaud, and Martin Gronbaek, a trinity of great doctors friendly to red wine consumption, aided by wine drinker Morley Safer (the interviewer) presented their case to the receptive American nation, which is not, however, a wine drinking culture. Red wine sales and advertising for it went up significantly.[51] The puritan patriarchs and matriarchs of the federal bureaucracy in BATF and the FDC were not amused. (The federal government, that is BATF, recently gave wine producers permission to put two neutral statements on wine labels to the effect that for information on health benefits of wine consumption the buyers should consult their family doctor and send for the federal department of agriculture's dietary guidelines.[52]) The French paradox is sometimes said to be that the French indulge in a dangerously high saturated fat-loaded diet, smoke more cigarettes, and drink more alcohol than Americans, but live longer and have fewer heart attacks than Americans because they drink more red wine. The conservative version, put forward by Criqui and Ringel in *Lancet* in 1994, merely states that France has a low rate of CHD 'compared with other developed countries [data from twenty one developed countries were analysed] with comparable dietary intake' and goes on to 'conclude that ethanol, particularly wine ethanol, is inversely related to CHD but not to longevity in populations.' Individuals who drink moderately may live longer, but the high level of alcohol abuse in wine drinking countries 'sharply reduces longevity' for the general population. 'Thus while the risk/benefit ratio varies for individuals, the use of alcohol for cardioprotective purposes should not be encouraged as a public health measure.'

Serge Renaud ruthlessly defends his thesis that wine protects the heart and skilfully uses statistics to get rid of the protective properties of food and, what is more outrageous for fans of Dean Ornish (the present American 'guru of heart health'), states that wine drinking counteracts 'the effects of dairy fats and cigarette smoking. Southern French farmers and Scottish farmers have similar HDL cholesterol levels but the French have a lower aggregation of platelets, which is explained by the higher level of French alcohol consumption.[53] Unless for the French it is the beneficial effect of eating more foie gras made from goose liver, which is rich in heart protective fatty acids. It seems that the paradox argument is based on a minority of the French population, for only twenty eight per cent of French men and eleven per cent of French women drink wine regularly, and only half of French adults drink wine at all.[54] The argument about better French health is, at most, a seductive hypothesis. Americans may eat more fat, though the French are catching up but because of their growing love of junk food and increasing appetite. More meat and less wine as well. Fortunately for researchers, this gastronomic horror story provides a new paradox. White Americans now live longer than most other people and, according to the latest public health propaganda, are the healthiest people on earth.[55] In any case, statistics for various well fed national groups having different eating habits show that longevity seems little affected by what is eaten, including saturated fatty acids.[56] In talking about the effects of food and drink on health, one cannot escape controversy and confusion, as is the case, to a lesser extent, in the discourse generated over different systems of medical care.

According to a survey published in the *Nouvel observateur* in January 1985, heart disease is worst in the Nord, Pas-de-Calais, Lorraine, Alsace, the Auvergne, and Brittany; the 'hearts of steel' are in the Poitou-Charentes and the Centre, although the Ile-de-France, Languedoc-Roussillon, and the Midi-Pyrénées shelter many strong hearts too. Death from alcoholism was highest in the Morbihan and lowest in the Haute-Garonne. Recent life expectancy at birth is 74 years for French men and 81.9 years for women. In the Ile-de-France, one of the world's richest regions, the figures are 74.5 for men and 82.3 for women. People live even longer in the Gers, though it hardly seems worthwhile. A lot of the added time is spent in the hospitals that make the Gers the hospital capital of the eight departments of the Midi-Pyrénées.

The argument that the French have fewer heart attacks – forty per cent fewer, it has been said – seems to rest on a flimsy statistical basis. A report at an international cardiology convention in 1994 debunked the claim on the grounds that many French death certificates are notorious for their lack of precision and state the cause of death in the Belgian beer-like language of 'sudden death' (*mort subite*). This may make it impossible to rely on statistics about the cause of French deaths, or at least make it difficult to believe that the French have less heart disease than other national groups. (American death certificates are also flawed, with 'coronary artery disease the default diagnosis for the death certificate when doctors are not sure of the cause of death,' which is true in thirty to forty per cent of the cases.[57] So does this mean that American figures are too high, perhaps by fifty per cent for people who died after age 85?) Though it is true that French drinkers consume much more alcohol than is needed for the heart protection benefit, 'there has been a decline in French per capita consumption – from 18.3 litres of pure alcohol a year in 1965 to 13.1 litres in 1988. Alcohol consumed as wine has also dropped to 9.1 litres of pure alcohol from 13.3. At the same time, however, coronary death rates have fallen, to 71.3 per 100,000 in 1988 from 94.9 per 100,000 in 1965, and deaths from cirrhosis have fallen even more sharply, to 37.9 per 100,000 in 1988 from 68.5 per 100,000 in 1975.'[58] In the twenty one countries studied by Criqui and Ringel, the total mortality of the French improved from the eighth lowest in 1980 to the sixth lowest in 1988. So the pro-wine argument is not helped by the fact that in recent years as the French have been drinking less they are living longer, with lower coronary and especially lower cirrhosis death rates. Uffe Ravnskov states bluntly that there is no French paradox; all we are talking about, without really knowing it, is the French data being situated 'at the extreme corner of a scatter diagram that includes most combinations of saturated fatty acids or serum cholesterol and mortality from coronary heart disease.'[59] The French comedian Patrick Marc summed up wine drinkers' regrets in observing that he had always doubted the argument about the medical virtues of red wine because 'it was too good to be true,' a judgment that might be applied to many medical miracles.

Numerous epidemiological studies exist showing that moderate consumption of alcohol gives the consumer some health advantages over the non-drinker, chiefly in cardiovascular fitness. And wine is certainly the most pleasurable way of getting alcohol. Moderation is hard to define, ranging from an American conservative estimate of two four-once glasses of about twelve-degree wine, about thirty grams of alcohol, to the generous Danish estimate of three to five glasses of wine a day, presumably with meals. The Copenhagen city heart study, which included over thirteen thousand people between the ages of thirty and seventy nine, reported a reduction of forty nine per cent in mortality for the wine drinkers.[60] If we take into account the increased alcoholic content of most contemporary wine, the Danish claim that the greatest health benefits are derived from three to five glasses a day is similar to the old French medical recommendation of somewhat less than a litre a day with meals.

Wine buffs may have been pleased to learn that in Denmark over a period of about twenty years wine drinking went up by thirty per cent and heart disease decreased by thirty per cent, but it is easy to leap to the wrong conclusion. Roy Porter points out that in the United States CHD 'dropped by half between 1970 and 1990 – a reduction of around 300,000 deaths a year – and there was also a substantial decline in strokes.'[61] Changes in life style and diet among the educated classes probably explain most of the mortality reduction, though the modest increase in wine consumption by the same people who are living longer is probably not a negligable factor. Nor can we ignore the positive if modest effects of advances in cardiology.

The results of a mega-study of the death rates over a nine-year period of 490,000 people between the ages of thirty and 104 indicates that subjects who had a daily drink of wine (5 ounces), beer (twelve ounces), or hard liquor had a lower death rate than non drinkers. The optimistic headline in *The New York Times* was that a 'Drink a Day Can Lower Death Rate By 20 Percent.' And 'the rates of death from all cardiovascular diseases were 30 to 40 per cent lower among men ... and women reporting about one drink daily than among non-drinkers, with little relation to the level of consumption. The overall death rates were lowest among men and women reporting about one drink daily.' One conclusion of the study was that 'In this middle-aged and elderly population, moderate alcohol consumption slightly reduced overall mortality.' The news was better for men than for women. 'The mortality from breast cancer was 30 percent higher among women reporting at least one drink daily than among non-drinkers.' Since cardiovascular disease is a much more serious killer of women than breast cancer, it can be argued that the general female population still benefits from one drink a day.[62] In spite of the evidence in favour of moderate drinking, especially wine, many physicians are reluctant to endorse any level of drinking, and are certainly against recommending that non-drinkers start drinking. The risks of alcohol abuse are simply too high: cardiotoxic effects, cerebral infarction, cirrhosis, and hypertension, accidents, and serious social problems. 'Men and women who drink alcoholic beverages regularly have, in comparison with abstainers, higher death rates from injuries, violence, suicide, poisoning, cirrhosis, certain cancers, and possibly haemorrhagic stroke, but lower death rates from coronary heart disease and thrombotic stroke.' It does seem, however, that moderate drinkers at least may stop worrying about that widely believed scientific old wives' tale that drinking alcohol kills brain cells.[63] Even the risk of heart disease can be handled by diet, physical exercise, and weight control. A recent major study by a Canadian team of the epidemiological literature over the past fifteen years produced very conservative guidelines for drinking, especially for women, and included a recommendation of total abstinence for one or two days a week.[64]

It may be that serious beer and liquor drinkers, like teetotallers, do not enjoy the same cardiovascular benefits as wine drinkers; perhaps beer drinkers tend to indulge in the unhealthy practice of a weekend binge rather than spreading the consumption over the week.[65] A valuable review of twelve ecological, three case-control, and ten separate prospective cohort studies concluded that the evidence shows that the reduction of risk in CHD comes from the alcohol.[66] A study of Kaiser Permanente's data on 128,934 men and women for the years 1978-1985, found that white wine and any other alcoholic beverage was just as good as red wine in reducing heart disease.[67] J. Michael Graziano (Harvard Medical School) found that beer, liquor, and wine have the same beneficial effect on the heart, raising artery-protecting, high-density lipoprotein cholesterol about ten per cent. But the Danish study found that beer and liquor, unlike wine, had no significant effect on mortality. And a number of other studies have found that 'wine seems to have a stronger protective effect for CHD than either beer or spirits.'[68] One of the problems we have in talking about the health effects of different beverages comes from the research itself. 'Epidemiologic studies on the effects of beverage type are plagued with lack of control for confounding different factors (e.g., wine consumption with social class.)'[69] A recent Danish study of 'social inequalities in risk of ischaemic heart disease' (IHD) suggested strongly that 'low social class,' increases the risk of IHD.[70] Lower class status is associated with 'a low serum selenium concentration [lower than that of the upper classes, who eat more fish and vegetables], and a low intake of wine and spirits (as compared with higher classes). Many American middle class consumers get 200-250 mcg. of selenium in their daily general vitamin pill, which does at least as much good as the pink mixture that kept up Mrs. Mawmsey of Middlemarch.

In their *Lancet* article Criqui and Ringel noted that though the findings of ecological or epidemiological studies 'are consistent with a large and growing number of case-control and cohort studies within populations that show a protective effect for CHD morbidity and mortality' for people who take one or two drinks a day, the cohort studies show that wine gives the best protection. Why is there this discrepancy between ecological and cohort studies? A second paradox! Is this just a statistical distortion reflecting differences in countries studied? Or might it be that wine-drinking countries 'have better nutrition, including foods such as olive oil and other components of the Mediterranean diet'? That diet is often praised and commercially exploited. Crete has provided the most famous version of that diet. It has been convincingly argued that the French paradox (a part of the European paradox) may be explained in terms of the high level of d-alpha-tocopherol component of vitamin E present in the French diet, seventy one per cent greater than in the U. K. The French source of this heart protective vitamin is not olive oil but sunflower seed oil, the leading oil consumed in France.[71] Or might wine have a better effect because it is traditionally drunk with meals, thus reducing 'some toxic effects of high alcohol consumption because of reduced absorption'? And wine with meals may 'have a favourable effect on post-prandial hyperlipidaemia.'[72] It looks like wine drinkers may be more affluent and better fed than other drinkers. And then there is family happiness, promoted some years ago in the guise of the model of the modest Italian family of the northeastern United States happily snarfing down pasta and *gros rouge*. Only recently *Lancet* presented us with the Albanian paradox, just as we were becoming tired of the French one with the inconclusive medical debates spinning out it. In spite of a high infant mortality rate, the adult mortality, including mortality from cardiovascular diseases, in southwest Albania, where the diet depends heavily on olive oil, vegetables, and carbohydrates, is similar to that in other Mediterranean countries.[73] 'Only one thing seems certain in the absence of a 'clinical trial of the wine hypothesis'[74]: the benefits of moderation.

The wine industry has always enjoyed much more support from medical practitioners and researchers than other alcohol industries. The medical community has also enjoyed the support of the wine industry. Nor should we forget that doctors have always made up an important part of the upper social level of wine drinking cultures. Wine drinking has always profited from a good social image deriving from the perception that the upper classes drink wine, and the higher the class of the drinker, the more famous the wine consumed. A picture of a pro-wine Harvard doctor in a recent issue of the *Wine Spectator* showed him tossing a bottle of 1990 Latour, rated by Parker 98+/100 the alarming praise that the wine has 'mouth-searing tannins that explode on the palate.' One could hardly ask for a better symbol of Bourdieu's view concerning class structure and consumption.[75]

The contemporary medical gurus of the wine therapy scene, such as R. Curtis Ellison (Boston University School of Medicine), Serge Renaud (much of whose career was spent with INSERM in Lyon), Arthur Klatsky (Kaiser Permanente Medical Center, Oakland, CA), Eric Rimm (Harvard School of Public Health) and their illustrious ilk, are the worthy successors of the European (especially French and British) pro-wine doctors who were the active propagandists for alcohol and wine therapy since the Enlightenment. They have much more serious epidemiological evidence than their ancestors could have even hoped for, but their conclusions are remarkably similar. They have more solid and specific physiological and biochemical evidence that moderate consumption of wine is good preventive medicine; the therapeutic use of wine, so important to the old doctors, has not yet made a return and is unlikely to do so. Both groups subscribe to the belief that scientific studies settle issues. Perhaps the moderns will have better luck here than their predecessors. Meanwhile, some medical mugwumps can only say that 'the stance that the medical community should take on alcohol consumption 'is seemingly a conundrum of the highest order'.'[76] From the viewpoint of preventive medicine, we seem to have ended up back with the ancient Greeks, though we have different and probably better wines, more scientific and medical knowledge justifying findings, and laboratory rats and transgenic mice to play with.

3. Cancer and life expectancy

Cancer was one of the subjects left untouched in the *Repertory of New Treatments* (1936) devised by Portmann and Eylaud. Perhaps the evidence did not lend itself to saying anything strikingly favourable for wine in the treatment of cancer. And until recently the disease was not a particularly French obsession. 'Cancer became the modern disease *par excellence* ... above all the American disease,' dominated by glitzy research and ... prima donnas.'[77] Although it was a disease of some medical interest by mid-nineteenth century, cancer slowly became a matter of general concern in the second half of the century. In 1904 W. Roger Williams examined the cancer death rate in the U.K. between 1840 and 1900 in order to refute the conclusion of the Imperial Cancer Research Fund that there had not been a real increase in cancer. He found an impressive increase.

Year	Cancer death rate per 1,000,000 living
1840	**177**
1860	**343**
1880	**502**
1900	**828**

Williams identified a disproportionate increase for men, though the rate was still 597 for males compared with 903 for females. He blamed the general context of urbanisation, which affected 'men more than women in altering ancestral habits.' The population of Britain had grown from nearly sixteen million to over thirty two million in the period under scrutiny. Among urban conditions responsible for moving men closer to the cancer mortality rate for women were 'want of proper exercise and excess of food.' Some French doctors would have included in this speculative but reasonable etiology the absence of moderate consumption of good wine.[78]

In 1903 Arthur Newsholme noted that statistics showed that cancer mortality is much higher among alcoholics; this raised the question of a connection between the consumption of alcohol and 'excessive mortality from cancer'.[79] Some other researchers jumped on this cause-of-cancer bandwagon. Tsurumi added to the anxiety of the drinker by pointing out that in Japan drinkers of saké had a high rate of cancer of the esophagus. The relation was explained by assuming that continual irritation causes cancer. But in 1916 Tsurumi found that ethyl alcohol did not directly influence the development of cancer in mice, or at least the influence of alcohol on the development of tumours remained obscure. Appearing in the *Annales de l'Institut Pasteur*, his article was used in pro-wine circles as an effective counter to that of Newsholme in the *British Medical Journal*. The problem was that Tsurumi was writing of mice, not men. Tsurumi made the difference clear in pointing out that the exoneration of alcohol involved extrapolating his findings from mice to men.[80]

Wine interests were not so scrupulous as researchers. Indulging in their favourite statistical game of comparative departmental mortalities, the defenders of wine drinking showed to their complete satisfaction that wine drinking decreases one's chances of getting cancer.[81] In 1928 the annual French death rate from cancer was ninety six per 100,000 inhabitants. One could take the departments producing sixty per cent of the grape crop and be impressed by the fact that they had cancer death rates below the national level.

Department	No. of deaths per 100,000
Alpes-Maritimes	**87**
Hérault	**73**
Pyrénées-Orientales	**66**
Aude	**64**
Var	**60**
Gard	**59**
Bouches-du-Rhône	**53**
Corsica	**26**

Then one can take non-viticultural departments, which for reasons that are not too clear, had higher cancer death rates.

Department	No. of deaths per 100,000
Aisne	**106**
Oise	**109**
Mayenne	**113**
Eure-et-Loir	**115**
Nord	**124**
Seine	**138**
Seine-Inférieure	**141**

It had to be admitted that there were wine producing departments where the cancer death rate (1929) was higher than the national rate: Moselle – 168, Haut-Rhin – 140, Saône-et-Loire – 131, Indre-et-Loire – 117, Loir-et-Cher – 108, Gironde – 102, Drôme – 99. It could be said, and it was, that these were the only viticultural departments where the death rate was higher than the average general mortality for the country as a whole.[82] Sceptics concluded that so much conflicting evidence and so many variables made it impossible to come to any scientific conclusion about wine and cancer. In 1937 L. Dieulafé, of the medical faculty in Toulouse, took on the role of the great simplifier: *You Can Avoid Cancer* was the title of a pamphlet in which he studied the evolution of cancer to show that in regions where wine is not the standard drink annual cancer mortality varied between 106 and 141 per 100,000 inhabitants, and in the other regions it was between 59 and 73.[83] No closure of the debate seemed possible, which is about where we are now.

In January 1985 *Le Nouvel Observateur* presented 'La France des records' by regions. At the top of the cancer hit list, presented as male mortality per 100,000 inhabitants: Seine-Saint-Denis – 314.53, Haut-Rhin – 310.18, and Finistère – 308.92; at the bottom: Corsica – 199.70, Ariège – 183.25, and Alpes-Maritimes – 153.16. Paris had a respectably low mortality – 270.71. Among the big wine-producing departments: the Gironde – 263.03, Côte d'Or – 255.96, Hérault – 227.52, and Aude – 218.79. Although French women live longer than other most female nationals in the European community, the gap between French male and female life expectancy is the widest in the European Union. One explanation of the difference is probably to be found in the more irrational behaviour of the male, whose lifestyle includes, in addition to more accidents, more cancer-related and coronary heart disease-related behaviour, especially smoking and drinking, than the female lifestyle. Since a large part of the alcohol consumed in France is from the grape, wine appears to be as dangerous as any other kind of medicine. In excess, wine becomes part of the large, classic empire of iatrogenesis. The wisdom of the body is found in the banal Aristotelian prescription of moderation, a moral quality seriously damaged by testosterone and machismo. The human animal and its diseases are not yet fully understood, but we do know that it craves alcohol, often likes wine, and is tempted to accept any piece of evidence showing that wine is good preventive and possibly curative medicine.

One piece of recent research does indicate that wine drinkers are less subject to some types of cancer. A 'large population-based, case-controlled study of esophageal and gastric cardia adenocarcinomas revealed ... a 40% reduced risk ... associated with wine drinking.' And the risk of developing esophageal squamous cell carcinoma was found to be three times higher among liquor drinkers. Of course the risk doubled for smokers and ex-smokers, including 'a non-significant decrease in risk associated with higher incomes.' But for the four tumour types included in this study 'risks were higher among those with low income or education.'[84] Studies using an animal model support the idea that red wine offers some protection against cancer. In tumour-prone transgenic mice the development of tumours was delayed when the creatures were fed red wine solids, with a clearly identified absorption of 'the major polyphenol of red wine (catechin) in the blood.[85] Until the mechanisms involved are discovered, what this means for humans remains speculative.

Presumably a glass of red wine with a meal can't hurt. Susan Ebeler and Mary Ann Weber insist that 'there is increasing evidence that wine may contain components that provide a health protective effect.' This is good news because there is strong evidence that alcohol acts as a cocarcinogen in the body. Even in the controversial case of breast cancer, where consumption of beer and spirits increase the risk, there are studies showing that there is a decrease in risk for moderate wine drinkers.[86] The propaganda put out by the Washington based Center for Science in the Public Interest disagrees, of course, and throws wine in with the rest of booze. Its *Booze News* was able to exploit the 'pooled analysis of cohort studies,' including over three hundred thousand women followed over a period of eleven years, which concluded that 'alcohol consumption is associated with a linear increase in breast cancer incidence in women even at a level of less than a drink a day.[87] What drinking only wine would mean for cancer risk is unknown. And the women studied did not belong to wine drinking cultures. This particular salvo from the CSPI did not mention the effect of wine on heart disease, which kills ten times more women annually than breast cancer; pro-wine people never miss that opportunity. And one can play it safe in this argument, as Martin Gronbæk did on 'Sixty Minutes' by recommending extreme moderation for women in their thirties and forties, when the risk of developing breast cancer is more of a concern than when women enter into their fifties, when the risk of cardiovascular disease increases. Alcohol-related breast cancer accounts for only two per cent of breast cancer cases, and yet 'another round in [the] drink-a-day debate' indicates that there is no evidence that women who consume up to one and a half drinks daily increase their risk of developing breast cancer, and the risk may even decline.[88] The metaphor of science as endless frontier has a Sisyphean subtext, which is frustrating to physician and patient. Nor do epidemiological investigations help in the short run, for they 'are never capable of determining specific causes for observed effects.'[89] Frustrated by the distance between epidemiology and the doctor's real activity, James Le Fanu has suggested closing all departments of epidemology.[90] A glass of cabernet sauvignon or pinot noir for everyone is a more reasonable prescription.

Notes

1. Docteur E. Maury, *La médecine par le vin ou le vin comme remède universelle* (Paris: J'ai Lu, 1996). Maury also published *Soignez-vous par le vin. Les caractéristiques de tous les vins et leurs vertus thérapeutiques* (Paris, Marabout, 1983; 1992). On the healing virtues of champagne, see François Bonal, Docteur Tran Ky, Docteur F. Drouard, *Les vertus thérapeutiques du champagne. Historique, tradition, biologie, diététique* (Paris: Artulen, 1990). Docteur Jean-Michel Guilbert joined Tran Ky and Drouard to produce a volume on *Les vertus thérapeutiques du Bordeaux. Histoire naturelle et culturelle, diététique, biologie* (Paris: Artulen, 1991) Bonal included a chapter on 'Le champagne et la santé' in *Le Livre d'or du Champagne* (Lausanne: Ed. Grand Pont, 1984). The Wine Advisory Board, 'an agricultural industry administrative agency established and operating pursuant to the Marketing Order for Wine, issued and made effective under the authority of the California Marketing Act of 1937,' published a pamphlet of about fifty pages on the *Uses of Wine in Medical Practice* (San Francisco, 1967, 5th edn.).
2. See the historical survey by Christopher Hoolihan, 'Wine and

Regimen from Hippocrates to the Renaissance,' *Caduceus*, 9 (Spring 1993), 5–16.

3. Lewis Thomas, *The Lives of a Cell* (New York: Bantam Books, 1975), 89.
4. Lewis Thomas, 'Medical Lessons from History,' in *The Medusa and the Snail* (New York: Bantam Books, 1980), 132–146.
5. W. F. Bynum, *Science and the Practice of Medicine in the Nineteenth Century* (Cambridge: Cambridge University Press, 1994), 86.
6. Emile Mauriac, *Le vin au point de vue médical* (Paris: Doin, 1903), 24. Mauriac says that 'le baume de Samaritain' is composed of equal parts of olive oil and red wine. Dr. Ferran (Lyon) recommended a mixture of glycerine and wine. See also Dr P. Carles, 'Le vin et la fièvre typhoïde,' *Journal de médecine de Bordeaux* (*JMBX*) 37 (1907), 373–4.
7. Jean-Claude A. Desenclos and others, 'The protective effect of alcohol on the occurrence of epidemic oyster-borne hepatitis A,' *Epidemiology*, 3 (July 1992), 371–4.
8. See Gert H. Brieger, 'Carl-Joseph Eberth,' in C.C. Gillispie (ed), *Dictionary of Scientific Biography* (New York: Scribner, 1970-80), IV, 275–77.
9. Pick, *Arch. f. Hygien.*, 19 (1893); Hélène-Germaine-Suzanne Jensen, *Recherches sur le pouvoir bactéricide des vins rouges* (Bordeaux: Thesis, Faculté des Sciences, 1954), a thesis for the Doctorat de l'Université in pharmacy. Jensen gives a succinct review of much of the literature done before her research; a summary of the work on wine and bugs is given by Salvatore Lucia, *A History of Wine as Therapy* (Philadelphia: Lippincott, 1963), ch. 14.
10. L. Taverni, in *Rivista d'igiene e sanità pubblica* (1900), 238.
11. Dr. P. Carles, 'le vin et la fièvre typhoïde,' *JMBX*, 37 (1907), 374.
12. J. Sabrazès et A. Marcandier, 'Action du vin sur le bacille d'Eberth,' *Annales de l'Institut Pasteur*, 21 (1907), 312–320.
13. Discussion in the Société de médecine de Paris, reported in *JMBX*, 38 (1908), 181-4.
14. *La Journée vinicole* of Montpellier, No. of 22 juin, reprinted in *Bulletin de l'organisation internationale du vin* (BIV), no. 152 (1942), 76–77.
15. *Liber de vinis*, quoted in Lucia, *op. cit.* (note 9), 103.
16. Mauriac, *op. cit.* (note 6), 26–7.
17. Auguste Bécart made constipation one of his specialities: *La constipation, son traitement* (Paris: Doin, 1931); *Hygiène du constipé* (Paris: Doin, 1932); and with Gaehlinger and Victor Pauchet, *La constipation – comment l'éviter – comment la guérir?* (Paris: Doin,

1926; 2d edn, 1933) and *Savez votre intestin; conseils aux constipés* (Paris: Doin, 1933; rev. and expanded, 1953). See also *La gastrophotographie* (Paris: Maloine, 1931). Bécart was an expert on haematology: *Le sang; abrégé d'hématologie* (Paris: Doin, 1927); *Hématologie clinique* (Paris: Maloine, 1943). With Gaehlinger he published a book on *La vaccination par voie buccale dans l'infection intestinale* (Paris: Doin, 1927). Gaehlinger, a consulting doctor at Châtel-Guyon who worked mineral water cures as well, turned *la colibacillose* into a new plague with his book on *La colibacillose; la maladie du siècle* (Paris: Oliven, 1934; 3d edn, 1954).

18. The pH (potential of hydrogen) scale is 'a logarithmic scale for expressing the acidity or alkalinity of a solution. ... A pH below 7 indicates an acid solution; one above indicates an alkaline solution. Oxford's *Concise Science Dictionary* (Oxford and New York: Oxford University Press, 1987), 533.
19. William Kissick, quoted in the John Walton and others (eds), *Oxford Medical Companion* (Oxford: Oxford University Press, 1994), 360.
20. MM. Gaehlinger and A. Bécart, 'Influence favourable du vin dans le traitement des colibacilloses urinaires,' BIV, no. 60 (1933), 45–46. See also H. Gaehlinger, *La maladie du siècle: la colibacillose* (2d edn, Paris: J. Oliven, 1950), 9, 11, 58–61.
21. F. Ramond, G. Guittonneau, Nicolas et Chevalier, 'Action thérapeutique du vin en injections et en lavements,' *Le progrès médical*, (12 août 1933), cited in J.-F.-N. Dougnac, *Le vin...* (2d edn, Bordeaux: Delmas, 1935), 242.
22. Dr. R. Scherb, 'Sur le pouvoir bactéricide du vin,' BIV, no. 197 (1947), 85–88.
23. Lucia, *op. cit.* (note 9), 179–180, draws attention to the work in the 1950s and 1960s of American researchers. John Gardner isolated an unidentified compound from red wine that 'completely inhibited the growth of *Staphylocooccus aureus* and *Bacillum megatherium*, and John J. Powers confirmed the anti-bacterial power of wine substances.
24. Hélène Jensen's *Recherches sur le pouvoir bactéricide des vins rouges* (1954). The work was done in the laboratory of zoology and parasitology of the faculty of medicine and pharmacy of the University of Bordeaux.
25. On the anthocyanin pigments in grapes, see M. A. Amerine and M. A. Joslyn, Table Wines. *The Technology of their Production* (Berkeley, CA.: University of California Press, 1970), 255–69, and on anthocyans (including anthocyanins) and phenolics, see Jancis Robinson (ed), *The Oxford Companion to Wine* (Oxford: Oxford

University Press, 1994), 37–8, 722–3.

26. See ch. 14 of Lucia, 'The Demonstration of the Physiologic Effects of Wine,' *op. cit.* (note 9), 174–214.
27. Lucia, *ibid.*, 186–189. Goetzl's work was done at the Kaiser Permanente Foundation Institute of Medical Research in Oakland and the study *Alcohol in Italian Culture* by Giorgio Lolli and others at the Yale Center of Alcohol Studies.
28. Lucia, *op. cit.* (note 9), 182, reporting on work done between 1906 and 1946 at Yale (Laboratory of Applied Physiology), Christiania University, the Pharmacological Institute of Jena, the Institute of Pathology in Berlin, and the University of California. Definition of congeners from *The New Shorter Oxford English Dictionary*; the more familiar scientific definition is that of elements belonging to the same group in the periodic table – see Oxford's *Concise Science Dictionary* (note 18).
29. A. F. Morgan and others, 'Utilization of calories from alcohol and wines and their effects on cholesterol metabolism,' *American Journal of Physiology*, 189 (1957), 290–96.
30. Agnes Fay Morgan, 'Wine in the normal diet,' *Bulletin of the Society of Medical Friends of Wine*, v, no. 2 (1962).
31. M. Seigneur and others (including Pascal Ribéreau-Gayon), 'Effect of the consumption of alcohol, white wine and red wine on platelet function and serum lipids,' *Journal of Applied Cardiology*, v (1990), 215–22.
32. Robyn Bullard, 'Wine may help coronary health,' *The Wine Spectator* (Dec. 31, 1990); M. Seigneur and others. 'Effect of the consumption of alcohol, white wine, and red wine on platelet function and serum lipids,' *Journal of Applied Cardiology*, v (1990), 215–222.
33. Andrew L. Waterhouse, 'Wine and heart disease,' *Chemistry and Industry* (1 May 1995), 339, which refers to a study by Hertog and others, published in *Lancet*, 342 (1993), 1007–11. Some work on green tea has been done by Lester Mitscher (Univ. Of Kansas), who doesn't make any claims for it except as 'an insurance policy for those who eat a healthy diet and exercise. 'Chemical helps green tea beat wine in health stakes,' on the web - http://www.ads.co.za/strathealth/19970812-124845.hltm
34. See Jennifer R. C. Bell and others (including Waterhouse), '(+)-Catechin in human plasma after ingestion of of a single serving of reconstituted red wine,' *American Journal of Clinical Nutrition* 71 (2000), 67–74; and Rima Abu-Amsha Caccetta and others, 'Ingestion of red wine significantly increases plasma phenolic acid

concentrations but does not acutely affect ex vivo lipoprotein,' *ibid.*, 103–8.

35. Barry Gehm and colleagues, report published in the *Proceedings of the National Academy of Sciences*, 94 (9 Dec. 1998), 14138.
36. E. H. Siemann and L. L. Creasy, 'Concentration of the phytoalexin resveratrol in wine,' *American Journal of Enology and Viticulture*, 43 (1992), 49–52.
37. R. Bessis and others (Laboratoire des sciences de la vigne, Institut Jules Guyot, Université de Bourgogne), 'Resvératrol, défenses naturelles de la vigne et image santé du vin,' *Revue des Œnologues*, no. 85 (Oct. 1997), 5–8.
38. Waterhouse, *Chemistry and Industry* (1 May 1995), 338–41.
39. E. N. Frankel and others, 'Inhibition of oxidation of human low-density lipoprotein by phenolic substances in red wine,' Lancet, 341 (1993), 454-7; see also Frankel, Waterhouse, and Pierre-Louis Teissedre, 'Principal phenolic phytochemicals in selected Californian wines and their antioxidant activity in inhibiting oxidation of human low-density lipoproteins,' *Jour. Agric. Food Chemistry*, 43 (1995), 890–4.
40. Lucia, *op. cit.* (note 9), 201–202; Jane E. Brody, 'Red Wine May Have Potential as Potion for the Blood's Ills,' *The New York Times* (14 August 1991); J. Michael Gaziano and others, 'Moderate alcohol intake, increased levels of high-density lipoprotein and its subfractions, and decreased risk of myocardial infarction,' *The New England Journal of Medicine*, 329 (1993), 1829 ff.; Thomas Matthews, 'Wine: prescription for good health,' *Wine Spectator* (15 March 1994), 36–44; and 'A drink a day may be an aid against clots,' *The New York Times* (28 Sept. 1994).
41. Andrew L. Waterhouse, 'Antioxidants in Chocolate,' document on the www at: winserver.ucdavis.edu/chocolate; see also his letter with same title in *Lancet*, 348 (1996), 834.
42. See the cover story 'Special report on wine and good health' in the *Wine Spectator* (15 March 1994). The reader's confidence is encouraged by the picture on the cover of a man in a white coat holding half a glass of red wine; his M.D. tag is clearly visible.
43. Waterhouse, *loc. cit.* (note 38), 340.
44. M. H. Criqui and Brenda L. Ringel, 'Does diet or alcohol explain the French paradox?,' *Lancet*, 344 (Dec. 24/31, 1994), 1722. For a convenient list of antioxidants, see James F. Scheer, 'Twelve Key Antioxidants,' *Better Nutrition* (Jan. 1999), 58-60.
45. On the benefits of vitamin C for the heart and in reducing cholesterol levels, see Linus Pauling, *How to live longer and feel better*

(New York: Freeman, 1986), 145–52. On the experiments done by Folts, see John D. Folts and others, 'Red wine, atherosclerosis, and coronary thrombosis,' in *Wine in Context: Nutrition, Physiology, Policy* (Davis, CA.: American Society for Enology and Viticulture, 1996), the proceedings of the symposium on wine and health of June 24 and 25, 1996 held in Reno, Nevada, edited by Andrew L. Whitehouse and JoAnne M. Rantz. I found the Baptist blast, 'Grape juice study debunks wine's health claims,' which ignores the wine benefits found in Folts' research, in the Tabernacle Baptist Home Page on the net. But the *Wine Enthusiast*, vii (April 1994), 11, reported on Folts' study quite differently, emphasising that 'red wine reduces cardiovascular risk by significantly decreasing platelet aggregration ....' The wine journal also noted that the wine was more effective when the meal contained garlic (*Allium sativum*). Another study published in 1996 found no cardiovascular benefits from garlic, but some recent studies are more favourable to this bulbous plant of the lily family. For the Zutphen study, see M. G. L. Hertog and others, 'Dietary antioxidant flavonoids and risk of coronary heart disease: the Zutphen elderly study,' *Lancet*, 342 (1993), 1007–11.

46. Lucie Randoin (1885-1960) became director of the Laboratoire de physiologie du Centre de recherches sur la nutrition of the ministry of agriculture in 1924. In addition to an impressive research career she was an institution builder, creating and organising an Ecole supérieure technique de diététique, which had by 1960 trained nearly 11,000 students for hospitals, school canteens, etc., the Service de contrôle des produits vitaminés, des aliments et des rations, and the Service d'enquêtes scientifiques sur l'alimentation. In 1945 she succeeded Gabriel Bertrand as president of the French society of biological chemistry, and later was even elected to the Académie de médecine, a rare honour for a woman.
47. Baglioni, 'Ce que l'on fait en Italie pour la défense scientifique du vin,' *JMBX*, 37 (30 Nov. 1937), 838–9. Baglioni praised Mussolini because the fascist government had created a sub-commission for the study of wine by various approaches: chemistry, physics, food science, hygiene, and therapy.
48. Eric B. Rimm and others, 'Folate and vitamin B6 from diet and supplements in relation to risk of coronary heart disease among women,' *Journal of the American Medical Association*, 279 (4 Feb. 1998), 359–93. Folic acid or B9 now appears as a panacea-like element, preventing cervical dysplasia, and neural tube defect, as well as being a regulator of serum levels of homosysteine (a toxic amino-

acid breakdown product of protein metabolism), thus possibly giving some protection against heart attacks, arterial disease, and cancer. One hardly needs wine at all, except to get drunk.

49. Homeostasis is 'the regulation by an organism of the chemical composition of its blood and body fluids and other aspects of its internal environment so that physiological processes can proceed at optimum rates.' Oxford's *Concise Science Dictionary*, 326. Rutin and bioflavonoid are recent linguistic concoctions. The 1941 edition of Starling's *Principles of Human Physiology* (London, 1912; rev. ed., 1941, by C. Lovett Evans), 863, uses the general designation 'vitamin P': 'found together with ascorbic acid, ... its lack is largely responsible for the capillary haemorrhages which occur in scurvy. It is also called citrin ... a mixture of two flavone pigments ....The human requirement is said to be 50 mg. daily.' See also J. Masquelier, 'Identification et dosage des facteurs vitaminiques P dans diverses boissons fermentées,' *Bulletin de la Société de chimie biologique*, xxxviii (1956), 65–70.
50. Research done at the Zurich University Hospital by Wilhelm Vetter found that alcohol reduces the growth of arterial muscle cells that would normally occur after ... [a person ate] a high-fat meal.' This seems to be a sort of mechanism, but perhaps not at the explanatory level desired by scientists at U.C. Davis. Vetter's article was published in the *American Journal of Clinical Nutrition* and reported by Jane Brody in the 'Health Watch' of *The New York Times* (7 April 1998.
51. R. Curtis Ellison, M. D., professor at the Boston University School of Medicine, where he founded the Institute on Lifestyle & Health, convincingly explained 'Why wine is good for you' in the *Wine Spectator* (Oct. 31, 1998), 34–46.
52. David Stout, 'Government allows labels about wine's benefits,' *The New York Times* (6 Feb. 1999), A12.
53. Criqui and Ringel, *Lancet*, 344 (1994), 1719–23. The earlier article by S. Renaud and M. De Lorgeril, 'Wine, alcohol, platelets and the French paradox for coronary heart disease,' was in *Lancet*, 339 (1992), 1523-26. See also Renaud's letter on 'the French paradox: vegetables or wine' in *Circulation*, vi (1994), 3118–9.
54. See Frank J. Prial, 'Wine Talk,' *The New York Times* (Dec. 1991), section B, 14.
55. Everything optimistic you want to know about the French paradox can be gleaned from Lewis Perdue and others, *The French Paradox and Beyond - Live Longer with Wine and the Mediterranean Lifestyle* (Sonoma, CA.: Renaissance Pub., 1992). The technical medical

arguments can be obtained from journals such as *Lancet, Circulation,* the *American Journal of Clinical Nutrition, British Medical Journal, New England Journal of Medicine,* and the *European Journal of Clinical Nutrition* in recent years. The *Wine Institute News* eagerly carries all the good news on wine consumption; the issue for May/June 1993 has a useful list of 'Key studies on wine and the heart,' but there is no substitute for searching under 'wine' in the *Index medicus.*

56. Consider the following figures, pulled from the *World Almanac* 1994 by I. Herbert Gordon in a letter to New York Times (8 May 1997): Japan – 77 years for males and 82 for females, Switzerland – 76 and 83, France – 74 and 82, Italy – 74 and 81, Greece – 75 and 80. Uffe Ravnskov, letter to the *British Medical Journal,* 319 (24 May 1999), points out that the results of some controlled randomised trials 'contradict the suggestion that consumption of dietary saturated fatty acids has any influence on atherosclerosis or coronary heart disease.' See Ravnskov's relevant article in *J. Clin. Epidemiol.*, 51 (1998), 443–60.
57. Lawrence Altman, M.D., 'Getting it right on the facts of death,' *The New York Times* (22 dec. 1998), D7. Information from researchers at the Framingham Heart Study in Mass., which began in in 1948 and included some 10,000 people. No autopsy, no accuracy: the autopsy rate has dropped from fifty per cent in the 1960s to ten per cent. See also Altman's article 'Diagnoses and the Autopsies are found to differ greatly,' *The New York Times* (14 Oct. 1998), A14, reporting on an article in the *Journal of the American Medical Association* (13 Oct. 1998) showing that 'the disparity between the diagnosis of cancer before and after death was 44 per cent.' The study was based on 1105 autopsies done at the Medical Center of Louisiana in New Orleans.
58. Jane E. Brody, 'Wine for the heart: benefits may be costly,' T*he New York Times* (Dec. 28, 1994), B8, using the data in Criqui and Ringel, *Lancet,* 344 (1994), 1723.
59. Uffe Ravnskov, letter to the *British Medical Journal,* 319 (24 May 1999).
60. Jane E. Brody, 'Danish study shows wine aiding longevity,' *The New York Times* (5 May 1995), which also includes typical medical doubts about the study and also warnings about following the drinking habits of the 13,000 Danes who were studied. See M. Gronbæk and others, 'Mortality associated with moderate intakes of wine, beer and spirits,' *British Medical Journal,* 310 (1995), 1165–9. Brewers have not given up hope, however, for the Danish Brewers

Association made good use of a study of 2000 German beer drinkers showing that beer is as good a preventive medicine as wine. *Und so weiter...*

61. Roy Porter, *The Greatest Benefit to Mankind. A Medical History of Humanity* (London: HarperCollins, 1997), 585.
62. Michael J. Thun and others, 'Alcohol consumption and mortality among middle-aged and elderly U.S. adults,' *The New England Journal of Medicine*, 337 (1997), 1705–14 . See 'Drink a day can lower death rate by 20 percent,' *The New York Times* (Dec. 11, 1997), A17. In 1996 breast cancer killed 44,300 women – prostate cancer kills about the same number of men; lung cancer killed 158,000 women; heart attacks killed nearly 500,000 women. See Lisa Belkin, on 'How breast cancer became this year's cause,' *The New York Times Magazine* (Dec. 22, 1996), 42. In 'Sixty Minutes' (Nov. 5, 1995) Morley Safer gave a figure of 46,000 for female deaths annually from breast cancer. In 1998 there were 43,500 deaths and 178,700 new cases; breast cancer does kill more women from their mid-thirties to mid-fifties than heart disease. See Denise Grady, 'In breast cancer data, hope, fear and confusion,' *The New York Times* (26 January 1999), D1, 4.
63. Thun and others, 'Alcohol Consumption,' *The New England Journal of Medicine*, 337 (1997), 1705. *The New York Times* (10 June 1997) reported on the article by O. F. Dent and others, 'Alcohol consumption and cognitive performance in a random sample of Australian soldiers who served in the second world war,' *British Medical Journal* 314 (1997), 1655–7, arguing that a study of 209 old men, 178 of whom drank, showed that alcohol does not adversely affect brain function. But a representative of the Center for Science in the Public Interest quickly fired back a rebuttal (14 June 1997) pointing out 'a significant shortcoming of the study' was that ' 28 per cent of the men died during the study and 11 per cent were lost to follow up,' and that neuropsychological tests 'have identified three categories of organic brain disease associated with chronic alcoholism: Wernicke-Korsakoff syndrome, alcoholic dementia and 'nonamnesic disorder.' Which may all be beside the point if chronic alcoholism is not at issue.
64. Mary Jane Ashley and others, 'Moderate drinking and health: implications of recent evidence,' *Canadian Family Physician*, 43 (April 1997), 687–94, and editorial, 592–4.
65. See *The New York Times* (17 Nov. 1995), A17. On wine versus alcohol, see the *British Medical Journal*, 313 (1996), 365, 1179–80.
66. Eric B. Rimm and others, 'Review of moderate alcohol consumption

and reduced risk of coronary heart disease: is the effect due to beer, wine, or spirits?,' *British Medical Journal*, 312 (1996), 731–6.

67. Arthur L. Klatsky, Mary Anne Armstrong, and Gary D. Friedman, 'Red wine, white wine, beer, and risk of coronary artery disease hospitalization,' *American Journal of Cardiology*, 80 (1997), 416–20.
68. Criqui and Ringel, *Lancet*, 344 (1994), 1722.
69. Ashley and others, *Canadian Family Physician*, 43 (1997), 689.
70. Poul Suadicani and others, 'Strong mediators of social inequalities in risk of ischaemic heart disease: a six-year follow-up in the Copenhagen male study,' *International Journal of Epidemiology*, 26 (1997), 516–22.
71. M. C. Bellizzi and others, 'Vitamin E and coronary heart disease: the European paradox,' *European Journal of Clinical Nutrition*, 48 (1994), 822–31.
72. Criqui and Ringel, *Lancet*, 344 (1994), 1722.
73. Arjan Gjonça and Martin Bobak, 'Albanian paradox, another example of protective effect of Mediterranean lifestyle?' in *Lancet*, 350 (Dec. 20/27, 1997), 1815–17.
74. Sabine Artaud-Wild and others, letter, *Circulation*, vi (Dec. 9, 1994), 3118-9.
75. Pierre Bourdieu, *Distinction. A social critique of the judgement of Taste* (Cambridge, Mass., 1984), 53. Translated by Richard Nice.
76. 'A drink a day may be an aid against clots,' *The New York Times* (28 September 1994), quoting Thomas A. Pearson and Paul Terry.
77. Quotations from Porter, *op. cit.* (note 61), 574, 579.
78. W. Roger Williams, 'The Prevalence of Cancer and its Increase,' *Lancet* (Aug. 13, 1904), 445–7.
79. A. Newsholme, 'The possible association of the consumption of alcohol with excessive mortality from cancer,' *British Medical Journal*, xi (1903),1529; see the relevant chapter in Victor Horsley and M. D. Sturge (eds), *Alcohol and the Human Body* (London: Macmillan, 1915).
80. M. Tsurmi, 'L'influence de l'alcool éthylique sur le développement des cancers de souris', *Annales de l'Institut Pasteur*, 30 (1916), 346–356.
81. *BIV*, no. 43 (1932), 28.
82. *BIV*, no. 60 (1933), 67.
83. L. Dieulafé, *On peut éviter le cancer* (Paris: Béziers, 1937).
84. Marilie D. Gammon and others, 'Tobacco, alcohol, and socioeconomic status and adenocarcinomas of the esophagus and gastric cardia,' *Journal of the National Cancer Institute*, 89 (Sept. 3, 1997), 1277–88.

85. Andrew J. Clifford and others, 'Delayed tumour onset in transgenic mice fed an amino acid-based diet supplemented with red wine solids,' *American Journal of Clinical Nutrition*, 64 (1996), 748–56, and Susan E. Ebeler and others, 'An in vivo experimental protocol for identifying and evaluating dietary factors that delay tumour onset,' in Tom R. Watkins (ed), *Wine: Nutritional and Therapeutic Benefits* (American Chemical Society symposium series 661, 1997. I thank Susan Ebeler and Andrew Waterhouse for these references).
86. Susan E. Ebeler and Mary Ann Weber, 'Wine and Cancer,' in Waterhouse and Rantz, (eds), *op. cit.* (note 47), 16–18.
87. The study, by Stephanie A. Smith-Warner and others, was published in the *Journal of the American Medical Association* on 18 Feb. 1998 and put to good use in *Booze News* (CSPI's Alcohol Policies Project) on 20 Feb., in a letter to the director of BATF attacking the machinations of the California Wine Institute. More amunition has been given to the CSPI in recent research by Mamoru Maeda and colleagues, published in *Cancer*, 83 (1998), 1483–8, indicating that in colorectal cancer patients drinkers are more likely to get liver cancer than non-drinkers.
88. Jane E. Brody, 'Another round in drink-a-day debate,' *The New York Times* (2 Feb. 1999), D7, reporting on Y. Zhang and others, 'Alcohol consumption and risk of breast cancer,' *American Journal of Epidemology*, 149 (Jan. 15, 1999), 93–101, followed by discussion. The careful conclusion of the researchers was 'that the light consumption of ... any type of alcoholic beverage is not associated with increased breast cancer risk.' Data was from the Framingham (Mass.) study, in which 2764 women were followed for over forty years (1948-93) and 2284 women in the offspring cohort followed for up to twenty four years (1971-93).
89. Waterhouse, *loc. cit.* (note 38), 339.
90. Iain Bamforth, review of James Le Fanu, *The Rise and Fall of Modern Medicine* (1999) in the *Times Literary Supplement* (Dec. 31, 1999), 3–4.

11

Wine Therapy: The future of another illusion?

The role of wine in therapy is mostly all history now. This judgment does not exclude the return of a modest role for moderate wine consumption in preventive medicine. Much of our contemporary medicine is based on less scientific evidence than the evidence for the health benefits of a daily glass of wine. In a generation or so after Mlle la doctoresse Poudensan's eulogy of the seduction of French virgins by Bacchus, the French would be top contenders for being the most medicalised people on earth, consuming two and a half times more antibiotics than Germans and three times more tranquillisers and sleeping pills than the English and Germans, with French women gulping 'down mood-changing drugs at twice the rate of [French] men.'[1] Who needs wine? The fall of wine therapy seems universal, unimpeded by the favourable results of scientific research. Lucia delivered a rash threnody, which is not entirely devoid of nostalgic myth.

> By 1900 new medicines were appearing: aspirin, the alleviant of pain and fever, soon followed by the [barbiturates, central nervous system depressant drugs, largely supplanted later by the benzodiazepines]; by the vitamins, which relieved deficiency diseases and then became a fetish; by the hormones, potent and dangerous; by the numerous sulfa drugs, which later faded; by the antibiotics, which paralyzed bacteria; by the tranquillisers; and by the swelling stream of newly developed synthetics and purported specifics, each crowding its predecessors into obsolescence. Each new product was accompanied by a deluge of elaborately designed laboratory and clinical data attesting dramatically to its marvelous efficacy.
>
> For wine, such proofs, by measurable criteria, were generally lacking. The only conclusive evidence of its value was the test of centuries – as a harmless stomachic, diuretic, and sedative, gently beneficial in virtually all ailments, in all segments of the population, uniformly effective despite the biologic variations which so frequently nullify and often violently repulse treatment by modern drugs.... A whole

> generation of physicians entered practice without knowledge of the time-tested remedies safely employed by their predecessors. And wine, besmirched by the prohibitionists, erased from the pharmacopoeia despite its magnificent record as a therapeutic agent, was gradually dismissed from most medical practice.[2]

It may be as difficult for the contemporary mind to regret the passing of wine therapy as to give much credence to nineteenth century medicine and its doctors. Some people probably believe that Pasteur's outburst is still relevant: 'Certains des ces médecins sont des misérables, vous entendez!'[3] Some people might even agree with the statement that in the 1930s it was discovered that the greater part of medicine was nonsense.[4] The statement itself may be nonsense, but our constitutional whiggism makes it difficult to avoid such condescending anachronisms and merely to remain content with the more insidious kind inherent in normal historical reconstruction. A historical understanding of the role of wine in medicine cannot escape the basic difficulties of a somewhat theoretical and perhaps even esoteric nature that must be faced by anyone wishing to explain, let alone justify, medical practice and research, past or present.

Science wears a halo of certainty but produces a great deal of controversy. About the nature of the universe, cells, fluoridation of drinking water, consumption of soy-derived isoflavones (phytoestrogens), genetic engineering, dinosaurs, and human evolution as well as about science's own 'criteria for making observations and performing competent experiments' and about the relation between reality and scientific representations of it.[5] Few debates seem susceptible of closure on the basis of conclusive experiments. How do scientific quarrels end? It seems that often it is a matter of the majority's exercising its tyranny. An exercise of power by a scientific group capable of making alliances, often with vested interests, based on the knowledge socially useful to the group, to render their opponents impotent. Science may not be gay but it is all too human.[6] There may never be an end to explanations of how science explains and how scientists achieve agreement in their communities. There will never be an end to explanations of diseases and cures. But we seem to get better at it all – well, some of it.[7]

Medicine has not escaped this kind of scrutiny, corrosive of both experimental and clinical certainties. Evelleen Richards has done an analysis of the shaky basis of the objective science on which cancer therapy is based; her conclusions may be applied to therapy in general. In an ambitious blend of macro and micro analysis she argues 'that the assessment of medical therapies is inherently a social and political process; that the idea of neutral appraisal is a myth; that clinical trials, no matter how rigorous their methodology, inevitably embody the professional values or commitments of the assessors; and that judgements about experimental findings may be structured by wider social interests, such as consumer choice or market forces.'[8] So much for 'the privileged epistemological status of medical knowledge.' If sick people were to read Richards on the politics of therapeutic evaluation, they might be tempted if not to replace then at least to complement biomedicine with popular medicine or alternative medicine, which might mean trying, for example, the ecumenical medicine of Andrew Weill, M.D.[9] Alternatives are not easy to find, for since the nineteenth century, scientific medicine in alliance with government, bureaucracy, higher education, and the community of the diseased, has effectively eliminated nearly all competitors. In the end, the patient may have the choice of dying after treatment by doctors in league with drug companies or after a non-orthodox treatment (called quackery by the establishment), neither of which has any statistically demonstrated superiority over the other.

Biomedicine has become traditional medicine in the west, and the tradition is science. Even an unorthodox therapy, like that of Pauling and Cameron advocating the use of vitamin C as a help in managing cancer, bases itself on science. A large part of Pauling's squabble with the cancer establishment was over the proper way to do scientific experiments. Unfortunately, one cannot hope for epistemological salvation through science because experimental design 'cannot be divorced from the commitments of the communities that frame and evaluate experiments.'[10]

Wine therapy seems to have been a form of ethnomedicine, that is, 'embedded within a system of social relations,' giving 'concrete form to assumptions about reality drawn from the wider culture, which in turn influence the wider culture.'[11] Wine was a part of the symbolic, social, and emotional context of healing. Pro-wine doctors reinforced the values of French culture (and part of British culture), which repaid the debt by giving authority and legitimation to therapeutic relations between doctors and patients. Wine and science were prominent parts of French culture. Medicine made healing strategies much more successful by including wine in the therapy, and since medicine had become scientific, this cultural value had to be reinforced by experimental proof of its efficacy, the hallmark of scientific medicine.

As a result of the nineteenth-century recognition of alcoholism, some doctors went logically from a recognition of the dangers of alcohol to a questioning of the therapeutic value of wine and the ethical wisdom of prescribing it. Nor was there any problem in questioning the scientific basis of wine therapy. Practices that had been widely accepted as self-evident, popular medicine in the mask of science, now came under attack on scientific and medical grounds. Believers in wine therapy had to take to the defence of their nostrum, and in so doing they actually created a coherent body of doctrine that had not really existed before in such a rigorously organised and scientifically proven form. The trouble was that the results of the testing did not seem to be convincing to the opposing camps, solidly entrenched behind their ideological banners and cultural walls, not to mention their scientific proofs. This is where one is tempted to agree with the Australian school on the reality of scientific myths: 'that method discourse should be treated as 'myths' which systematically mask processes of social construction and control. They serve rhetorical and political purposes and are resources in the power struggles within and between scientific communities and wider social forces.'[12]

Whigs may impatiently ask if wine has any medical value? It is easier now than it was a few years ago to find a respectable doctor to give a positive answer, in French or in English. Some years ago Jack Pickleman, of Loyola Medical Center in Maywood, Illinois, summed up, with the skill one expects of a surgeon, 'the beneficial effects of wine (not alcohol) on upper and lower G.I. function, the cardiovascular, renal and neurologic systems.' He listed 'the following effects in regular moderate wine drinkers.

1. A decrease in the number of heart attacks and deaths secondary to cardiovascular disease.
2. A decrease in the frequency of angina and leg claudication.
3. An increase in appetite with protein sparing and improved nitrogen balance in cachectic patients.
4. Alterations in lower G.I. function with improved bowel movements or colostomy emptying.
5. A decreased secretion of antidiuretic hormone (ADH) promoting diuresis in patients with excess fluid.
6. An increased sense of well-being and a decreased need for psychotropic medications among elderly patients.'[13]

In the latest books on wine therapy the argumentative strategy of authors seems to be to impress the reader with a vast amount of respectable medical and scientific information, culled from orthodox mainline journals and books on the functioning and healing of body and mind, all of which is then linked to moderate wine consumption, with the strong implication that there is a causal relation between the healthy body and mind and wine drinking. Even Lewis Purdue's book *The Wine Paradox* follows this strategy to the extent possible for pablum-loving readers. The French masters of the genre are François Drouard and Tran Ky.[14] The complexity of wine makes it amenable to this kind of treatment. An enormous amount of fodder for speculation can be gotten from the fact that wine contains hundreds if not thousands of esters, organic acids, higher alcohol, aldhehydes, phenols, flavanoids, amino acids and so on. And virtues can be found in minimum quantities. Wine has little vitamin content, but it is argued that even half a glass a day can promote health because of the quality of the vitamins in wine as well as the importance of the action of small amounts of some of them. Wine being hardly acceptable as a food any more, the argument in its favour has shifted to its total effect on the organism during meals, without excluding the beneficial effect of individual substances.

What the medical wine buffs say may be true; it sounds reasonable and seems consistent with what we know about the physiological functioning of the human organism. Take for example an organ on which the French consider themselves particularly expert: the brain. The discourse of doctors bristles with information on neurotransmitters, the movement of positive and negative ions, excited neurons, and how the presence of mineral salts such as magnesium and lithium in wine operate in the brain to get rid of an attack of anxiety. Somewhere in the argument one needs to comment on the wisdom of our great-grandparents, who took a little bordeaux to get rid of anxiety. There is no point in objecting that a small drink of wine contains only a tiny amount of the minerals, which may or may not make it to the receptors on the neurotransmitters, for it can be assumed that wine acts in nearly homeopathic doses. A similar argument can be made for counteracting exhaustion and worry by supplying the sugar-loving brain with immediately usable glucose and the other sugars that enable the glucose to cross the organ's protective barrier. Classic men of literature can be cited in favour of this pleasant and quick fix for a tired brain: Baudelaire and Pierre Loti.[15] It would be nice to know the intimate workings of this 'bundle of billions of neurons' well enough to be as certain about the moderate use of wine as we are about its abuse. But given the brain's complexity (and wine's), it is hardly possible to hope that wines could ever be designer drugs clearly affecting one receptor protein of brain cells. We just have to be happy with wine as a 'dirty' medication that has been the treacherous and indispensable companion of western man since Noah, one of our first psychopharmacologists, got drunk on his version of Beaujolais nouveau.[16]

Before rushing off to buy a case of Château Chasse-Spleen to take as medicine, the non-drinker may wish to ponder one of the latest careful conclusions of experimental science on these issues. Of course, it is yet another study with tentative results and guarded conclusions – the essence of solid science – but full of Turnerian 'fallacious hope' for the optimistic wine buff.

> The results of several epidemiological studies have suggested that coronary heart disease mortality can be decreased by moderate consumption of alcohol, especially red wine. It is conceivable that resveratrol plays a role in the prevention of heart disease because it has been reported to inhibit platelet aggregation and coagulation, alter eicosanoid synthesis, and modulate lipoprotein metabolism.
>
> Our results suggest that resveratrol merits further investigation as a cancer chemopreventive agent in humans. In light of the adverse health effects of long-term alcohol consumption, however, foods and nonalcoholic beverages derived from grapes should be considered as alternative dietary sources.[17]

Even if the flavonoids in wine and foods turn out to be as important as we hope, it is well to keep in mind that at present we have only begun to 'provide a foundation to assess the nutritional significance of ... flavonoids in foods and wines.'[18]

Wine is a gift of Dionysus or Bacchus, the god of wine, who can be 'kind and beneficient' or 'cruel and drive men on to frightful deeds.' He can drive men mad. He is 'the tragic god.'[19]

Notes

1. Marlise Simons, 'Gluttons for Sedatives, the French Ask Why,' *The New York Times* (Jan. 21, 1991), A12. The article contains a piece of nonsense – that the French do not like to consult psychiatrists. On the French as champion drug consumers, see also Edouard Zarifian, *Le prix du bien-être. Psychotropes et société* (Paris: O. Jacob, 1996), and Fabien Gruhier, 'La France médaille d'or des pilules du bonheur,' *Le Nouvel Observateur* (5-11 Sept. 1996), 38–40.
2. Lucia, *A History of Wine as Therapy* (Philadelphia: Lippincott, 1963),

171–172. In the period 1790-1860 American wine and alcohol medical consumption declined (after 1800) and then rose again; see Sarah E. Williams, 'The Use of Beverage Alcohol as Medicine, 1790-1860,' *Journal of Studies on Alcohol*, 41 (1980), 543–66.

3. Pasteur, in Sacha Guitry, *Pasteur* (Paris: Paris-Théâtre, 1919), 50.
4. Lewis Thomas, *The Medusa and the Snail* (New York: Bantam Books, 1980), 132–146.
5. Steven Shapin, 'History of Science and its Sociological Reconstructions,' *History of Science, 20* (1982), 162. This article is the classic epitaph for the faith of our fathers in the objectivity and certainty of their own phallic science with its corollary of the impossibility of the sociology of scientific knowledge.
6. Consider, e.g., the line-up of 'principalities and powers' in the contemporary dispute over the safety of fluoridation: 'Rat study reignites dispute on fluoride,' *The New York Times* (March 13, 1990), B5/8.
7. Paul Thagard, *How Scientists Explain Disease* (Princeton, NJ: Princeton University Press, 1999) promises to deliver some hard knocks to both 'traditional philosophy of science ... and contemporary sciences studies,' and really explain how those Prometheans do it.
8. Evelleen Richards, 'The Politics of Therapeutic Evaluation: The Vitamin C and Cancer Controversy,' *Social Studies of Science*, 18 (1988), 653–701; quotation from 653. See Evelleen Richards, *Vitamin C and Cancer: Medicine or Politics?* (New York: St. Martin's Press, 1991).
9. See Andrew Weill, *Natural Health. Natural Medicine* (New York: Houghton Mifflin, 1995 and 1998).
10. Richards, 'The Politics of Therapeutic Evaluation,' 672, quoting Shapin, 'History of Science and Its Sociological Reconstructions,' 162, who goes on to conclude that 'there is no possibility of avoiding a sociological account of fact-production by appealing to the impersonal rules of experimental procedure.'
11. See Steven Feierman, 'Struggles for Control: The Social Roots of Health and Healing in Modern Africa,' *African Studies Review*, 28 (1985), 73-147.
12. Richards, 'The Politics of Therapeutic Evaluation,' 676, which draws upon the brazen theses of J. Schuster and R. Yeo, *The Politics and Rhetoric of Scientific Method* (Dordrecht: Reidel, 1986).
13. Jack Pickleman, M.D., 'A glass a day keeps the doctor...,' presidential address to Midwest Surgical Association (1989), *The American Surgeon*, 56 (1990), 395–7.

14. See, for example, Tran Ky, François Drouard, and Jean-Michel Guilbert, *Les vertus thérapeutiques du Bordeaux – Histoire naturelle et culturelle – Diététique, biologie* (Paris: Artulen, 1991).
15. *Ibid.*, 124–7.
16. See Daniel Goleman, 'Research on brain leads to pursuit of designer drugs,' *The New York Times* (19 Nov. 1996), B1 and 9, and Jean-Pierre Changeux, 'Chemical Signaling in the brain,' *Scientific American* (Nov. 1993), 58-62.
17. Meishiang Jang and others, 'Cancer chemopreventive activity of resveratrol, a natural product derived from grapes,' *Science*, 275 (1997), 219.
18. See Jennifer R. C. Bell and others (including Waterhouse), '(+)-Catechin in human plasma after ingestion of of a single serving of reconstituted red wine,' *American Journal of Clinical Nutrition* 71 (2000), 67–74.
19. Edith Hamilton, *Mythology* (New York: The New American Library, 1953), 56, 62.

Bibliography

Journals

American Journal of Clinical Nutrition; American Journal of Enology and Viticulture; American Journal of physiology; The American Surgeon; Annales de chimie et de physique; Annales de l'Ecole nationale d'agriculture de Montpellier; Annales de l'Institut Pasteur; Archives générales de médecine; Booze News; British Medical Journal; Bulletin de l'académie de médecine; Bulletin de la société de chimie biologique; Bulletin [*Revue,* 1904-10] *de la société scientifique d'hygiène alimentaire; Bulletin de l'organisation internationale du vin; Bulletin du ministère de l'agriculture; Bulletin of the History of Medicine; Caduceus; Canadian Family Physician; Cancer; Circulation; La Clinique; Chemical and Engineering News; Chemistry and Industry; La Chronique médicale; Clio Medica; Epidemiology; European Journal of Clinical Nutrition; International Journal of Epidemiology; Journal of the American Medical Association; Journal of Applied Cardiology; Journal of the History of Medicine and Allied Sciences; Journal of the National Cancer Institute; Journal de médecine de Bordeaux; Journal de pharmacie et de chimie; Journal of the Science of Food and Agriculture; The Lancet; La Médecine populaire; The New England Journal of Medicine; Le Progrès médical; Revue philanthropique; Revue de viticulture; Science; Scientific American; The Wine Spectator; Wines and Vines.*

Books and some key articles

Ackerknecht, Erwin H. *Medicine at the Paris Hospital* (Baltimore: The Johns Hopkins Univ. Press, 1967); *A Short History of Medicine* (rev. edn, Baltimore: The Johns Hopkins Univ. Press, 1982).

Alibert, J.-L. *Nouveaux élémens de thérapeutique et de matière médicale...* (5th edn, 3 vols., Paris: Béchet jeune, 1826).

Amerine, Maynard A., and Singleton, Vernon L. *Table Wines: the Technology of their Production* (Berkeley, CA: The Univ. of California Press, 1951).

Barrows, Susanna, and Room, Robin (eds). *Drinking Behavior and Belief in Modern History* (Berkeley, CA: The Univ. of California Press, 1991).

Barry, Edward. *Observations historical, critical, and medical on the wines of the Ancients...* (London: T. Cadell, 1775).

Black, William George. *Folk Medicine; A Chapter in the History of Culture* (London: Elliot Stock, 1883).

Blanchet, Bernard. *Code du vin et textes viti-vinicoles français et communitaires* (Montpellier: Ed. de la Journée viticole, 1970).

Blumgarten, A. S. *Textbook of Materia Medica* (4th edn, New York: Macmillan, 1927).

Bonal, François, and others. *Les vertus thérapeutiques du champagne* (Paris: Artulen, 1990).

Bouchardat, A. *Traité d'hygiène publique et privée basée sur l'étiologie* (3d edn, Paris: Alcan, 1887).

Bourdel, A. *Du plâtrage des vins. Expériences cliniques sur l'homme soumis à l'usage du vin platré* (4th edn, Montpellier: Coulet, 1888).

Bourke, John C. *Scatologic Rites of All Nations* (Washington, D. C.: W. H. Lowdermilk, 1891).

Bouteiller, Marcelle. *Médecine populaire d'hier et d'aujourd'hui* (Paris: Maisonneuve et Larose, 1987).

Buchan, William. *Domestic Medecine* (1769; 18th edn, London and Edinburgh: J. Smith, 1803).

Bynum, W. F. *Science and the Practice of Medicine in the Nineteenth Century* (Cambridge: Cambridge Univ. Press, 1994). See pages 227–50 for an excellent "Bibliographical Essay" on the nineteenth-century.

Bynum, W. F., and Porter, Roy (eds). *Brunonianism in Britain and Europe* (London: Wellcome Institute for the History of Medicine, 1988).

Chevallier, Alphonse, and Baudrimont, E. *Dictionnaire des altérations et falsifications des substances alimentaires* (4th edn, Paris: P. Asselin, 1875).

Cheyne, George. *An Essay on Health and Long Life* (2d edn, London: G. Strahan and Leake, 1735).

Codex medicamentarius gallicus — pharmacopée française (Paris: Béchet jeune, 1837, 1866; 1884; 1908; 1911; etc.).

Conrad, Lawrence I., and others. *The Western Medical Tradition 800 B. C. To A.D. 1800* (Cambridge: Cambridge Univ. Press, 1995).

(*Dictionnaire encyclopédique des sciences médicales,* edited by Raige-Delorme et A. Dechambre with L. Lereboullet taking over in 1886, when the monster work was in its fifth series (Paris: Victor Masson, 1864-).

Doléris, J.-A. *Le vin et les médecins: le pour et le contre* (Paris: Vigot, 1907; 1931).

Dougnac, J.-F.-N. *Le vin au points de vue physico-chimique, physiologique, hygiénique et thérapeutique* (Bordeaux: Delmas, 1933; 2d edn, 1935).

Ellis, Jack D. *The physician-legislators of France. Medicine and politics in the early Third Republic, 1870-1914* (Cambridge: Cambridge Univ. Press, 1990).

Emch-Deriaz, Antoinette. *Tissot: Physician of the Enlightenment* (New York: Peter Lang, 1992).

Fleury, Maurice de. *Les grands symptômes neurasthéniques — pathogénie et traitement* (2d edn, Paris: Alcan, 1901).

Gautier, Armand. *La sophistication des vins* (3d edn, Paris: Baillière, 1884).

Gillispie, C. C. (ed). *Dictionary of Scientific Biography* (16 vols., New York: Scribner, 1970-80).

Gingeot, Paul. *Essai sur l'emploi thérapeutique de l'alcool chez les enfants et en général le rôle de cet agent dans le traitement des maladies aiguës fébriles* (Paris: A. Delahaye, 1867).

Goldstein, Jan. *Console and Classify. The French Psychiatric Profession in the Nineteenth Century* (Cambridge: Cambridge Univ. Press, 1987)

Hecquet, Philippe. *La médecine, la chirurgie et la pharmacie des pauvres* (3 vols., Paris: Clousier, 1742).

Herpin, Jean-Charles. *De l'acide carbonique, de ses propriétés physiques, chimiques et physiologiques; de ses applications thérapeutiques* (Paris: Baillière, 1864).

Hillemand, Bernard. *L'alcoolisme* (Paris: Presses universitaires de France, 1999).

Hoolihan, Christopher. "Wine and Regimen from Hippocrates to the Renaissance," *Caduceus*, 9 (1993).

Huguet, Françoise. *Les professeurs de la Faculté de médecine de Paris — Dictionnaire biographique 1794-1939* (Paris: Editions du C.N.R.S., 1991).

James, Robert. *A Medicinal Dictionary* (3 vols., London: T. Osborne, 1743-5); translated into French as *Dictionnaire universelle de médecine...* (6 vols., Paris: J. A. Brosson, 1746-8).

Jeffs, Julian. *Sherry* (4th edn, London: Faber & Faber, 1992).

Jensen, H.-G.-S. *Recherches sur le pouvoir bactéricide des vins rouges* (Bordeaux: Thesis, Faculté des sciences, 1954).

Jouanna, Jacques. "Le vin et la médecine dans la Grèce ancienne," *Revue des études grecques*, 109 (1996), 410-34.

Lancereaux, E. *De l'alcoolisme* (Paris: Doin, 1878); *Traité des maladies du foie et du pancréas* (Paris: Doin, 1899).

Laporte, Dominique. *Histoire de la merde* (2d edn, Paris: Christian Bourgeois, 1993).

Levet-Gautrat, Maximilienne, and others. *La médecine familiale au début du siècle* (Paris: Ed. Heures de France, 1978).

Lévy, Michel. *Traité d'hygiène publique et privée* (2 vols., 6th edn, Paris: Baillière, 1879).

Loebenstein-Loebel, Eduard Leopold. *Traité sur l'usage et les effets des vins dans les maladies dangereuses et mortelles, et sur la falsification de cette boisson* (Strasbourg: Levrault, 1817). Translated from the German (*Die Anwendung und Wirkung des Weine in lebensgefährlichen Krankeiten, und deren Verfälschungen; nach eigenen Ansichten und Erfahrungen*, Leipzig: Brockhaus, 1816) by J. Fr. Daniel Lobstein.

Loubère, Leo A. *The Red and the White. The History of Wine in France and Italy in the Nineteenth Century* (Albany, NY: State Univ. of N. Y. Press, 1978).

Loux, Françoise. *Sagesses du Corps. La santé et la maladie dans les proverbes français* (Paris: Maisonneuve et Larose, 1978).

Lucia, Salvatore P. *A History of Wine as Therapy* (Philadelphia: Lippincott, 1963).

Marty, H. *Le plâtrage des vins* (Paris: Masson, 1888).

Marvaud, Angel. *Etude de physiologie thérapeutique: l'alcool, son action physiologique, son utilité et ses applications en hygiène et en thérapeutique* (Paris: V. Rozier, 1872).

Mauriac, Emile. *La défense du vin et la lutte contre l'alcoolisme* (Paris: Doin, 1901); *Le vin au point de vue médical* (Paris: Doin, 1903); *Les vins de Bordeaux, leurs qualités hygiéniques et curatives* (Bordeaux: Féret et fils, 1907).

Maury, E. *La médecine par le vin ou le vin comme remède universelle* (Paris: J'ai Lu, 1996) ; *Soignez-vous par le vin* (Paris: Marabout, 1983).

Montignac, Michel and Robert, Hervé. *Boire du vin pour rester en bon santé* (Paris: Flammarion, 1997).

Murchison, Charles. *Clinical Lectures on Diseases of the Liver, Jaundice and Abdominal Dropsy* (London: Longmans, Green, 1868); *On Functional Derangements of the Liver* (2d edn, London: Smith, Elder, 1879).

Nouveau dictionnaire de médecine et de chirurgie pratiques, edited by Bernutz, Richet, Tardieu, Troussseau, etc. (39 vols., Paris: Baillière, 1864-1886).

Nysten, P.-H. *Traité de matière médicale* (2 vols., 3d edn, Paris: J. A. Brosson, 1818).

Paul, Harry W. *Science, Vine, and Wine in Modern France* (Cambridge: Cambridge Univ. Press, 1996).

Porter, Dorothy, and Porter, Roy. *Patient's Progress. Doctors and Doctoring in Eighteenth-Century England* (Stanford, CA: Stanford Univ. Press, 1989).

Porter, Roy. *The Greatest Benefit to Mankind. A Medical History of Humanity* (London and New York: HarperCollins; Norton 1997). See pages 719-64 for a splendid bibliography in the history of medicine.

Porter, Roy (ed). *The Popularization of Medicine 1650-1850* (London: Routledge, 1992).

Prestwich, Patricia E. *Drink and the Politics of Social Reform: Antialcoholism in France Since 1870* (Palo Alto, CA: The Society for the Promotion of Science and Scholarship, 1988).

Ramsey, Matthew. *Professional and Popular Medicine in France, 1770-1830* (Cambridge: Cambridge Univ. Press, 1988).

Renouil, Yves (ed). *Dictionnaire du vin* (Bordeaux: Féret et fils, 1988).

Ribéreau-Gayon, Pascal. *Le vin* (2d ed, rev., Paris: Presses universitaires de France, 1994).

Richards, Evelleen. *Vitamin C and Cancer: Medicine or Politics?* (New York: St. Martin's Press, 1991).

Richerand, A. *Des erreurs populaires relatives à la médecine* (Paris: Caille et Ravier, 1812).

Robinson, Jancis (ed), *The Oxford Companion to Wine* (Oxford: Oxford Univ. Press, 1994).

Salvy, P. *Traité de thérapeutique clinique* (3d ed, Paris: Masson, 1940).

Schmitt, Jean. *Etude oenologique, médicale et philosophique du vin et particulièrerment du vin du Languedoc* (Paris: Thesis, Faculté de médecine, 1949).

Simonis, Pierre. *L'hygiène du vin d'Alsace* (Strasbourg: Thesis, Faculté de médecine, 1977).

Starling, Ernest Henry. *Principles of Human Physiology* (8th edn, London: J. & A. Churchill, 1941).

Sprengel, Kurt. *Histoire de la médecine depuis son origine jusqu'au dix-neuvième siècle* (5 vols., Paris: Béchet jeune, 1815-). Translated from the German by Dr. A.-J.-L. Jourdan.

Sydenham, Thomas. *The Entire works of Dr. Thomas Sydenham* (London: E. Cave, 1742). Translated by Dr. John Swan.

Thudichum, J. L. W. *A Treatise on Wines* (London: G. Bell and sons, 1896); *On Wines, their Production, Treatment and Use* (London: Trounce, 1873)

Thudichum, J. L. W. and Dupré, August. *A Treatise on the Origin, Nature and Varieties of Wine, being a Compleat Manual of Viticulture and Oenology* (London: Macmillan, 1872).

Tran Ky, and others. *Les vertus thérapeutiques du bordeaux* (Paris: Artulen, 1991).

Walton, John, and others (eds). *The Oxford Medical Companion* (Oxford: Oxford Univ. Press, 1994).

Warner, John Harley. "Physiological theory and therapeutic explanation in the 1860s: the British debate on the medical uses of alcohol," *Bulletin for the History of Medicine,* 54 (1980), 235–57.

Waterhouse, Andrew, and Rantz, JoAnne M. (eds.), *Wine in Context: Nutrition,Physiology, and Policy* (Reno, Nevada: Symposium on wine health, 1996).

Weiner, Dora B. *Raspail, Scientist, and Reformer* (New York: Columbia Univ. Press, 1968).

Weisz, George. *The Medical Mandarins. The French Academy of Medicine in the Nineteenth and Early Twentieth Centuries* (Oxford and New York: Oxford Univ. Press, 1995).

Williams, Sarah E. "The Use of Beverage Alcohol as Medicine, 1790-1860," *Journal of Studies on Alcohol,* 41 (1980), 543–566.

Index of Wines and Grape-based Drinks

V

W

Y

Subject Index

A

B

C

D

G

H

M

N

O

Q

R

S